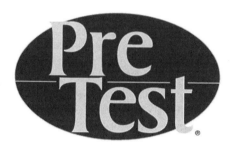

Obstetrics and Gynecology

PreTest® Self-Assessment and Review

Notice

Medicine is an ever-changing science. As new research and clinical experience broaden our knowledge, changes in treatment and drug therapy are required. The authors and the publisher of this work have checked with sources believed to be reliable in their efforts to provide information that is complete and generally in accord with the standards accepted at the time of publication. However, in view of the possibility of human error or changes in medical sciences, neither the authors nor the publisher nor any other party who has been involved in the preparation or publication of this work warrants that the information contained herein is in every respect accurate or complete, and they disclaim all responsibility for any errors or omissions or for the results obtained from use of the information contained in this work. Readers are encouraged to confirm the information contained herein with other sources. For example and in particular, readers are advised to check the product information sheet included in the package of each drug they plan to administer to be certain that the information contained in this work is accurate and that changes have not been made in the recommended dose or in the contraindications for administration. This recommendation is of particular importance in connection with new or infrequently used drugs.

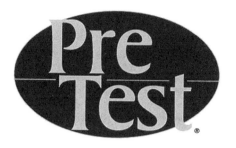

Obstetrics and Gynecology

PreTest® Self-Assessment and Review

14th Edition

Shireen Madani Sims, MD
Associate Professor and Clerkship Director
Department of Obstetrics and Gynecology
University of Florida College of Medicine
Gainesville, Florida

New York   Chicago   San Francisco   Athens   London   Madrid   Mexico City
Milan   New Delhi   Singapore   Sydney   Toronto

Obstetrics and Gynecology: PreTest® Self-Assessment and Review, 14th Edition

2 3 4 5 6 7 8 9 0   LCR   20 19 18 17

ISBN 978-1-259-58555-5
MHID 1-259-58555-7

This book was set in Minion pro by Cenveo® Publisher Services.
The editors were Catherine A. Johnson and Cindy Yoo.
The production supervisor was Richard Ruzycka.
Project management was provided by Tanya Punj, Cenveo Publisher Services.
RR Donnelley was printer and binder.

This book is printed on acid-free paper.

Library of Congress Cataloging-in-Publication Data

Names: Sims, Shireen Madani, author. | Schneider, Karen M. Obstetrics and gynecology.
    Preceeded by (work):
Title: Obstetrics and gynecology : PreTest self-assessment and review /
    Shireen Madani Sims.
Description: 14th edition. | New York : McGraw-Hill Education, [2016] |
    Preceeded by Obstetrics and gynecology : PreTest self-assessment and review / Karen M.
        Schneider, Stephen K. Patrick. 13th ed. c2012. |
    Includes bibliographical references and index.
Identifiers: LCCN 2015040563| ISBN 9781259585555 (pbk. : alk. paper) |
    ISBN 1259585557 (pbk. : alk. paper)
Subjects: | MESH: Gynecology—Examination Questions. |
    Obstetrics—Examination Questions.
Classification: LCC RG111 | NLM WP 18.2 | DDC 618.10076—dc23 LC record available
    at http://lccn.loc.gov/2015040563

International Edition ISBN 978-1-259-25123-8; MHID 1-259-25123-3.
Copyright © 2016. Exclusive rights by McGraw-Hill Education for manufacture and export.
This book cannot be re-exported from the country to which it is consigned by McGraw-Hill Education. The International Edition is not available in North America.

McGraw-Hill Education books are available at special quantity discounts to use as premiums and sales promotions or for use in corporate training programs. To contact a representative, please visit the Contact Us pages at www.mhprofessional.com.

Student Reviewers

Samantha Baer
Third-Year Medical Student
University of Florida
Class of 2016

Alexandra Monaco
Third-Year Medical Student
University of Florida
Class of 2016

Cheri Mostisser
Third-Year Medical Student
University of Florida College of Medicine
Class of 2016

Amelia Schaub
Third-Year Medical Student
University of Florida
Class of 2016

Ali Strochak
Third-Year Medical Student
University of Florida
Class of 2016

Contents

Introduction

Obstetrics and Gynecology: PreTest® Self-Assessment and Review, 14th Edition, is intended to provide medical students, as well as physicians, with a convenient tool for assessing and improving their knowledge of obstetrics and gynecology. The 504 questions in this book are similar in format and complexity to those included in Step 2 of the United States Medical Licensing Examination (USMLE). They may also be a useful study tool for Step 3.

Each question in this book has a corresponding answer, a reference to a text that provides background for the answer, and a short discussion of various issues raised by the question and its answer. A listing of references for the entire book follows the last chapter. For multiple-choice questions, the **one best** response to each question should be selected. For matching sets, a group of questions will be preceded by a list of lettered options. For each question in the matching set, select **one** lettered option that is **most** closely associated with the question.

To simulate the time constraints imposed by the qualifying examinations for which this book is intended as a practice guide, the student or physician should allot about 1 minute for each question. After answering all questions in a chapter, as much time as necessary should be spent reviewing the explanations for each question at the end of the chapter. Attention should be given to all explanations, even if the examinee answered the question correctly. Those seeking more information on a subject should refer to the reference materials listed or to other standard texts in medicine.

Obstetrics

Preconception Counseling, Genetics, and Prenatal Diagnosis

Questions

1. After an initial pregnancy resulted in a spontaneous loss in the first trimester, your patient is concerned about the possibility of this recurring. Which of the following is the most appropriate answer regarding the risk of recurrence after one miscarriage?

a. It depends on the genetic makeup of the prior abortus.
b. It is no different than it was prior to the miscarriage.
c. It has increased to approximately 50%.
d. It does not increase regardless of number of prior miscarriages.
e. It depends on the gender of the prior abortus.

2. A 24-year-old woman presents with a history of one first-trimester spontaneous abortion. Which of the following is the single most common specific chromosome abnormality associated with first trimester miscarriage?

a. 45 X (Turner syndrome)
b. Trisomy 21 (Down syndrome)
c. Trisomy 18
d. Trisomy 16
e. 46 XXY (Klinefelter syndrome)

3. A 29-year-old G3P0 presents to your office for preconception counseling. All of her pregnancies were lost in the first trimester. She has no significant past medical or surgical history. She should be counseled that without evaluation and treatment her chance of having a live birth is which of the following?

a. < 20%
b. 20% to 35%
c. 40% to 50%
d. 70% to 85%
e. > 85%

4. A 26-year-old G3P0030 has had three consecutive spontaneous abortions in the first trimester. As part of an evaluation for this problem, which of the following tests is most appropriate in the evaluation of this patient?

a. Hysterosalpingogram
b. Chromosomal analysis of the couple
c. Endometrial biopsy in the luteal phase
d. Postcoital test
e. Cervical length by ultrasonography

Questions 5 to 8

A 30-year-old G1P0 at 8 weeks' gestation presents for her first prenatal visit. She has no significant past medical or surgical history. A 29-year-old friend of hers just had a baby with Down syndrome and she is concerned about her risk of having a baby with the same problem. The patient reports no family history of genetic disorders or birth defects.

5. You should tell her that she has an increased risk of having a baby with Down syndrome in which of the following circumstances?

a. The age of the father of the baby is 40 years or older.
b. Her pregnancy was achieved by induction of ovulation and artificial insemination.
c. She has an incompetent cervix.
d. She has a luteal phase defect.
e. She has had three first-trimester spontaneous abortions.

6. You offer her a first trimester ultrasound looking for ultrasound markers associated with Down syndrome. Which of the following ultrasound markers is most closely associated with Down syndrome?

a. Choriod plexus cyst
b. Ventriculomegaly
c. Increased nuchal translucency (NT)
d. Intracardiac echogenic focus
e. Echogenic bowel

7. In order to increase the detection rate for Down syndrome in the first trimester, you may also offer her which of the following tests *in addition to the NT measurement*?

a. α fetoprotein (AFP) serum screening
b. First trimester screen, which includes biochemical testing with serum markers PAPP-A and free or total β-hCG, along with maternal age
c. Amniocentesis
d. Inhibin level serum screening
e. Fetal echocardiogram

8. The patient has an abnormal first trimester screen with increased risk of Down syndrome reported. What is the most appropriate next step?

a. Offer termination of the pregnancy.
b. Tell the patient that the baby will have Down syndrome.
c. Refer the patient to a high-risk specialist.
d. Refer the patient to genetic counseling.
e. Refer the patient to genetic counseling, and offer her diagnostic testing by CVS or a second-trimester genetic amniocentesis.

9. A 20-year-old woman presents to your office for routine well-woman examination. She has a history of acne, for which she takes minocycline and isotretinoin on a daily basis. She has a history of epilepsy that is well-controlled on valproic acid. She also takes a combined oral contraceptive birth control pill containing norethindrone acetate and ethinyl estradiol. She is a nonsmoker but drinks alcohol on a daily basis. She is concerned about the effectiveness of her birth control pill, given all the medications that she takes. She is particularly worried about the effects of her medications on a developing fetus in the event of an unintended pregnancy. Which of the following substances that she ingests has the lowest potential to cause birth defects?

a. Alcohol
b. Isotretinoin (accutane)
c. Tetracyclines
d. Progesterone
e. Valproic acid (Depakote)

10. A 24-year-old woman is in a car accident and is taken to an emergency room, where she receives x-ray examinations of her neck, chest, and lower spine. It is later discovered that she is 10 weeks pregnant. Which of the following is the most appropriate statement to make to the patient?

a. The fetus has received 50 rads of x-ray exposure and will likely abort.
b. Either chorionic villus sampling (CVS) or amniocentesis is advisable to check for fetal chromosomal abnormalities.
c. At 10 weeks, the fetus is particularly susceptible to derangements of the central nervous system (CNS).
d. The fetus has received less than the assumed threshold for radiation damage.
e. The risk that this fetus will develop leukemia as a child is raised.

Questions 11 to 12

A 25-year-old G0 presents to your office for preconception counseling. She is a long-distance runner and wants to continue to train should she conceive. She wants to know whether there are any potential adverse effects to a developing fetus if she were to pursue a program of regular exercise during her pregnancy.

11. You provide her with the following counseling about exercise during pregnancy?

a. During pregnancy, she should stop exercising because such activity is commonly associated with intrauterine growth retardation in the fetus.
b. She should perform exercises in the supine position to maximize venous return and cardiac output.
c. She may continue to exercise throughout pregnancy as long as her heart rate does not exceed 160 beats per minute.
d. She should only perform nonweight-bearing exercises because they minimize the risks of maternal and fetal injuries.
e. She should reduce her daily exercise routine by one-half during the pregnancy but following delivery, she may resume her activities to pre-pregnancy levels.

12. She asks you what other exercises would be appropriate during pregnancy. You counsel her that which of the following exercises would also be safe during pregnancy?

a. Riding a stationary bicycle
b. Horseback riding
c. Downhill skiing
d. Ice hockey
e. Scuba diving

13. Your patient presents for her first prenatal visit. She is 27-year-old and this is her first pregnancy. She is an achondroplastic dwarf. Her husband is of normal stature. Which of the following statements should you tell her regarding achondroplasia?

a. The inheritance pattern is autosomal recessive therefore there is a one-in-four chance that her child will be affected.
b. Achondroplasia is caused by a new genetic mutation therefore it cannot be passed on to her child.
c. Because she has achondroplasia she has a low risk of cesarean section for delivery.
d. She is fortunate to have lived to reproductive age.
e. She likely has some degree of spinal stenosis which could present a difficulty with spinal or epidural anesthesia.

14. A 25-year-old G3P0 presents for preconception counseling. She has had three first-trimester pregnancy losses. As part of her evaluation for recurrent abortion, she had karyotyping done on herself and her husband. Her husband is 46, XY. She carries a balanced 13;13 translocation. What is the likelihood that her next baby will have an abnormal karyotype?

a. < 5%
b. 10%
c. 25%
d. 50%
e. 100%

15. A 31-year-old G1P0 presents to your office at 22 weeks' gestation for a second opinion. She was told that her baby has a birth defect. She has copies of the ultrasound films and asks you to review them for her. The ultrasound image shows the birth defect. Which of the following is the most likely defect?

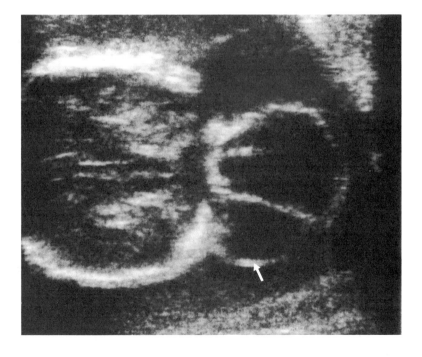

a. Cystic hygroma
b. Encephalocele
c. Hydrocephaly
d. Anencephaly
e. Omphalocele

Questions 16 to 18

A 24-year-old white woman has a maternal serum α-fetoprotein (MSAFP) level at 17 weeks' gestation of 6.0 multiples of the median (MOM). She had an ultrasound the same day that appeared normal.

16. Which of the following is the most appropriate next step in management?
a. Offer her a second MSAFP test
b. Reassure her that the baby does not have a neural tube defect (NTD)
c. Recommend an amniocentesis
d. Perform an amniography
e. Offer her termination of pregnancy due to a lethal fetal anomaly

17. The fetus is confirmed to have an open NTD with a diagnosis of spina bifida. What is the most appropriate counseling for this woman regarding future pregnancies?
a. She has a 50% risk of having an affected child in the future, because anencephaly is an autosomal dominant trait.
b. She has a decreased risk of having another baby with anencephaly because she is younger than 30 years of age.
c. When she becomes pregnant, she should undergo diagnostic testing for fetal NTDs with a first-trimester CVS.
d. Prior to becoming pregnant again she should begin folic acid supplementation.
e. She has a recurrence risk of having another baby with a NTD of less than 1%.

18. The patient asks how the diagnosis of spina bifida will impact her obstetric management and delivery. You should counsel her that:
a. She should be delivered by cesarean to prevent damage to the open NTD.
b. She should be delivered preterm to improve fetal neurologic outcomes.
c. She should be delivered in a tertiary care facility with a neonatal intensive care unit and personnel capable of managing the spinal defect and any immediate complications.
d. She should plan to deliver vaginally, even if the fetus is breech, as this will limit trauma to the defect.
e. She should be referred to a specialized center to undergo fetal surgery to close the NTD.

19. A 41-year-old woman had a baby with Down syndrome 10 years ago. She is anxious to know the chromosome status of fetus in her current pregnancy. She is currently at 8 weeks of gestation. Which of the following tests will provide the most rapid and reliable diagnosis of Down syndrome?

a. Amniocentesis
b. Multiple maternal serum marker analysis (Quad Screen)
c. Chorionic villi sampling (CVS)
d. First trimester screening using nuchal fold measurements and maternal serum markers
e. Cell free fetal DNA testing

20. A 44-year-old pregnant woman is trying to choose CVS versus amniocentesis for prenatal diagnosis due to her increased risk of having a child with a chromosomal anomaly. Which of the following is an advantage of amniocentesis over CVS?

a. Amniocentesis can be performed earlier in pregnancy than CVS.
b. First-trimester amniocentesis has a lower complication rate than CVS.
c. A second-trimester diagnosis of an abnormal karyotype afforded by amniocentesis allows for safer options for termination of pregnancy if desired by the patient.
d. Mid-trimester amniocentesis has a lower complication rate than CVS.
e. Amniocentesis in any trimester is less painful than CVS.

21. A patient presents for prenatal care in the second trimester. She was born outside the United States and has never had any routine vaccinations. Which of the following vaccines is contraindicated in pregnancy?

a. Injectable influenza vaccine
b. Tetanus toxoid
c. Reduced diphtheria toxoid and acellular pertussis (Tdap)
d. Hepatitis B
e. Measles, mumps, and rubella (MMR)

22. A patient presents to your office at term with no prenatal care. An ultrasound is performed and shows the fetus to be in the third trimester and to have multiple congenital anomalies, including microcephaly, cardiac anomalies, and growth retardation. You should question the patient if she has abused which of the following substances during her pregnancy?

a. Alcohol
b. Benzodiazepines
c. Heroin
d. Methadone
e. Marijuana

23. Your 25-year-old patient is pregnant at 36 weeks' gestation. She has an acute urinary tract infection (UTI). Which of the following antibiotics is contraindicated in the treatment of this patient?

a. Ampicillin
b. Nitrofurantoin
c. Trimethoprim/sulfamethoxazole
d. Cephalexin
e. Amoxicillin/clavulanate

24. You diagnose a 21-year-old woman at 12 weeks' gestation with gonorrhea cervicitis. Which of the following is the most appropriate treatment for her infection?

a. Doxycycline
b. Chloramphenicol
c. Tetracycline
d. Minocycline
e. Ceftriaxone

25. An obese, 25-year-old G1P0 comes to your office at 8 weeks' gestational age for her first prenatal visit. She is currently 5 ft 2 in tall and weighs 300 lb. Which of the following is the best advice to give this patient regarding obesity and pregnancy?

a. Marked obesity in pregnancy does not cause any additional risks.
b. She should gain at least 25 lb during the pregnancy because, although she is obese, nutritional deprivation can result in impaired fetal brain development and intrauterine fetal growth retardation.
c. She should try not to gain weight because obese women still have adequate fetal growth in the absence of any weight gain during pregnancy.
d. She should immediately initiate a vigorous exercise program to improve her health and help her lose weight.
e. She should try to lose weight during the pregnancy in order to limit the size of her baby, because obesity places her at an increased risk of requiring a cesarean delivery for fetal macrosomia.

26. A 26-year-old G2P1 presents to your office for her first prenatal visit. Social history reveals that she smokes one pack of cigarettes each day. Which of the following statements is true regarding tobacco and pregnancy?

a. Consuming small amounts of tobacco is probably safe; only heavy smokers incur increased risk of complications with their pregnancy.
b. Pregnant women are often motivated to stop smoking, so this is a good opportunity to provide counseling regarding smoking cessation.
c. Pregnant women should be encouraged to stop smoking during their pregnancy, but can be reassured they may restart as soon as the baby is born.
d. Tobacco use has been associated with an increased risk of congenital anomalies.
e. Tobacco use in pregnancy is a common cause of mental retardation and developmental delay in neonates.

27. A 36-year-old G0 who has been epileptic for many years is contemplating pregnancy. She wants to stop taking her phenytoin because she is concerned about the adverse effects that the medication may have on her unborn fetus. She has not had a seizure in the past 5 years. Which of the following is the most appropriate statement to make to the patient?

a. Babies born to epileptic mothers have an increased risk of structural anomalies even in the absence of anticonvulsant medications.
b. She should see her neurologist to change from phenytoin to valproic acid because valproic acid is not associated with fetal anomalies.
c. She should discontinue her phenytoin because it is associated with a 1% to 2% risk of spina bifida.
d. Vitamin C supplementation reduces the risk of congenital anomalies in fetuses of epileptic women taking anticonvulsants.
e. The most frequently reported congenital anomalies in fetuses of epileptic women are limb defects.

Questions 28 to 30

A 26-year-old P0 who works as a nurse in the surgery intensive care unit comes to see you for her annual gynecologic examination. She tells you that she plans to discontinue her oral contraceptives because she wants to become pregnant in the next few months. She has many questions regarding the immunizations required by her hospital and whether or not she can do this while pregnant.

28. Which of the following is the most appropriate recommendation regarding MMR vaccination?

a. She should be checked for immunity against the rubella virus prior to conception and vaccinated at least 28 days prior to conception because the rubella vaccine contains a live virus and should not be given during pregnancy.
b. She can receive the MMR vaccine after completion of the first trimester.
c. The MMR vaccine has been clearly associated with development of congenital fetal anomalies when given during the first trimester.
d. The MMR vaccine is an inactivated virus, and therefore can be given during any trimester of pregnancy.
e. The MMR vaccine may be safely given in third trimester, after completion of organogenesis.

29. What is the most appropriate counseling regarding the tetanus toxoid, reduced diphtheria toxoid, and acellular pertussis (Tdap) vaccine during pregnancy?

a. The Tdap should be avoided during pregnancy because whooping cough is not a major health issue.
b. The Tdap should be avoided during pregnancy because it is a live virus.
c. The Tdap is an inactivated vaccine that may be given during pregnancy during any trimester.
d. The Tdap is an inactivated vaccine that is currently recommended in each pregnancy between 27 and 36 weeks' gestation.
e. Family members do not need to receive Tdap.

30. What should you tell this patient about the annual influenza vaccine that is required by her hospital?

a. Pregnant women may receive the influenza vaccine during any trimester of pregnancy.
b. She should defer the influenza vaccine this year if she becomes pregnant.
c. Pregnant women are not at risk for severe complications from influenza, and therefore she should not receive this vaccine if pregnant or planning to become pregnant soon.
d. Influenza vaccine is a live virus that has been associated with fetal congenital anomalies.

31. An Ashkenazi Jewish couple comes in to see you for preconception counseling. They are concerned that they might be at an increased risk for certain genetic disorders because of their ethnic background. The woman is 28 years old and tells you that neither side of the family has a history of any genetic disorders. Which one of the following statements is the best advice for this couple?

a. They are at an increased risk of having a child with β-thalassemia.
b. They are at an increased risk of having a baby born with a NTD.
c. They do not need to undergo additional screening if there is no history of affected children in either family.
d. They should be screened for cystic fibrosis only if there is a known family history.
e. Tay-Sachs disease has a carrier frequency of 1/30 in the Jewish population, and the couple therefore should be screened for this genetic disease.

32. You have a patient who is very health conscious and regularly ingests several vitamins in megadoses and herbal therapies on a daily basis. She recently became a strict vegetarian because she heard it is the best diet for the developing fetus. She is going to attempt pregnancy and wants your advice regarding her diet and nutrition intake. Which of the following should you recommend during her pregnancy?

a. Because herbal medications are natural, she may continue these dietary supplements during pregnancy.
b. She should resume an omnivorous diet during pregnancy since animal sources provide the most desirable combination of proteins.
c. She should continue to take large doses of vitamin A supplements during pregnancy because dietary intake alone does not provide sufficient amounts needed during pregnancy.
d. During pregnancy, her vegetarian diet provides sufficient amounts of vitamin B_{12} needed for the developing fetus.
e. She should avoid vitamin C supplementation in pregnancy because excessive levels can result in fetal malformations.

Questions 33 to 37

Match each clinical situation described with the appropriate inheritance pattern. Each lettered option may be used once, more than once, or not at all.

a. Autosomal dominant
b. Autosomal recessive
c. X-linked recessive
d. Codominant
e. Multifactorial

33. An African-American woman presents to your office for her annual examination. She reports she was just released from the hospital after being treated for acute pain requiring narcotics.

34. A pregnant patient presents to you for prenatal care. Her parents are from Greece. She has a 2-year-old son, who was diagnosed with hemolytic anemia after he was treated for otitis media with a sulfonamide antibiotic. Her pediatrician gave her a list of antibiotics and foods that may trigger her son's anemia.

35. A patient presents to you for a well-woman examination. On physical examination she has a café au lait lesion on her back, along with multiple smooth, flesh-colored, dome-shaped papules scattered over her entire body.

36. A patient has a 2-year-old son with chronic pulmonary disease. His recent sweat test showed an elevated chloride level.

37. Your patient's father was just diagnosed with dementia associated with emotional disturbances and choreiform body movements. She was told his disease is hereditary.

Questions 38 to 46

For each sonographic image, select one diagnosis or diagnostic indicator. Each lettered option may be used once, more than once, or not at all.

a. Obstructed urethra and bladder
b. Nonspinal marker for spina bifida
c. Blighted ovum
d. Marker for Down syndrome (trisomy 21)
e. Cystic hygroma
f. Osteogenesis imperfecta
g. Mesomelic dwarfism
h. Anencephaly
i. Prune belly syndrome
j. Hydrocephalus
k. Spina bifida with meningocele

38.

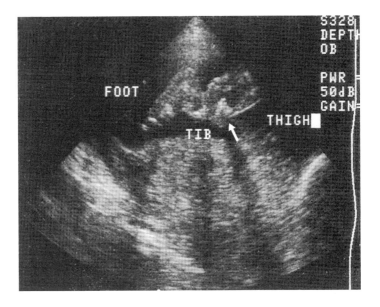

39.

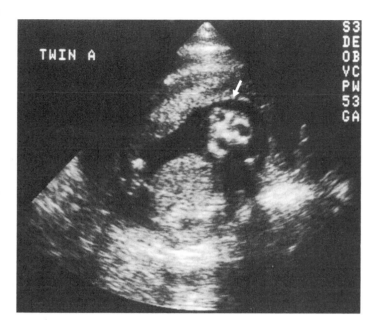

40.

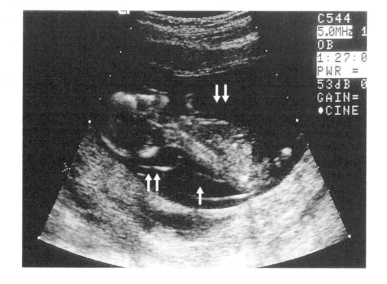

41.

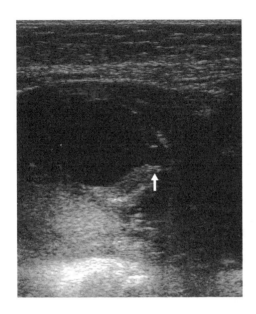

42.

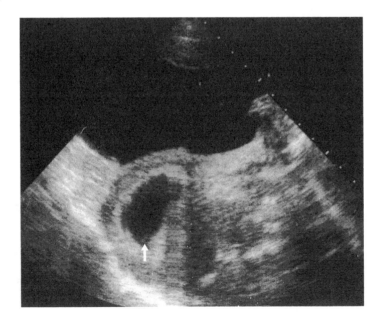

43.

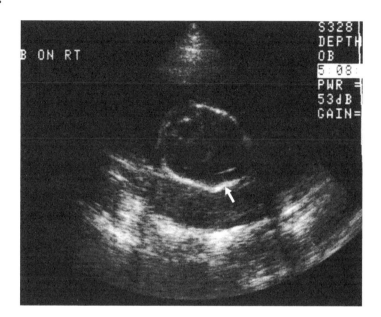

44.

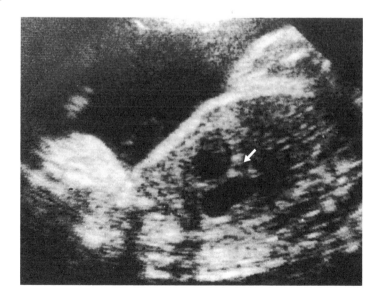

45.

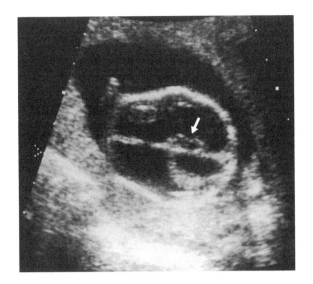

46.

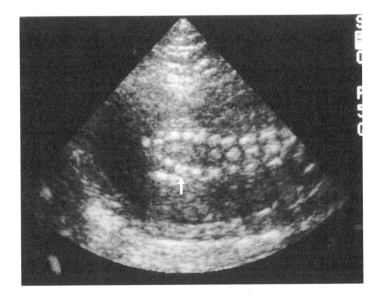

Questions 47 to 50

Match the appropriate scenario with the antibiotic most likely responsible for the clinical findings presented. Each lettered option may be used once, more than once, or not at all.

a. Tetracycline
b. Streptomycin
c. Nitrofurantoin
d. Chloramphenicol
e. Sulfonamides

47. At 1 year of age, a child has six deciduous teeth, which are discolored and have hypoplasia of the enamel.

48. A 1-week-old baby boy is brought in to the emergency department by his mother. For the past few days he has been lethargic. The day before he did not eat well and in the morning of the day of presentation he started vomiting. On the way to the hospital the baby had a seizure. On examination, the baby is jaundiced.

49. During routine auditory testing of a 2-day-old baby, the baby failed to respond to high-pitched tones.

50. A 2-week-old neonate who was delivered at 28 weeks' gestation developed pallid cyanosis, abdominal distension, and vascular collapse after exposure to an antibiotic. A few days later the baby died.

Questions 51 to 55

For each disease, select the recommendation regarding vaccination during pregnancy. Each lettered option may be used once, more than once, or not at all.

a. Recommended
b. Recommended after known exposure or before travel to endemic areas
c. Recommended if the patient is at high risk for the disease
d. Not recommended
e. Contraindicated

51. Varicella

52. Measles, mumps, and rubella (MMR)

53. Influenza

54. Hepatitis B

55. Human papillomavirus (HPV)

Preconception Counseling, Genetics, and Prenatal Diagnosis

Answers

1. The answer is b. An initial spontaneous abortion, regardless of the karyotype or gender of the child, does not change the risk of recurrence in a future pregnancy. The rate is commonly quoted as 15% of all known pregnancies.

2. The answer is a. Chromosomal abnormalities are found in approximately 50% of spontaneous abortions in the first trimester. Chromosome abnormalities become less common in advancing pregnancy, and are found in approximately one-third of second trimester losses and 5% of third trimester losses. Autosomal trisomy is the most common group of chromosomal anomalies leading to first trimester miscarriage. However, 45 X (Turner syndrome) is the most common single abnormality found.

3. The answer is c. Miscarriage risk rises with the number of prior spontaneous abortions. Without treatment, the live birth rate approaches 50%. With treatment, successful pregnancy rates of 70% to 85% are possible in a patient with a diagnosis of habitual abortion, depending on the underlying cause. When cervical incompetence is present and a cerclage is placed, success rates can approach 90%.

4. The answer is b. A major cause of spontaneous abortions in the first trimester is chromosomal abnormalities. Parental chromosome anomalies account for 2% to 4% of recurrent losses; therefore, karyotype evaluation of the parents is an important part of the evaluation. The causes of losses in the second trimester are more likely to be uterine or environmental in origin. Patients should also be screened for thyroid function, diabetes mellitus, and collagen vascular disorders. There is also a correlation between patients with a positive lupus anticoagulant and recurrent miscarriages. For recurrent second-trimester losses, a hysterosalpingogram should be ordered to rule out uterine structural abnormalities, such as bicornuate uterus, septate uterus, or unicornuate uterus. Endometrial biopsy is performed to rule out an insufficiency of the luteal phase or evidence of chronic endometritis. A postcoital test may be useful during an infertility evaluation for couples who cannot conceive, but does not address postconception losses. Measuring the cervical length by ultrasonography is helpful in the management of patients with recurrent second-trimester losses caused by cervical incompetence.

5. The answer is e. The risk of aneuploidy is increased with multiple miscarriages not attributable to other causes such as endocrine abnormalities or cervical incompetence. Paternal age does not contribute significantly to aneuploidy until around age 55, and most risks of paternal age are for point mutations. A 45 X karyotype results from loss of chromosome material and does not involve increased risks for nondisjunctional errors. Similarly, induced ovulation does not result in increased nondisjunction, and hypermodel conceptions (triploidy) do not increase risk for future pregnancies.

6. The answer is c. All of the markers listed are associated in some degree with Down syndrome as well as other genetic abnormalities, but increased NT is most closely and consistently associated. Increased NT is an early presenting feature of Down syndrome. Guidelines for systemic measurement of NT are standardized. Specific training and ongoing audits of examination quality are required for screening programs in order to ensure the expected detection rate. The optimal time to schedule NT measurement is between 12 and 13 weeks, but results are considered valid between 10 4/7 and 13 6/7 weeks. This results in Down syndrome detection rates of 72% at a screen positive rate of 5%. Most centers use a thickness of >/= 3 mm to define abnormal.

7. The answer is b. Several large, multicenter trials have shown that, in the first trimester, a combination of NT measurement, maternal age, and serum markers (PAPP-A and free or total β-hCG) is a reliable test for Down syndrome, with a detection rate of approximately 84%. Serum AFP is available as a screen for NTDs, and should be ordered after 15 weeks. Inhibin level alone is not a screen for Down syndrome, but may be part of a Quad screen. Amniocentesis cannot be offered until the second trimester. Fetal echocardiogram is not reliable in the first trimester, may not show cardiac defects in the first trimester, and is not considered a screening test for Down syndrome. It may be ordered in fetuses suspected to have Down syndrome based on abnormal diagnostic testing.

8. The answer is e. The patient should be referred for genetic counseling and offered a diagnostic test such as CVS or amniocentesis. Genetic counseling alone is not adequate, and referral to a high-risk specialist is not indicated at this time. The patient should not be told that the baby has Down syndrome, as the first trimester screen has a 5% false positive rate, and requires follow-up diagnostic testing. The patient should not be offered termination at this point, but it would be reasonable to offer termination if diagnostic testing confirmed Down syndrome.

9. The answer is d. Alcohol is an enormous contributor to otherwise preventable birth defects. Sequelae include retardation of intrauterine growth, craniofacial abnormalities, and mental retardation. The occasional drink in pregnancy has not been proved to be deleterious, but is still not recommended. Isotretinoin (accutane) is a powerful drug for acne that has enormous potential for producing congenital anomalies when ingested in early pregnancy; it should never be used in pregnancy. Tetracyclines interfere with development of bone and can lead to stained teeth in children. Progesterones have been implicated in multiple birth defects, but controlled studies have failed to demonstrate a significant association with increased risk. Patients who have inadvertently become pregnant while on birth control pills should be reassured that the incidence of birth defects is no higher for them than for the general population. Valproic acid is used for epilepsy and can be associated with a spectrum of abnormalities, including NTDs and abnormal facial features.

10. The answer is d. While a 50-rad exposure in the first trimester of pregnancy would be expected to entail a high likelihood of serious fetal damage and wastage, the anticipated fetal exposure for chest x-ray and one film of the lower spine would be less than 1 rad. This is well below the threshold for increased fetal risk, which is generally thought to be 10 rads. High doses of radiation in the first trimester primarily affect developing organ systems such as the heart and limbs; in later pregnancy, the brain is more sensitive. The chromosomes are determined at the moment of conception. Radiation does not alter the karyotype, and determination of the karyotype is not normally indicated for a 24-year-old patient. The incidence of leukemia is raised in children receiving radiation therapy or those exposed to the atomic bomb, but not from such a minimal exposure as here.

11. The answer is d. Women with uncomplicated pregnancies can continue to exercise during pregnancy if they had previously been accustomed to exercising prior to becoming pregnant. Studies indicate that well-conditioned women who maintain an antepartum exercise program consisting of aerobics or running have improved pregnancy outcomes in terms of shorter active labors, fewer cesarean section deliveries, less meconium-stained amniotic fluid, and less fetal distress in labor. On average, women who run regularly during pregnancy have babies that weigh 310 g less than women who do not exercise during pregnancy. Even though birth weight is reduced in exercising pregnant women, there is not an increased incidence of intrauterine growth retardation. The American College of Obstetricians and Gynecologists recommends that women avoid exercising while in the supine position to avoid a decrease in venous return to the heart, which results in decreased cardiac output. In addition, women should modify their exercise based on symptoms. There is no set pulse above which exercise is to be avoided; rather, women should decrease exercise intensity when experiencing symptoms of fatigue. Nonweight-bearing exercises will minimize the risk of injury. Since the physiologic changes associated with pregnancy will persist from 4 to 6 weeks following delivery, women should not resume the intensity of pre-pregnancy exercise regimens immediately following delivery.

12. The answer is a. There are many recreational activities that are considered to be safe during pregnancy. Riding a stationary bike, swimming, and walking are examples. Participation in sports with a high risk of abdominal trauma due to contact or due to falling is not recommended. These sports include competitive ice hockey or soccer, horseback riding, and downhill skiing. Scuba diving should be avoided during pregnancy because it places the fetus at an increased risk for decompression sickness due to the inability of the fetal pulmonary circulation to filter bubble formation.

13. The answer is e. Achondroplasia, a congenital disorder of cartilage formation characterized by dwarfism, is associated with an autosomal dominant pattern of inheritance. However, new mutations account for 90% of all cases of the disorder. Affected women almost always require cesarean delivery due to the distorted shape of the pelvis. Achondroplastic fetuses, when prenatally diagnosed, should also be delivered by cesarean to minimize trauma to the fetal neck. Women who have achondroplasia and receive adequate treatment for its associated complications generally have a normal life expectancy. The most common medical complaint in adulthood in patients with achondroplasia is symptomatic spinal stenosis.

14. The answer is e. Carriers of balanced translocations of the same chromosome are phenotypically normal. However, in the process of gamete formation (either sperm or ova), the translocated chromosome cannot divide, and therefore the meiosis products end up with either two copies or no copies of the particular chromosome. In the former case, fertilization leads to trisomy of that chromosome. Many trisomies are lethal in utero. Trisomies of chromosomes 13, 18, and 21 lead to classic syndromes. In the latter case, a monosomy is produced, and all except for monosomy X (Turner syndrome) are lethal in utero.

15. The answer is b. An encephalocele is a version of a NTD that involves an outpouching of neural tissue through a defect in the skull. A cystic hygroma, with which encephalocele can often be confused on ultrasound, emerges from the base of the neck with an intact skull present. Hydrocephalus is related to the size of the lateral ventricles. Anencephaly would require absence of a much larger proportion of the skull with diminished neural tissues. An omphalocele is a defect in the abdominal wall at the insertion of the umbilical cord, which may lead to herniation of the abdominal contents. Omphaloceles are associated with various other birth defects and chromosomal abnormalities.

16. The answer is c. The MSAFP may be performed between 15 and 21 weeks' gestation to screen for NTDs. The screen positive cut-off is usually set at 2.5 MoM, which results in a screen positive rate of 5% or less, and identifies 85% of NTDs. In the past, if the patient had only a moderately elevated value, a second MSAFP value could be drawn, as a small number of these patients will have a normal test and therefore drop back into the "low risk" category. Ultrasound evaluation may have high sensitivity and specificity in detecting fetal NTDs in specialized centers; however, in less experienced hands, there is a higher false negative rate. Therefore, you cannot reassure the patient that the fetus does not have a NTD. Ultrasound will help identify other reasons for elevated MSAFP, such as anencephaly, twins, wrong gestational age of the fetus, or fetal demise. The traditional diagnostic test to offer women with positive MSAFP results is genetic amniocentesis. Testing may be done to evaluate for elevated AFP in the amniotic fluid, as well as elevated acetylcholinesterase. In the setting where both of these amniotic fluid levels are elevated, this test has been shown to identify 100% of cases of anencephaly and open NTDs, as well as 20% of ventral wall defects. The other benefit of amniocentesis is that amniotic fluid may be used for karyotype assessment, as several studies have shown that elevated MSAFP independently increases the risk of fetal aneuploidy. Amniography is an outdated procedure in which radiopaque dye is injected into the amniotic cavity for the purpose of taking x-rays. Termination of pregnancy should not be recommended on the basis of MSAFP testing alone. MSAFP is a screening test used to define who is at risk, and requires further diagnostic testing in order to confirm or rule out a diagnosis.

17. The answer is d. The incidence of NTDs in the general population is approximately 1.4 to 2.0/1000. It is a multifactorial defect and is not influenced by maternal age. Women who have a previously affected child have a NTD recurrence risk of about 3% to 4%. This patient is at increased risk of having another child with a NTD and, therefore, should be offered prenatal diagnosis with an amniocentesis and targeted ultrasound. A CVS will determine a fetus' chromosomal makeup but will give no information regarding AFP levels or risk for a NTD. Woman with a previously affected fetus should take 4 mg of folic acid daily before conception and through the first trimester, as this has been shown to result in a 72% reduction in the recurrence risk. The neural tube is almost formed by the time of a missed period, and therefore, beginning supplementation with folic acid when a woman finds out she is pregnant is not sufficient to decrease the risk of NTDs. Women with no prior history of NTD who are of childbearing age should be encouraged to take 400μg of folic acid daily.

18. The answer is c. There is good data that outcomes are better when these neonates are delivered in settings that offer specialized personnel and neonatal intensive care facilities. Delivery at term is preferred, and preterm delivery is not known to improve neurologic outcomes. Breech presentation is common in pregnancies complicated by fetal spina bifida, resulting from either hydrocephalus with an enlarged head, or from fetal neurologic compromise. These infants should be delivered by cesarean. The best delivery route for a cephalic fetus is controversial, but several studies suggest that vaginal delivery does not adversely impact fetal outcome. The role of fetal surgery for repair of spina bifida is considered investigational. The studies in this field were not randomized and were largely limited to fetuses with lesions at or below the thoracic spine. Data suggested no improvement in bowel or bladder function or ambulatory ability. There may be a modest improvement in the degree of hindbrain herniation.

19. The answer is c. Amniocentesis and CVS are techniques of obtaining fetal cells for cytogenetic analysis. Amniotic fluid cells (obtained by amniocentesis at 15-20 weeks) require tissue culture to obtain adequate cell numbers for analysis. CVS at 10 to 13 weeks, either by transcervical or transabdominal access to the placenta, will provide the earliest results in order to diagnose Down syndrome. Multiple maternal serum marker analysis (Quad screen) may be done between 15 and 21 weeks, but it is primarily used for screening otherwise low-risk women for Down syndrome. Similarly, first trimester screening with NT measurements and maternal serum markers is not a diagnostic test. Neither of these tests are the most correct choice in this patient of advanced maternal age with a prior affected child. Cell free fetal DNA testing may be ordered as early as 10 weeks' gestation, and has a sensitivity of 98% with low false positive rates (< 0.5%), but is still a screening test. A normal screen would be reassuring, but an abnormal screen would still require diagnostic testing. Therefore, CVS is the best choice in this setting.

20. The answer is d. CVS has many advantages over amniocentesis, including its earlier performance and quicker results. Normal results provide early reassurance, while abnormal results may allow for earlier and safer options for pregnancy termination. However, CVS does have a higher complication rate. Mid-trimester amniocentesis carries a procedure-related fetal loss rate of 1 in 300 to 500. This may be even lower in experienced hands. The procedure-related loss rate for CVS is probably similar to that of amniocentesis; however, the overall pregnancy loss rate for CVS is higher than for amniocentesis due to the increased baseline loss rate between 9 and 16 weeks' gestation. First-trimester amniocentesis has a complication rate higher than that for CVS, and has been shown to have an increased risk of amniotic fluid culture failures and membrane rupture. For these reasons, early amniocentesis should not be offered.

21. The answer is e. There is a benefit for some women to be vaccinated against certain conditions during pregnancy. Live, attenuated virus vaccines, such as the MMR or the nasally delivered influenza vaccine, are not recommended during pregnancy. Vaccines that contain killed antigens, virus-like particles, or noninfectious components of bacteria, are considered safe in pregnancy. Examples include tetanus toxoid, Tdap, and the injectable influenza vaccine. Pregnancy is not a contraindication to the hepatitis B vaccine, and pregnant women identified as being at high risk for HBV infection should be vaccinated.

22. The answer is a. Chronic alcohol abuse, which can cause liver disease, folate deficiency, and many other disorders in a pregnant woman, also can lead to the development of congenital abnormalities in the child. Ethyl alcohol is one of the most potent teratogens known. The chief abnormalities associated with the fetal alcohol syndrome (FAS) are cardiac anomalies and joint defects FAS may also be associated with growth problems (either before or after pregnancy), mental or behavioral problems, and abnormal facial features. There is no known "safe" amount of alcohol that a woman may drink during pregnancy. Women who drink heavily both before and during pregnancy are at the highest risk of giving birth to a child with FAS. Heroin, benzodiazepines, marijuana, and methadone are not major teratogens.

23 and 24. The answers are 23-c, 24-e. These two questions address the question of the teratogenicity of antibiotics. Tetracycline may cause fetal dental anomalies and inhibition of bone growth if administered during the second and third trimesters, and it is a potential teratogen to first-trimester fetuses. Administration of tetracyclines can also cause severe hepatic decompensation in the mother, especially during the third trimester. Chloramphenicol may cause the gray baby syndrome (symptoms of which include vomiting, impaired respiration, hypothermia, and, finally, cardiovascular collapse) in neonates who have received large doses of the drug. No notable adverse effects have been associated with the use of penicillins or cephalosporins. Trimethoprim-sulfamethoxazole (bactrim) should not be used in the third trimester because sulfa drugs can cause kernicterus.

25. The answer is c. Women who are markedly obese are at increased risk of developing complications during pregnancy. Obese women are more likely to develop gestational diabetes and preeclampsia during pregnancy.

In addition, these women are more likely to develop fetal macrosomia and require cesarean delivery, which is associated with an increased risk of infectious and operative morbidity. This may include problems establishing and recovering from anesthesia, prolonged operating times, increased blood loss, higher rates of wound infection, and thromboembolism. Obese patients are less likely to have a successful vaginal birth after a cesarean delivery. Maternal obesity also has implications for the fetus, including increased risk of congenital anomalies, growth abnormalities, miscarriage, and stillbirth. Morbidly obese women who do not gain weight during pregnancy are not at risk for having a fetus with growth abnormalities, and therefore they do not need to gain the 25 lb to 35 lb recommended for women of normal weight. Although it is not recommended that obese women gain weight during pregnancy, diet restriction and weight loss are to be avoided. In addition, as with all women, it is not recommended that obese women initiate a rigorous exercise program during pregnancy.

26. The answer is b. There are many potential teratogens in cigarette smoke, including nicotine, carbon monoxide, cadmium, lead, and hydrocarbons. Smoking has been shown to cause fetal growth restriction and to be related to increased incidences of subfertility, spontaneous abortions, placenta previa, abruption, and preterm delivery. The mechanisms for these adverse effects include increased fetal carboxyhemoglobin levels, reduced uteroplacental blood flow, and fetal hypoxia. Most studies do not indicate that tobacco use is related to an increased risk of congenital malformations, mental retardation, or developmental delay. Almost half of women who smoke quit directly before or during pregnancy. An office-based protocol that offers treatment or referral for smoking cessation has been proven to increase quit rates. The 5A's is an office based intervention to help pregnant women quit smoking. These are as follows: (1) Ask the patient about smoking, (2) Advise the patient to stop, (3) Assess the patient's willingness to attempt to quit, (4) Assist the patient who is interested by providing smoking cessation materials, (5) Arrange follow-up visits to track the progress of the patient's attempt to stop smoking. Patients should be encouraged to remain smoke free. Children born to mothers who smoke are at an increased risk of asthma, obesity, and colic.

27. The answer is a. Offspring of women with epilepsy have two to three times the risk of congenital anomalies even in the absence of anticonvulsant medications, because seizures cause a transient reduction in uterine blood flow and fetal oxygenation. When anticonvulsant medications are used, pregnant women have an even greater risk of congenital malformations. It is recommended that women undergo a trial of being weaned off their medications prior to becoming pregnant. If antiseizure medications must be used, monotherapy is preferred to minimize the risk to the fetus, since the incidence of fetal anomalies increases as additional anticonvulsants are consumed. Many anticonvulsants have been found to impair folate metabolism, and folate supplementation in pregnancy has been associated with a decreased incidence of congenital anomalies in epileptic women taking antiseizure medications. Fetal exposure to valproic acid has been associated with a 1% to 2% risk of spina bifida.

28. The answer is a. In general, it is ideal for women to be up to date on routine adult vaccines before becoming pregnant. Live vaccines, such as MMR, should be given at least 1 month before pregnancy, due to theoretic risks to the fetus. Women should be offered testing for immunity to rubella during preconception counseling visits, and offered immunization prior to pregnancy if needed. Pregnant women who are found to be rubella nonimmune may be given the MMR vaccine immediately postpartum.

29. The answer is d. The Tdap should be offered to all pregnant women during each pregnancy between 27 and 36 weeks, regardless of the patient's prior history of receiving Tdap. Pertussis, or whooping cough, is a common vaccine-preventable disease that can be very serious for newborns. The level of pertussis antibodies decreases over time, hence the recommendation to administer during every pregnancy. In addition, all family members and caregivers of infants should be vaccinated with Tdap. Vaccinating pregnant women helps prevent the mother from acquiring the disease and passing it to her newborn, and also provides passive immunity to the infant. Tdap is an inactivated vaccine.

30. The answer is a. Influenza is an inactivated vaccine that is recommended for all women who are pregnant or who may be pregnant during flu season. It may be given in any trimester. Pregnant women who get the flu are at increased risk for severe complications requiring hospitalization. Flu season in the United States is generally from early October to late March.

31. The answer is e. Certain autosomal recessive diseases are more common in individuals of Eastern European Jewish ancestry. ACOG recommends carrier screening for Tay-Sachs disease (carrier frequency 1/30), Canavan disease (carrier frequency 1/40), familial dysautonomia (carrier frequency 1/32), and cystic fibrosis (carrier frequency 1/29). Carrier screening tests are also available for several diseases that are less common, such as Fanconi anemia, Niemann-Pick disease, Bloom syndrome, and Gaucher disease. When only one partner is of Ashkenazi Jewish descent, that partner should be screened first. If this individual is found to be a carrier, then the partner should be offered screening. β-Thalassemias are hemoglobinopathies especially prevalent in individuals of Mediterranean or Asian heritage. The couple described is not at an increased risk of β-thalassemia and therefore does not need to undergo screening with hemoglobin electrophoresis. Based on ethnic background, this couple is not at increased risk of having a baby with a NTD. NTD follows a multifactorial inheritance pattern.

32. The answer is b. The use of herbal remedies is not recommended during pregnancy because such products are classified as dietary supplements and therefore are not FDA-regulated for purity, safety, and efficacy. In fact, the actual ingredients of many herbal substances are not even known. There is almost no data regarding the teratogenic potential of herbal medications in humans. Although a carefully planned vegetarian diet provides sufficient amino acids for pregnancy, it is not recommended that women assume a vegetarian diet during pregnancy. Animal sources of protein such as meat, poultry, fish, and eggs contain amino acids in the most desirable combinations. Strict vegetarians can give birth to infants who are low in vitamin B_{12}, because vitamin B_{12} occurs naturally only in foods of animal origin. Pregnant women do not need to take vitamin A supplements because adequate amounts can be obtained in the diet; in addition, a very high intake of vitamin A has been associated with the type of congenital malformations seen with oral accutane use. Adequate vitamin C levels needed for pregnancy can be provided in a reasonable diet. No known fetal anomalies have been reported with vitamin C supplementation in pregnancy.

33 to 37. The answers are 33-b, 34-c, 35-a, 36-b, 37-a. Sickle cell anemia is an autosomal recessive condition that is common in people of African origin. In low-oxygen conditions, the red cells become distorted (sickle), and this can lead to vasoocclusive crisis causing severe pain. Glucose-6-phosphate dehydrogenase (G6PD) deficiency is X-linked recessive and is found predominantly in males of African and Mediterranean origin.

Although the causes of clinical manifestations in G6PD deficiency are multifactorial (eg, sulfa drugs), the inheritance is not. Neurofibromatosis, whose occurrence is often sporadic (ie, a spontaneous mutation in 50%), is inherited as an autosomal dominant trait once the gene is in a family. The severity of the condition can be quite variable even within the same family. Cystic fibrosis is the most common autosomal recessive disorder in the white European population. Huntington disease is autosomal dominant.

38 to 46. The answers are 38-f, 39-h, 40-e, 41-a, 42-c, 43-b, 44-d, 45-j, 46-k. The diagnosis of osteogenesis imperfecta can be made by visualizing fractures in utero by ultrasound. The ultrasound in question 38 shows a crumpling of the tibia and fibula and curvature of the thigh such that proper extension of the foot does not occur.

The sonographic image in question 39 was done at approximately 15 weeks' gestation and shows two orbits, a mouth, and a central nose, but there is clearly no forehead and no cranial contents. Anencephaly is incompatible with life.

The sonographic image in question 40 shows a 13-week-old fetus with a large NT (double arrows) and early hydrops, sometimes called a cystic hygroma. In the second and third trimesters, cystic hygromas are commonly associated with Turner syndrome (45, X). In early pregnancy, however, 50% of cases will be associated with a trisomy, usually trisomy 21, trisomy 18, or trisomy 13. Of those cases that are chromosomally normal, most of these nuchal translucencies disappear, and the fetus goes on to have perfectly normal development.

In question 41, the transverse cut through the bladder shows megacystis (ie, the bladder is markedly enlarged) and the distal portion of the urethra can be visualized up to the point of urinary blockage. The blocked urethra acts as a dam that causes the bladder to fill up, then the ureters, and finally the kidneys (hydronephrosis). There is oligohydramnios noted in this picture because by 16 weeks—the gestational age at which this picture was taken—the vast majority of amniotic fluid comes from fetal urine. These pregnancies are usually associated with fetal death due to pulmonary hypoplasia, because the early oligohydramnios does not allow for proper lung development.

The sonographic image in question 42 was performed at approximately 8 weeks after the last menstrual period and shows a placenta but no fetal pole—the classic blighted ovum. Traditionally, 50% of first-trimester spontaneous abortions are said to be chromosomally abnormal. However, more recent evidence suggests that, particularly with advancing age of the mother (ie, in women who are likely to have early ultrasonography for potential CVS), the risk of fetal chromosomal abnormalities is in fact much higher, in many cases approaching even 90% of first-trimester spontaneous abortions.

The cross-section through the fetal head in question 43 shows a classic lemon sign; that is, there is a frontal bossing of the forehead such that the sides of the forehead are actually pulled in. This is because of the pull on the cisterna magna from spina bifida that is distorting the intracranial contents. This so-called lemon sign has a very high degree of sensitivity, although it is not perfect. The lemon sign disappears in the third trimester and is therefore not useful late in pregnancy.

The longitudinal sonographic image in question 44 shows the double bubble sign indicating duodenal atresia. The two bubbles are the stomach and the jejunum. This finding is classic for trisomy 21. Approximately one-third of fetuses who have this finding will be found to have trisomy 21, and in this situation, prenatal diagnosis should be offered to document the chromosomes regardless of any other indication the patient may have.

The ultrasound in question 45 demonstrates dilation of the lateral ventricles consistent with hydrocephalous. In question 46 the ultrasound shows splaying of the lumbar spine consistent with spina bifida.

47 to 50. The answers are 47-a, 48-e, 49-b, 50-d. The teratogenicity of antibiotics after fetal exposure depends on many factors such as gestational age, protein binding, lipid solubility, pH, molecular weight, degree of ionization, and concentration gradient. Some antibiotics are even concentrated in the fetal compartment. Tetracycline is contraindicated in all three trimesters. It has been associated with skeletal abnormalities, staining and hypoplasia of budding fetal teeth, bone hypoplasia, and fatal maternal liver decompensation. Sulfonamides are associated with kernicterus in the newborn. They compete with bilirubin for binding sites on albumin, thereby leaving more bilirubin free for diffusion into tissues. Sulfonamides should be withheld during the last 2 to 6 weeks of pregnancy. With prolonged treatment of tuberculosis (TB) in pregnancy, streptomycin has been associated with fetal hearing loss. Its use is restricted to complicated cases of TB. Nitrofurantoin can cause maternal and fetal hemolytic anemia if glucose 6-phosphate dehydrogenase deficiency is present. Chloramphenicol is noted for causing the gray baby syndrome. Infants are unable to properly metabolize the drug, which reaches toxic levels in about 4 days and can lead to neonatal death within 1 to 2 days.

51 to 55. **The answers are 51-e, 52-e, 53-a, 54-c, 55-d.** Pregnant women should not be vaccinated against varicella or MMR during pregnancy, because the effects on the fetus are unknown. Women should wait 1 month after vaccination to become pregnant. Influenza vaccine is recommended for all pregnant women during all trimesters, due to the potential severe effects of the disease on pregnant women. Pregnancy is not a contraindication to hepatitis B vaccination. Limited data suggest that there are not adverse fetal effects due to this vaccine. It should be considered in pregnant women who are at increased risk for hepatitis B. HPV vaccination is not recommended during pregnancy. If a women is found to be pregnant during administration of the vaccine (which requires three doses), the remainder of the series should be delayed until pregnancy is complete.

Suggested Readings

American College of Obstetricians and Gynecologists. *Bariatric Surgery and Pregnancy.* Practice Bulletin Number 105, June 2009, reaffirmed 2013.

American College of Obstetricians and Gynecologists. *Exercise During Pregnancy and the Postpartum Period.* Committee Opinion Number 267, January 2002, reaffirmed 2009.

American College of Obstetricians and Gynecologists. *Invasive Prenatal Testing for Aneuploidy.* Practice Bulletin Number 88, December 2007, reaffirmed 2014.

American College of Obstetricians and Gynecologists. *Neural Tube Defects.* Practice Bulletin Number 44, July 2003, reaffirmed 2014.

American College of Obstetricians and Gynecologists. *Noninvasive Prenatal Testing for Fetal Aneuploidy.* Committee Opinion Number 545, December 2012.

American College of Obstetricians and Gynecologists. *Preconception and Prenatal Carrier Screening for Genetic Diseases in Individuals of Eastern European Jewish Descent.* Committee Opinion Number 442, October 2009, reaffirmed 2014.

American College of Obstetricians and Gynecologists. *Screening for Fetal Chromosome Abnormalities.* Practice Bulletin Number 77, January 2007, reaffirmed 2013.

American College of Obstetricians and Gynecologists. *Smoking Cessation During Pregnancy.* Committee Opinion Number 471, November 2010, reaffirmed 2013.

Centers for Disease Control. *Guidelines for Immunizing Pregnant Women.* Atlanta (GA): CDC; 2012. http://www.cdc.gov/vaccines/pubs/preg-guide. htm, Accessed March 2014.

Cunningham FG, Leveno KJ, Bloom SL, et al. eds. Chapter 9: Abortion. *Williams Obstetrics.* 23rd ed. New York, NY: McGraw-Hill Education; 2010.

Malone FD, Canick JA, Ball RH, et al. First-trimester or second-trimester screening, or both, for Down's syndrome. *N Engl J Med.* 2005; 353:2001-2011.

Maternal-Fetal Physiology and Placentation

Questions

56. A 29-year-old Caucasian primigravida is 20 weeks pregnant with twins. Today, on her routine ultrasound for fetal anatomy, she found out that she is carrying two boys. In this patient's case, which of the following statements correctly describes the zygosity of this pregnancy?

a. The twins must be monozygotic since they are both the same gender.
b. If division of these twins occurred after formation of the embryonic disk, the twins will be conjoined.
c. She has a higher incidence of having monozygotic twins because she is Caucasian.
d. If the ultrasound showed two separate placentas, the twins must be dizygotic.
e. If the ultrasound showed two separate placentas, the twins cannot be monozygotic.

57. After delivery of a term newborn with Apgar scores of 2 at 1 minute and 7 at 5 minutes, you ask that blood from the umbilical arteries be collected for pH. The umbilical arteries carry which of the following?

a. Oxygenated blood to the placenta
b. Oxygenated blood from the placenta
c. Deoxygenated blood to the placenta
d. Deoxygenated blood from the placenta
e. Mixed oxygenated blood from the placenta

Questions 58 to 59

A 25-year-old P0 presents for routine anatomy ultrasound at 20 weeks' gestation. The only significant finding at the time of ultrasound is the presence of a single umbilical artery (SUA).

58. How should you counsel this patient about the finding of a SUA?

a. It is a very common finding and is insignificant.
b. Fetal karyotype should be determined, because this finding is associated with an increased risk of aneuploidy.
c. Careful anatomic survey should be performed, because it is an indicator of an increased incidence of congenital anomalies of the fetus.
d. It is equally common in newborns of diabetic and nondiabetic mothers.
e. Even if it is the only abnormality present, SUA is commonly associated with adverse pregnancy outcomes.

59. Targeted ultrasound does not demonstrate any other abnormalities. The patient asks you if this SUA will impact how you manage the rest of her pregnancy. What should you tell her?

a. Her pregnancy will not be managed any differently due to the isolated finding of SUA.
b. The next step in her management should be genetic amniocentesis.
c. She will require periodic assessments of fetal growth.
d. She should be delivered by 39 weeks' gestation at the latest.
e. She will require delivery by cesarean.

60. A 22-year-old G1P0 at 28 weeks' gestation by LMP presents to labor and delivery complaining of decreased fetal movement. She has had no prenatal care. On the fetal monitor there are no contractions. The fetal heart rate is 150 beats per minute and reactive, with no decelerations in the fetal heart tracing. An ultrasound demonstrates a 28-week fetus with normal anatomy and size consistent with menstrual dates. The placenta is implanted on the posterior uterine wall and its margin is well away from the cervix. A succenturiate lobe of the placenta is seen implanted low on the anterior wall of the uterus. Doppler flow studies indicate a blood vessel is traversing the cervix connecting the two lobes. This patient is most at risk for which of the following?

a. Premature rupture of the membranes
b. Fetal exsanguination after rupture of the membranes
c. Torsion of the umbilical cord caused by velamentous insertion of the umbilical cord
d. Amniotic fluid embolism
e. Placenta accreta

61. A healthy 25-year-old G1P0 at 37 weeks' gestational age comes to your office to see you for a routine obstetric visit. She reports that on several occasions she has experienced dizziness, light-headedness, and feeling as if she is going to pass out when she lies down on her back to take a nap. What is the most appropriate plan of management for this patient?

a. Perform an electrocardiogram
b. Monitor her for 24 hours with a Holter monitor to rule out an arrhythmia
c. Perform an arterial blood gas analysis
d. Refer her to a cardiologist
e. Reassure and encourage her not to lie flat on her back

62. A 22-year-old primigravida presents to your office for a routine OB visit at 34 weeks' gestational age. She voices concern because she has noticed an increasing number of spidery veins appearing on her face, upper chest, and arms. She is upset with the unsightly appearance of these veins and wants to know what you recommend to get rid of them. How should you counsel this patient?

a. Tell her that this is a condition which requires evaluation by a vascular surgeon.
b. Tell her that you are concerned that she may have serious liver disease and order liver function tests.
c. Tell her that you are going to refer her to a dermatologist for further workup and evaluation.
d. Tell her that the appearance of these blood vessels is a normal occurrence with pregnancy.
e. Tell her to wear an abdominal binder.

63. You are the third year medical student assigned to labor and delivery. A 29-year-old P3003 at 29 weeks with known placenta previa presents to the triage area with a report of vaginal bleeding. The fetal heart tracing is reactive and the bleeding is minimal. You take history and present her to your intern. You accompany the intern to triage to further evaluate the patient together. Your intern confirms the history and prepares to perform a digital cervical examination. What should your next step be in this situation?

a. Watch the intern perform a digital cervical examination
b. Ask if you may also perform a digital cervical examination
c. Remind the intern that the patient has a placenta previa and should not have a digital cervical examination
d. Suggest that the intern perform an ultrasound to evaluate the placenta
e. Do not say anything at the time, but afterward remind the intern that the patient has a placenta previa and should not have a digital cervical examination

64. A healthy 34-year-old G1P0 patient comes to see you in your office for a routine OB visit at 12 weeks' gestational age. She tells you that she has stopped taking her prenatal vitamins with iron supplements because they make her sick and she has trouble remembering to take a pill every day. A review of her prenatal laboratory tests reveals that her hematocrit is 39%. Which of the following statements is the best way to counsel this patient?

a. Tell the patient that she is not anemic, and therefore she will not need the iron supplied in prenatal vitamins.
b. Tell the patient that if she consumes a diet rich in iron, she does not need to take any iron supplements.
c. Tell the patient that if she fails to take her iron supplements, her fetus will be anemic.
d. Tell the patient that she needs to take the iron supplements, even though she is not currently anemic, in order to meet the iron demands of pregnancy.
e. Tell the patient that she needs to start her iron supplements if her hematocrit falls below 36%.

65. A 19-year-old P0 at 20 weeks' gestation presents to the emergency department (ED) with complaints of right flank pain. The ED physician orders a renal sonogram as part of a workup for a possible kidney stone. The radiologist reports that no nephrolithiasis is present, but reports the presence of bilateral mild hydronephrosis and hydroureter, which is greater on the right side than on the left. What is the most appropriate next step in management?

a. Order renal function tests, including BUN and creatinine, to evaluate the renal function.
b. These findings are consistent with normal pregnancy and are not of concern. No further evaluation is required.
c. Order an intravenous pyelogram to further evaluate the bilateral hydronephrosis.
d. Request a urology consult to obtain recommendations for further workup and evaluation.
e. The findings are concerning for bilateral ureteral obstruction, and the patient should be referred for stent placement.

66. During a routine return OB visit, an 18-year-old G1P0 patient at 23 weeks' gestational age undergoes a urinalysis. The dipstick done by the nurse indicates the presence of trace glucosuria. All other parameters of the urine test are normal. Which of the following is the most likely etiology of the increased glucose detected in the urine?

a. The patient has gestational diabetes.
b. The patient has a urinary tract infection.
c. The patient's urinalysis is consistent with normal pregnancy.
d. The patient's urine sample is contaminated.
e. The patient has underlying renal disease.

67. A 29-year-old G1P0 at 28 weeks' gestation presents to your office complaining of shortness of breath that is more intense with exertion. She has no significant past medical history and is not on any medication. The patient denies any chest pain. She is concerned because she has always been very athletic and cannot maintain the same degree of exercise that she was accustomed to prior to becoming pregnant. On physical examination, her pulse is 72 beats per minute. Her blood pressure is 90/50 mm Hg. Cardiac examination is consistent with a grade I systolic ejection murmur. The lungs are clear to auscultation. Which of the following is the most appropriate next step in management of this patient?

a. Refer the patient for a ventilation-perfusion scan to rule out a pulmonary embolism (PE)
b. Perform an arterial blood gas
c. Refer the patient to a cardiologist
d. Reassure the patient
e. Order an electrocardiogram

Questions 68 to 70

Match the descriptions with the appropriate placenta type. Each lettered option may be used once, more than once, or not at all.

a. Fenestrated placenta
b. Succenturiate placenta
c. Vasa previa
d. Placenta previa
e. Membranous placenta
f. Placenta accreta

68. A 33-year-old G2P1 is undergoing an elective repeat cesarean section at term. The newborn is delivered without any difficulties, but the placenta cannot be removed easily because a clear plane between the placenta and uterine wall cannot be identified. The placenta is removed in pieces. This is followed by uterine atony and hemorrhage.

69. A 22-year-old G3P2 undergoes a normal spontaneous vaginal delivery without complications. The placenta is spontaneously delivered and appears intact. The patient is later transferred to the postpartum floor where she starts to bleed profusely. Physical examination reveals a boggy uterus and a bedside sonogram indicates the presence of placental tissue.

70. A 34-year-old G6P5 presents to labor and delivery by ambulance at 33 weeks' gestational age complaining of the sudden onset of profuse vaginal bleeding. The patient denies any abdominal pain or uterine contractions. She denies any problems with her pregnancy to date but has had no prenatal care. She admits to smoking several cigarettes a day, but denies any drug or alcohol use. The fetal heart rate tracing is normal. There are no contractions on the tocometer.

Maternal-Fetal Physiology and Placentation

Answers

56. The answer is b. The incidence of monozygotic twinning is constant at a rate of one set per 250 births around the world. It is unaffected by race, heredity, age, parity, or infertility agents. The incidence of dizygotic twinning is influenced by all of these factors, and varies based on group. These twins of the same gender could be monozygotic or dizygotic. Two identifiable chorions can occur in monozygotic or dizygotic twinning. Dizygotic twins will always have two amnions and two chorions, since they result from fertilization of two eggs. Therefore, dizygotic twins may be of the same or different genders. The placentas of dizygotic twins may be totally separate, or intimately fused, depending on the location of the implantation of the two zygotes. Monozygotic twins are always of the same gender because they originate from the division of one zygote; however, they may be monochorionic or dichorionic depending on when the separation of the twins occurred. Twenty to thirty percent of monozygotic twins have dichorionic, diamniotic placentation (similar to dizygotic twins), which results from separation of the blastocyst within the first 72 hours after fertilization. Division that occurs between days 4 and 8 will result in monochorionic, diamniotic twins. One percent of monozygotic twins will be monochorionic, monoamniotic, which occurs with division after day 8 but before the embryonic disc is formed. Conjoined twins are always monozygotic, and occur with late division after formation of the embryonic disk.

57. The answer is c. Deoxygenated fetal blood is returned directly to the placenta through the umbilical branches of the two hypogastric arteries. The umbilical arteries exit through the abdominal wall at the umbilicus and continue by way of the umbilical cord to the placenta. Deoxygenated blood circulates through the placenta then returns, oxygenated, to the fetus via the umbilical vein. The umbilical arteries atrophy and obliterate within 3 to 4 days after birth; remnants are called *umbilical ligaments*.

58. The answer is c. The finding of a SUA occurs in approximately 1% of pregnancies, and 5% of at least one twin. The incidence of SUA is increased in diabetic mothers. The incidence of major fetal malformations when SUA is identified has been reported to be as high as 18%, and usually involves the cardiac or renal systems; therefore, a careful anatomic survey is indicated. The rate of aneuploidy in the setting of isolated SUA is not increased, so routine karyotype analysis is not needed unless there are other indications to offer this testing. In the absence of other findings, SUA is rarely associated with poor pregnancy outcomes.

59. The answer is c. The finding of SUA in the absence of other abnormalities does not require karyotype evaluation, early delivery, or delivery by cesarean. The timing and mode of delivery may be determined by routine obstetric indications. Patients with a fetus with SUA should undergo periodic growth assessments with ultrasound, as there is an increased risk of growth restriction in these fetuses.

60. The answer is b. This patient has a vasa previa. When fetal vessels cross the internal os (vasa previa), rupture of membranes may be accompanied by rupture of a fetal vessel leading to fetal exsanguination. Vasa previa does not increase the risk for placenta accreta or amniotic fluid embolism. With velamentous insertion of the cord, the umbilical vessels separate in the membranes at a distance from the placental margin which they reach surrounded only by amnion. Such insertion occurs in about 1% of singleton gestations but is quite common in multiple pregnancies. Fetal malformations are more common with velamentous insertion of the umbilical cord. An increased risk of premature rupture of membranes and torsion of the umbilical cord has not been described in association with velamentous insertion of the cord.

61. The answer is e. Late in pregnancy, when the mother assumes the supine position, the gravid uterus compresses the inferior vena cava and decreases venous return to the heart. This results in decreased cardiac output and symptoms of dizziness, light-headedness, and syncope. This significant arterial hypotension resulting from inferior vena cava compression is known as supine hypotensive syndrome or inferior vena cava syndrome. Therefore, it is not recommended that women remain in the supine position for any prolonged period of time in the latter part of pregnancy. When patients describe symptoms of the supine hypotensive syndrome, there is no need to proceed with additional cardiac or pulmonary workup.

62. The answer is d. Vascular spiders, or angiomas, are common findings during pregnancy. They form as a result of the hyper-estrogenism associated with normal pregnancies and are of no clinical significance. The presence of these angiomas does not require any additional workup or treatment, and they will resolve spontaneously after delivery. Reassurance to the patient is all that is required.

63. The answer is c. Patient safety has no hierarchy. Placenta previa is a condition where the placenta is implanted over the internal cervical os. Digital cervical examination is contraindicated in this setting due to the possibility of causing severe hemorrhage. The correct next step is to speak up to make sure the intern knows that the patient has a placenta previa and should not have a digital cervical examination.

64. The answer is d. The amount of iron that can be mobilized from maternal stores and obtained from the diet is insufficient to meet the demands of pregnancy. A pregnant woman with a normal hematocrit at the beginning of pregnancy who is not given iron supplementation will develop iron deficiency during the latter part of gestation, as iron requirements increase significantly during the second half of pregnancy. It is important to remember that the fetus will not have impaired hemoglobin production, even in the presence of maternal anemia, because the placenta will transport the needed iron at the expense of maternal iron store depletion. The hematocrit in pregnancy normally falls in pregnancy due to plasma volume expansion and therefore is not used as a parameter to determine when to begin iron supplementation.

65. The answer is b. Bilateral mild hydronephrosis and hydroureter are normal findings during pregnancy and do not require any additional workup or concern. When the gravid uterus rises out of the pelvis after 12 weeks, it presses on the ureters at the pelvic brim, causing ureteral dilatation and hydronephrosis. It is also likely that hormonal effect from progesterone contributes to the development of hydroureter and hydronephrosis of pregnancy. In the vast majority of pregnant women, ureteral dilatation tends to be greater on the right side as a result of the dextrorotation of the uterus and/or cushioning of the left ureter provided by the sigmoid colon.

66. The answer is c. The finding of glucosuria is common during pregnancy, and usually is not indicative of a pathologic condition. During pregnancy, there is an increase in the glomerular filtration rate, and a decrease in tubular reabsorption of filtered glucose. In fact, one in six women will spill glucose into the urine during pregnancy. If the patient has risk factors for gestational diabetes, such as obesity, previous macrosomic baby, advanced maternal age, or family history of diabetes, the physician may want to screen for diabetes with a glucose challenge test. If the patient has a urinary tract infection, the dipstick will be more likely to show an increase in WBCs, and the presence of nitrites and blood. A contaminated urine sample would not be a cause of isolated glucosuria.

67. The answer is d. The patient's symptoms and physical examination are most consistent with physiologic dyspnea, which is common in pregnancy. The increased awareness of breathing that pregnant women experience can occur as early as the end of the first trimester, and is caused by an increase in lung tidal volume. The increase in minute ventilation that occurs during pregnancy may make patients feel as if they are hyperventilating, and may also contribute to the feeling of dyspnea. The patient in this case needs to be reassured and counseled regarding these normal changes of pregnancy. She may have to modify her exercise regimen accordingly. There is no need to refer this patient to a cardiologist or to order an ECG. Systolic ejection murmurs are common findings in pregnant women and are caused by the normal increased blood flow across the aortic and pulmonic valves. The incidence of PE in pregnancy is about 1 in 6400, and in many of these cases there is clinical evidence of a DVT. The most common symptoms of a PE are dyspnea, chest pain, apprehension, cough, hemoptysis, and tachycardia.

68 to 70. The answers are 68-f, 69-b, 70-d. A placenta accreta occurs when the trophoblastic tissue invades the superficial lining of the uterus. In this instance, the placenta is abnormally adherent to the uterine wall and cannot be easily separated from it. A portion of the placenta may be removed, while other parts remain attached, resulting in hemorrhage. A succenturiate placenta is characterized by one or more smaller accessory lobes located in the membranes at a distance from the main placenta. A retained succenturiate lobe may cause uterine atony and result in postpartum hemorrhage. In placenta previa, the placenta is located very near or over the internal cervical os. Painless hemorrhage can occur without warning, and is caused by tearing of the placental attachments during formation of the lower uterine segment in the third trimester, or with cervical dilation during term or preterm labor. A history of previous cesarean delivery, grand multiparity, and maternal smoking have been associated with an increased risk of placenta previa. Vasa previa occurs when there is a velamentous insertion of the umbilical cord or a succenturiate lobe and the fetal vessels within the membranes traverse the internal cervical os. The fenestrated placenta is a rare anomaly where the central portion of the placenta is missing. In the membranous placenta, all fetal membranes are covered by villi, and the placenta develops as a thin membranous structure. This type of placenta is also known as placenta diffusa.

Suggested Readings

American College of Obstetricians and Gynecologists. *Fetal Growth Restriction*. Practice Bulletin Number 134, May 2013.

Cunningham FG, Leveno KJ, Bloom SL, et al. eds. Chapter 5: The placenta and fetal membranes; Chapter 8: Maternal adaptations to pregnancy; Chapter 30: Multifetal pregnancy; Chapter 32: Diseases and abnormalities of the placenta. In: *Williams Obstetrics*. 23rd ed. New York, NY: McGraw-Hill Education; 2010.

Antepartum Care and Fetal Surveillance

Questions

71. A patient presents in labor at term. Clinical pelvimetry is performed. She has an oval-shaped pelvis with the anteroposterior (AP) diameter at the pelvic inlet greater than the transverse diameter. The baby is occiput posterior. The patient most likely has what kind of pelvis?

a. A gynecoid pelvis
b. An android pelvis
c. An anthropoid pelvis
d. A platypelloid pelvis
e. An androgenous pelvis

72. Pelvic examination is performed in a 34-year-old P0101 at 34 weeks' gestation who is in labor. The patient is noted to be 6 cm dilated, and completely effaced with the fetal nose and mouth palpable. The chin is pointing toward the maternal left hip. This is an example of which of the following?

a. Transverse lie
b. Mentum transverse position
c. Occiput transverse position
d. Brow presentation
e. Vertex presentation

73. You are counseling a 36-year-old obese, Hispanic G2P1 at 36 weeks' gestation about route of delivery. During her first pregnancy, she was induced at 41 weeks' gestation for mild preeclampsia, and delivered by cesarean as a result of fetal distress during her induction. The patient would like to know if she can have a trial of labor after cesarean (TOLAC) with this pregnancy. Which of the following is the best response to this patient?

a. No, since she has never had a vaginal delivery.
b. Yes, but only if she had a low transverse uterine incision.
c. No, because once she has had a cesarean delivery, she must deliver all of her subsequent children by cesarean.
d. Yes, but only if her skin incision was a Pfannensteil.
e. Yes, but she must wait until she goes into labor spontaneously to have a repeat cesarean.

74. The patient wants to know about the probability of success if she chooses to undergo TOLAC. What can you tell her about factors that impact the probability of success in TOLAC?

a. The probability of successful TOLAC is increased for her because she is Hispanic.
b. She is likely to have a successful TOLAC because she has never had a vaginal delivery.
c. Her weight does not impact her chance for successful TOLAC.
d. Her age does not impact her chance for successful TOLAC.
e. If she goes into labor spontaneously before 40 weeks, her chance for successful TOLAC will be increased.

75. The patient has still not gone into spontaneous labor at 41 weeks' gestation. You see her in clinic and her blood pressure is 150/90 mmHg and she has +3 proteinuria on urine dipstick. You send her to labor and delivery for further evaluation, and her blood pressure remains elevated, consistent with a diagnosis of preeclampsia. You examine her cervix and find that it is closed and thick. She asks whether she can undergo induction of labor at this point. What should you tell her about induction of labor?

a. She may be induced after using a prostaglandin as a cervical ripening agent.
b. Her chance of successful VBAC is just as high with induction of labor as it is with spontaneous labor.
c. Prior cesarean delivery is a contraindication to induction of labor.
d. She may be induced with a mechanical cervical ripening agent such as a transcervical catheter.
e. Her unfavorable cervical exam does not impact her chance of successful TOLAC.

76. A 32-year-old poorly controlled diabetic G2P1 is undergoing amnio-centesis at 38 weeks for fetal lung maturity prior to having a repeat cesarean delivery. Which of the following laboratory tests results on the amniotic fluid would best indicate that the fetal lungs are mature?

a. Phosphatidylglycerol (PG) is absent
b. Lecithin/sphingomyelin (L/S) ratio of 1:1
c. Lecithin/sphingomyelin ratio of 1.5:1
d. Lecithin/sphingomyelin ratio of 2.0:1
e. Phosphatidylglycerol is present

77. A 26-year-old G1P0 patient at 34 weeks' gestation is being evaluated with Doppler ultrasound studies of the fetal umbilical arteries. The patient is a healthy smoker. Her fetus has shown evidence of intrauterine growth restriction (IUGR) on previous ultrasound examinations. The Doppler studies currently show that the systolic to diastolic ratio (S/D) in the umbilical arteries is much higher than it was on her last ultrasound 3 weeks ago, and there is now reverse diastolic flow. Which of the following is correct information to share with the patient?

a. The Doppler studies indicate that the fetus is doing well.
b. With advancing gestational age, the S/D ratio is expected to rise.
c. These Doppler findings are normal in someone who smokes.
d. Reverse diastolic flow is normal as a patient approaches full term.
e. The Doppler studies are worrisome, and indicate that the fetal status is deteriorating.

78. A 17-year-old primipara presents to your office at 41 weeks. Her pregnancy has been uncomplicated. Because her cervix is unfavorable for induction of labor, she is being followed with biophysical profile (BPP) testing. Which of the following is correct information to share with the patient regarding BPPs?

a. BPP testing includes assessment of amniotic fluid volume, fetal breathing, fetal body movements, fetal body tone, and contraction stress testing.
b. The false-negative rate of the BPP is 10%, so a reassuring BPP should be repeated in 48 hours.
c. False-positive results on BPP are rare even if the amniotic fluid level is low.
d. Spontaneous decelerations during BPP testing are associated with significant fetal morbidity.
e. A normal BPP should be repeated twice a week.

79. A patient comes to your office with her last menstrual period 4 weeks ago. She denies any symptoms such as nausea, fatigue, urinary frequency, or breast tenderness. She thinks that she may be pregnant because she has not had her period yet. She is very anxious to find out because she has a history of a previous ectopic pregnancy and wants to be sure to get early prenatal care. Which of the following actions is most appropriate at this time?

a. No action is needed because the patient is asymptomatic, has not missed her period, and cannot be pregnant.
b. Order a serum quantitative pregnancy test.
c. Listen for fetal heart tones by Doppler equipment.
d. Perform an abdominal ultrasound.
e. Perform a bimanual pelvic examination to assess uterine size.

80. A patient presents for her first OB visit after having a positive home pregnancy test. She reports her last menstrual period was about 8 weeks ago, but she is not entirely certain because she has a long history of irregular menses. Her urine pregnancy test in your office is positive. Which of the following is the most accurate way to date this patient's pregnancy?

a. Determination of uterine size on pelvic examination
b. Quantitative serum human chorionic gonadotropin (HCG) level
c. Crown-rump length on abdominal or vaginal ultrasound
d. Determination of progesterone level along with serum HCG level
e. Precise knowledge of the first day of her last menstrual period

Questions 81 and 82

A healthy 26-year-old G1P0 presents for her first OB visit at 10 weeks' gestation. She has no significant personal or family medical history.

81. When should she have her screening test for gestational diabetes?

a. She should do this test at her first prenatal visit.
b. She is at low risk, and therefore does not need to be screened for gestational diabetes.
c. She should be tested now, and again at 28 weeks.
d. The only screening test she needs is a HbA1c.
e. She should be screened between 24 and 28 weeks' gestation.

82. She fails her 1-hour glucose challenge test at 26 weeks. What is the next best step in management?

a. Repeat the test again at 28 weeks' gestation.
b. Refer her for nutritional counseling and diabetes education.
c. Prescribe insulin and instruct her how to check her blood sugars.
d. Order a 3-hour glucose tolerance test.
e. Prescribe glyburide and instruct her how to check her blood sugars.

83. A healthy 31-year-old G3P2002 patient presents at 34 weeks for a routine OB visit. She has had an uneventful pregnancy to date. Her baseline blood pressures were 100 mm Hg to 110/60 mm Hg to 70 mm Hg in the first trimester, and she has gained a total of 20 lb so far. During the visit, the patient complains of swelling in both her feet and ankles that sometimes causes her feet to ache at the end of the day. Her urine dip indicates trace protein, and her blood pressure in the office is currently 115/75 mm Hg. She has no other symptoms or complaints. On physical examination, there is pitting edema of both her feet and ankles extending to the lower one-half of her legs. There is no calf tenderness. Which of the following is the most appropriate response to the patient's concern?

a. Prescribe furosemide to relieve the painful swelling.
b. Send the patient to the radiology department to have venous Doppler studies done to rule out deep vein thromboses.
c. Admit the patient to labor and delivery to rule out preeclampsia.
d. Reassure the patient that this is a normal finding of pregnancy and no treatment is needed.
e. Tell the patient that her leg swelling is caused by too much salt intake and instruct her to follow a low-sodium diet.

84. A 28-year-old G1P0 presents to your office at 24 weeks' gestation for an unscheduled visit secondary to right-sided groin pain. She describes the pain as sharp and occurring with movement and exercise. She reports no change in urinary or bowel habits, and no fever or chills. Sitting down and putting her feet up helps alleviate the discomfort. As her obstetrician, what should you tell her is the most likely etiology of this pain?

a. Round ligament pain
b. Appendicitis
c. Preterm labor
d. Kidney stone
e. Urinary tract infection

85. A 19-year-old G1P0 presents to her obstetrician's office for a routine OB visit at 32 weeks' gestation. Her pregnancy has been complicated by gestational diabetes requiring insulin for control. She has been noncompliant with diet and insulin therapy. She has had two prior normal ultrasound examinations at 20 and 28 weeks' gestation. She has no other significant past medical or surgical history. During the visit, her fundal height measures 38 cm. Which of the following is the most likely explanation for the discrepancy between the fundal height and the gestational age?

a. Fetal hydrocephaly
b. Uterine fibroids
c. Polyhydramnios
d. Breech presentation
e. Undiagnosed twin gestation

86. A 43-year-old G1P0 who conceived via in vitro fertilization comes into the office for her routine OB visit at 38 weeks. She reports good fetal movement and reports no leakage of fluid, vaginal bleeding, or regular uterine contractions. She reports that sometimes she feels crampy at the end of the day when she gets home from work, but this discomfort is alleviated with getting off her feet. The fundal height measurement is 36 cm; it measured 37 cm the week before. Her cervical examination is 2 cm dilated and the fetal head is engaged. Which of the following is the most appropriate next step in the management of this patient?

a. Instruct the patient to return to the office in 1 week for her next routine visit.
b. Admit the patient for induction of labor for a diagnosis of fetal growth restriction.
c. Send the patient for an ultrasound to determine the amniotic fluid index.
d. Order the patient to undergo a nonstress test (NST).
e. Do a fern test in the office.

87. A pregnant woman who is 7 weeks from her LMP comes in to the office for her first prenatal visit. Her previous pregnancy ended in a missed abortion in the first trimester. The patient therefore is very anxious about the well-being of this pregnancy. Which of the following modalities will allow you to best document fetal cardiac activity?

a. Regular stethoscope
b. Fetoscope
c. Fetal Doppler stethoscope
d. Transvaginal ultrasound
e. Transabdominal pelvic ultrasound

88. A 30-year-old G2P1001 presents to your office at 37 weeks for her routine OB visit. Her first pregnancy resulted in a vaginal delivery of a 9-lb 8-oz baby boy after 30 minutes of pushing. On doing Leopold maneuvers during this office visit, you determine that the fetus is breech. Vaginal examination demonstrates that the cervix is 50% effaced and 2-cm dilated. The presenting breech is high out of the pelvis. The estimated fetal weight is about 7 lb. The patient reports no contractions. You send the patient for an ultrasound, which confirms a fetus with a double footling breech presentation. There is a normal amount of amniotic fluid present, and the head is hyperextended in the "stargazer" position. Which of the following is the best next step in the management of this patient?

a. Allow the patient to undergo a vaginal breech delivery whenever she goes into labor.
b. Send the patient to labor and delivery immediately for an emergent cesarean delivery.
c. Tell her to return in 1 week for reevaluation of fetal presentation.
d. Schedule an external cephalic version (ECV) in the next few days.
e. Allow the patient to go into labor and do an ECV at that time if the fetus is still in the double footling breech presentation.

Questions 89 to 91

A healthy 23-year-old G1P0 has had an uncomplicated pregnancy to date. She is disappointed because she is 40 weeks by a first-trimester ultrasound. She feels like she has been pregnant forever, and wants to have her baby now. The patient reports good fetal movement and no contractions. She has been doing kick counts for the past several days, and reports that the baby moves at least ten times in 2 hours. On physical examination, her cervix is firm, posterior, 50% effaced, and 1-cm dilated, and the vertex is at a-1 station.

89. As her obstetrician, which of the following should you recommend to the patient as the best next step in management?

a. She should be admitted for an immediate cesarean delivery.
b. She should be admitted for Pitocin induction.
c. She should be scheduled for a cesarean delivery in 1 week if she has not gone into labor by that time.
d. She should continue to monitor kick counts and to return to your office in 1 week to reassess her situation.
e. She should walk as much as possible to stimulate contractions.

90. The patient presents in 1 week for a follow-up visit. She is now 41 weeks' gestation. She reports that the baby is still passing the fetal kick count assessment, and she has been having intermittent contractions for several days. On physical examination, her cervix is 3 cm dilated, 70% effaced, anterior, soft, and the vertex is at 0 station. Now what is the next best step in management?

a. Allow her to continue the pregnancy and await spontaneous labor.
b. Schedule her for induction of labor, because now her cervix is favorable.
c. Strip her membranes, and if this does not work, instruct her to return in 1 week for reevaluation.
d. Since she has not gone into labor by 41 weeks, schedule her for a cesarean delivery the following day.
e. Order a NST to assess fetal well-being.

91. What would the next best step in management be if this patient were 41 weeks with an unfavorable cervix and oligohydramnios found on ultrasound?

a. Admit her to the hospital for cesarean delivery.
b. Admit her to the hospital for cervical ripening and induction of labor.
c. Write her a prescription for misoprostol to take at home orally every 4 hours until she goes into labor.
d. Perform stripping of the fetal membranes and perform a BPP in 2 days.
e. Administer a cervical ripening agent in your office and have the patient present to the hospital in the morning for induction with oxytocin.

92. A healthy 30-year-old P1001 at 24 weeks' gestation presents for a routine OB visit. She has no medical problems, and her pregnancy has been uncomplicated. Her last pregnancy was uncomplicated as well. However, she tells you that with her last pregnancy, her obstetrician performed an ultrasound at every visit to reassure her that "everything was alright." She requests that you also perform an ultrasound at every visit to provide her reassurance that the pregnancy is progressing normally. How should you counsel her regarding the safety of ultrasound during pregnancy?

a. Tell her that ultrasound is completely safe, and agree to perform one at every visit in order to provide her with reassurance.
b. Tell her that ultrasound is completely safe, but you do not have time to perform one at every visit. Recommend that she transfer her care to her previous obstetrician.
c. Tell her that having multiple ultrasounds has been associated with adverse fetal effects.

d. Counsel her that prenatal ultrasound should only be used when clinically indicated, for the shortest amount of time, and with the lowest level of acoustic energy compatible with an accurate diagnosis in order to maximize safety.
e. Tell her that ultrasound is completely safe, and recommend that she pay out-of-pocket for extra ultrasounds at a business that specializes in performing these studies in order to provide keepsake videos and photos.

93. A 27-year-old G3P2002, who is 34 weeks' gestational age, calls the on-call obstetrician on a Saturday night at 10:00 PM reporting decreased fetal movement. She says that the previous day her baby moved only once per hour. For the past 6 hours she has felt no movement. She is healthy, has had regular prenatal care, and reports no complications so far during the pregnancy. Which of the following is the best advice for the on-call physician to give the patient?

a. Instruct the patient to go to labor and delivery for a contraction stress test.
b. Reassure the patient that one fetal movement per hour is within normal limits and she does not need to worry.
c. Recommend the patient be admitted to the hospital for delivery.
d. Counsel the patient that the baby is probably sleeping, and that she should continue to monitor fetal kicks. If she continues to experience no fetal movement by morning, she should call you back for further instructions.
e. Instruct the patient to go to labor and delivery for a NST.

94. Your patient reports decreased fetal movement at term. You recommend a modified BPP test. NST in your office was reactive. The next part of the modified BPP is which of the following?

a. Contraction stress testing
b. Amniotic fluid index evaluation
c. Ultrasound assessment of fetal movement
d. Ultrasound assessment of fetal breathing movements
e. Ultrasound assessment of fetal tone

95. You are seeing a patient in the hospital for decreased fetal movement at 36 weeks' gestation. She is healthy and has had no prenatal complications. You order a BPP. The patient scores an 8 on the test. Two points were deducted for lack of fetal breathing movements. How should you counsel the patient regarding the results of the BPP?

a. The results are equivocal, and she should have a repeat BPP within 24 hours.
b. The results are abnormal, and she should be induced.
c. The results are normal, and she can go home.
d. The results are abnormal, and she should undergo emergent cesarean section.
e. The results are abnormal, and she should undergo umbilical artery Doppler velocimetry.

96. An 18-year-old G2P1001 presents for her first OB visit at 10 weeks. She reports that the first day of her last menstrual period was May 7. What is this patient's estimated date of delivery?

a. February 10 of the next year
b. February 14 of the next year
c. December 10 of the same year
d. December 14 of the same year
e. December 21 of the same year

97. A 36-year-old G1P0 presents to your office for her first prenatal visit. By her last menstrual period she is 11 weeks' pregnant. She has no medical problems. On physical examination, her uterus is palpable midway between the pubic symphysis and the umbilicus. No fetal heart tones are audible with the Doppler stethoscope. Which of the following is the best next step in the management of this patient?

a. Reassure her that fetal heart tones are not yet audible with the Doppler stethoscope at this gestational age.
b. Tell her the uterine size is appropriate for her gestational age and schedule her for routine ultrasonography at 20 weeks.
c. Schedule genetic amniocentesis because of her advanced maternal age.
d. Schedule her for a dilation and curettage, because she has a molar pregnancy since her uterus is too large and the fetal heart tones are not audible.
e. Schedule an ultrasound as soon as possible to determine the gestational age and viability of the fetus.

98. A healthy 30-year-old G2P1001 presents to her obstetrician's office at 34 weeks for a routine prenatal visit. She has a history of a low transverse cesarean delivery performed secondary to fetal malpresentation (footling breech). Her current pregnancy has been uncomplicated. She tells her physician that she would like to undergo a trial of labor during this pregnancy. However, the patient is interested in permanent sterilization and wonders if it would be better to undergo another scheduled cesarean so she can have a bilateral tubal ligation performed at the same time. How should the physician counsel this patient?

a. A history of a previous low transverse cesarean is a contraindication to TOLAC.
b. Her risk of uterine rupture with TOLAC after one prior low transverse cesarean is 4% to 9%.
c. Her chance of having a successful VBAC is less than 60%.

d. The patient should schedule an elective induction if not delivered by 38 weeks.
e. If the patient desires a bilateral tubal ligation, it is safer for her to undergo a vaginal delivery followed by a postpartum tubal ligation rather than an elective repeat cesarean with intrapartum bilateral tubal ligation.

99. A 16-year-old primigravida presents to your office at 38 weeks' gestation. Her first trimester blood pressure was 100/72 mm Hg. On the day of presentation it was 170/110 mm Hg and she has 4+ proteinuria on a clean catch specimen of urine. She has significant swelling of her face and extremities. She reports no contractions. Her cervix is closed and thick. The baby is breech by bedside ultrasonography. She reports the baby's movements have decreased in the past 24 hours. Which of the following is the best next step in the management of this patient?

a. Send her to labor and delivery for a BPP.
b. Send her home with instructions to stay on strict bed rest until her swelling and blood pressure improve.
c. Admit her to the hospital for enforced bed rest and diuretic therapy to improve her swelling and blood pressure.
d. Admit her to the hospital for induction of labor.
e. Admit her to the hospital for cesarean delivery.

100. While you are on call at the hospital covering labor and delivery, a 32-year-old G3P2002, at 35 weeks' gestation, presents with a chief complaint of lower back pain. You take her history, and learn that she had been lifting some heavy boxes while preparing the baby's nursery. The patient's pregnancy has been complicated by diet-controlled gestational diabetes. She reports no uterine contractions, rupture of membranes, vaginal bleeding, dysuria, fever, chills, nausea, or emesis. She states that the baby has been moving normally. She is afebrile and her blood pressure is normal. On physical examination, you note that she is obese. Her abdomen is soft and nontender, with no palpable contractions or uterine tenderness. No costovertebral angle tenderness can be elicited. On pelvic examination her cervix is closed and thick. The fetal heart tracing is reactive, and there are rare, irregular uterine contractions demonstrated on the tocometer. The patient's urinalysis shows trace glucose, but is otherwise negative. The patient's most likely diagnosis is which of the following?

a. Preterm labor
b. Musculoskeletal pain
c. Urinary tract infection
d. Chorioamnionitis
e. Round ligament pain

Questions 101 to 105

Match each description with the appropriate fetal heart rate tracing. If none of the tracings apply, answer e. (none). Each lettered option may be used once, more than once, or not at all.

a.

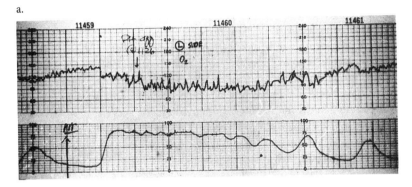

b.

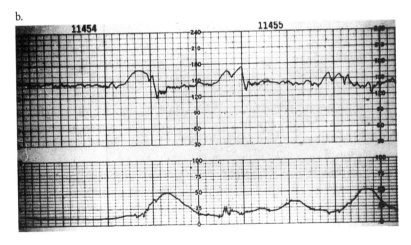

c.

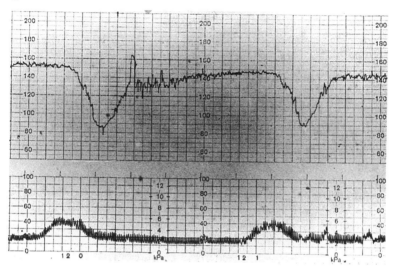

d.

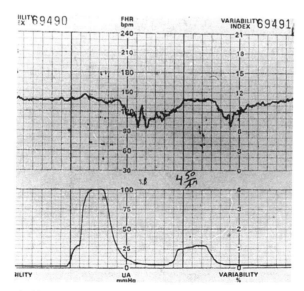

(Reproduced with permission from Cunningham FG, Leveno KL, Bloom SL, et al. *Williams Obstetrics*. 22nd ed. New York, NY: McGraw-Hill, 2005: 455)

e. None

101. A 23-year-old G1P0 at 42 weeks is undergoing induction of labor. She is receiving intravenous oxytocin. She complains that her contractions are very painful and seem to be continuous.

102. A laboring patient has an internal fetal scalp electrode in place. Pelvic examination shows the patient to be 7-cm dilated with the fetal vertex at +1 station. The fetal heart rate tracing is consistent with fetal head compression.

103. A patient at 41 weeks is undergoing NST. Her NST is reactive and reassuring.

104. A laboring patient at 40 weeks' gestation presents with spontaneous rupture of membranes. Bedside ultrasonography shows no measurable pockets of amniotic fluid. With each contraction, the fetal heart rate tracing shows evidence of umbilical cord compression.

105. A preeclamptic patient at 33 weeks' gestation with IUGR is undergoing induction of labor. The fetal heart rate tracing shows evidence of uteroplacental insufficiency and is nonreassuring.

Antepartum Care and Fetal Surveillance

Answers

71. The answer is c. By tradition, pelves are classified as belonging to one of four major groups, based on the shape of the pelvis. A line drawn through the greatest diameter of the pelvic inlet divides the pelvis into anterior and posterior sections, and the shape of these segments helps determine the pelvis type. The gynecoid pelvis is the classic female pelvis, with a posterior sagittal diameter of the inlet only slightly shorter than the anterior sagittal diameter. The posterior pelvis is rounded and wide, the sidewalls are straight, the spines are not prominent, and the pubic arch is wide. In the android pelvis, the posterior sagittal diameter at the inlet is much shorter than the anterior sagittal diameter, limiting the use of the posterior space by the fetal head. The sidewalls are convergent, the spines are prominent, and the pubic arch is narrowed. In the anthropoid pelvis, the AP diameter of the inlet is greater than the transverse diameter, resulting in an oval with large sacrosciatic notches, convergent side walls, prominent ischial spines, and a narrow pubic arch. The platypelloid pelvis is flattened with a short AP and wide transverse diameter. Wide sacrosciatic notches are common. The pelves of most women do not fall into a pure type and are blends of one or more of these types.

72. The answer is b. The lie of the fetus refers to the relation of the long axis of the fetus to that of the mother, and is classified as longitudinal, transverse, or oblique. The presentation, or presenting part, refers to the portion of the baby that is foremost in the birth canal. The presentation may be cephalic, breech, or shoulder. Cephalic presentations are further classified as vertex, brow, or face. The position is the relative relationship of the presenting part of the fetus to the mother. In this instance, the fetus is cephalic, with the face presenting. In a face presentation, the fetal head is hyperextended so that the occiput is in contact with the fetal back, and the chin (mentum) is presenting. The mentum is the point of reference of the fetus when describing the position of the face. Since the mentum is pointing toward the mother's left hip, the fetal position is described as mentum transverse. In vertex presentations, the occiput is the point of reference for determining position. In breech presentations, the sacrum is the point of reference.

73. The answer is b. A patient with a prior low transverse incision may attempt a TOLAC. Repeat cesarean and TOLAC both have inherent risks. The main risk of TOLAC that increases maternal and neonatal morbidity is uterine rupture, the risk of which is impacted significantly by the location of the uterine incision. A low transverse incision is made transversely through the lower uterine segment, which does not actively contract during labor. The risk of uterine rupture after prior low transverse incision is less than 1%. The skin incision does not reflect the location of the uterine incision, and therefore is not an indicator of the suitability of TOLAC for a patient. Although a prior vaginal delivery increases the success rate for a successful VBAC, a prior vaginal birth is not a prerequisite for a TOLAC. If the patient desires a repeat cesarean delivery, this should be performed at 39 weeks as a scheduled procedure.

74. The answer is e. Good candidates for TOLAC are women in whom the balance of risks and benefits are acceptable to the patient and health care provider. Decisions regarding TOLAC must be made on an individual basis while taking these factors into account. Most evidence suggests that most women with one prior low transverse cesarean should be counseled about vaginal birth after cesarean (VBAC) and offered TOLAC. Factors that increase the probability of success include prior vaginal delivery and spontaneous labor. Factors that predict a decreased probability of success include increased maternal age, Hispanic or African American ethnicity, postdates gestation, and maternal obesity. Therefore, spontaneous labor prior to 40 weeks would provide this patient with the greatest chance of successful TOLAC.

75. The answer is d. Induction of labor for maternal or fetal indications is an option for women undergoing TOLAC. However, the chance of successful TOLAC with induction versus spontaneous labor is lower, and her unfavorable cervical examination decreases the potential success rate. Data support use of mechanical ripening agents, such as transcervical catheter, in this setting of an unfavorable cervix. Prostaglandins are not used for cervical ripening due to concerns over increased risk of uterine rupture.

76. The answer is e. The lecithin-to-sphingomyelin (L/S) ratio in amniotic fluid is close to 1 until about 34 weeks of gestation, when the concentration of lecithin begins to rise. For pregnancies of unknown duration but otherwise uncomplicated, the risk of respiratory distress syndrome (RDS) is relatively low when the L/S is at least 2:1. Maternal hypertensive disorders and fetal growth retardation may accelerate the rate of fetal pulmonary maturation, possibly as a result of chronic fetal stress. A delay in fetal pulmonary maturation is observed in pregnancies complicated by maternal diabetes or erythroblastosis fetalis. A risk of RDS of 40% exists with an L/S ratio of 1.5:2; when the L/S ratio is less than 1.5, the risk of RDS is 73%. When the L/S ratio is greater than 2, the risk of RDS is slight. However, when the fetus is likely to have a serious metabolic compromise at birth (eg, diabetes or sepsis), RDS may develop even with a mature L/S ratio (> 2.0). This may be explained by lack of PG, a phospholipid that enhances surfactant properties. The identification of PG in amniotic fluid provides considerable reassurance (but not an absolute guarantee) that RDS will not develop. Moreover, contamination of amniotic fluid by blood, meconium, or vaginal secretions will not alter PG measurements.

77. The answer is e. Simple continuous-wave Doppler ultrasound can be used to display flow velocity waveforms as a function of time. With increased gestational age, in normal pregnancy there is an increase in end-diastolic flow velocity relative to peak systolic velocity, which causes the S/D ratio to decrease with advancing gestation. An increase in S/D ratio is associated with increased resistance in the placental vascular bed, as can be noted in preeclampsia or fetal growth restriction. Nicotine and maternal smoking have also been reported to increase the S/D ratio. Many studies document the value of umbilical Doppler flow studies in recognition of fetal compromise. The S/D ratio increases as the fetal condition deteriorates; this is most severe in cases of absent or reversed end diastolic flow.

78. The answer is d. The BPP is based on FHR monitoring with non-stress test (NST) in addition to four parameters observed on real-time ultrasonography—amniotic fluid volume, fetal breathing, fetal body movements, and fetal body tone. Each parameter gets a score of 0 or 2. A score of 8 or 10 is considered normal, a score of 6 is equivocal, and a score of 4 or less is abnormal and prompts delivery. The false-negative rate for the BPP is less than 0.1%, but false-positive results are relatively frequent, with poor specificity. Oligohydramnios is an ominous sign, as are spontaneous decelerations. In patients with profile scores of 8 but with spontaneous decelerations, the rate of cesarean delivery indicated for fetal distress has been 25%. There are no large clinical trials to guide the frequency of testing; however, when the maternal condition is stable and the testing is reassuring, the testing may be repeated at weekly intervals. Certain high risk conditions may prompt more frequent testing.

79. The answer is b. Nausea, fatigue, breast tenderness, and urinary frequency are all common symptoms of pregnancy; however, they are nonspecific symptoms, and are not consistently found in early pregnancy. On physical examination, the pregnant uterus enlarges and becomes more boggy and soft, but these changes are not usually apparent until after 6 weeks' gestation. In addition, other conditions such as adenomyosis or fibroids may result in an enlarged uterus. Abdominal ultrasound will not demonstrate a gestational sac until a gestational age of 5 to 6 weeks is reached, nor will it detect an ectopic pregnancy at the time of the missed menstrual period. It is therefore not indicated in this patient. A Doppler will detect fetal heart tones usually no sooner than 10 to 12 weeks. A sensitive serum quantitative pregnancy test can detect HCG levels by 8 to 9 days postovulation, and it is therefore the most appropriate next step in the evaluation of this patient.

80. The answer is c. Measurement of the fetal crown-rump length is the most accurate means of estimating gestational age. In the first trimester, this ultrasound measurement is accurate to within 3 to 5 days. Estimating the uterine size on physical examination can result in an error of 1 to 2 weeks in the first trimester. Quantification of serum HCG cannot be used to determine gestational age, because at any gestational age the HCG number can vary widely in normal pregnancies. A single serum progesterone level cannot be used to date a pregnancy; however, it can be used to establish that an early pregnancy is developing normally. Serum progesterone levels less than 5 ng/mL usually indicate a nonviable pregnancy, while levels greater than 25 ng/mL indicate a normal intrauterine pregnancy. Progesterone levels in conjunction with quantitative HCG levels are often used to determine the presence of an ectopic pregnancy. Early ultrasound is more reliable than precise knowledge of last menstrual period in determining dates.

81. The answer is e. Most organizations recommend universal screening for gestational diabetes for all pregnant women. A 1-hour glucose challenge test should be performed between 24 and 28 weeks' gestation. This screen involves administration of a 50 g oral glucose solution followed by a 1-hour venous glucose determination. Certain women at high risk for gestational diabetes should be screened earlier (ie, at the first prenatal visit). This includes women with a history of gestational diabetes, body mass index greater than 30, family history of diabetes, age older than 35 years, or a history of fetal macrosomia in a prior pregnancy. If gestational diabetes is not diagnosed during this early screen, the test should be repeated at 24 to 28 weeks' gestation.

82. The answer is d. The two-step approach to testing is based on first screening with a 1-hour glucose tolerance test (described earlier). Those individuals meeting or exceeding the screening threshold should then undergo a 100 g, 3-hour diagnostic oral glucose tolerance test. Two out of four elevated values results in a diagnosis of gestational diabetes. The 1-hour glucose tolerance test is a screening test, and must be followed up with a diagnostic test. In most cases, it would not be appropriate to offer therapy for gestational diabetes (such as diabetes education, insulin, or oral therapy) based on results of a screening test alone.

83. The answer is d. Increased fluid retention manifested by pitting edema of the ankles and legs is a normal finding in late pregnancy. During pregnancy, there is a decrease in colloid osmotic pressure and a fall in plasma osmolality. Moreover, there is an increase in venous pressure created by partial occlusion of the vena cava by the gravid uterus. These physiologic changes contribute to bilateral pedal edema. Diuretics are sometimes given to pregnant women who have chronic hypertension, but should not be given in pregnancy to treat physiologic pedal edema. More commonly, furosemide is used in the acute setting to treat pulmonary edema associated with severe preeclampsia. This patient is not hypertensive and does not have any other signs or symptoms of preeclampsia and therefore does not need to be admitted for further workup. Trace protein in the urine is common in normal pregnancies and is not of concern. Doppler studies of the lower extremities are not indicated in this patient since the history and examination (specifically, the lack of calf tenderness) are consistent with physiologic edema. The normal swelling detected in pregnancy is not prevented by a low-sodium diet or improved with a lower intake of salt.

84. The answer is a. This patient reports a classic description of round ligament pain. Each round ligament extends from the lateral portion of the uterus below the oviduct, travels in a fold of peritoneum downward to the inguinal canal, and inserts in the upper portion of the labium majus. During pregnancy, these ligaments stretch as the gravid uterus grows farther out of the pelvis, and can therefore cause sharp pain, particularly with sudden movements. Round ligament pain is more frequently experienced on the right side due to the dextrorotation of the uterus that commonly occurs in pregnancy. Usually this pain is greatly improved by avoiding sudden movements, changing position slowly, and by sitting and elevating the feet. Local heat and analgesics may also help with pain control. The diagnosis of appendicitis is not likely because the patient is not experiencing any fever or anorexia. In addition, because the gravid uterus pushes the appendix out of the pelvis, pregnant women with appendicitis often have pain located much higher than the groin area. The diagnosis of preterm labor is unlikely because the pain is localized to the groin area on one side, and is alleviated with elevation of her feet. Labor contractions generally cause generalized abdominal and low back pain. In addition, when labor occurs, the pains continue at rest, not just with movement. A urinary tract infection is unlikely because the patient has no urinary symptoms. A kidney stone is unlikely because this usually presents with pain in the back and flank—not low in the groin—and would persist at rest as well.

85. The answer is c. The fundal height in centimeters has been found to correlate with gestational age in weeks with an error of 3 cm from 16 to 36 weeks. Uterine fibroids, polyhydramnios (excessive amniotic fluid), fetal macrosomia, and twin gestation are all plausible explanations of why the uterine size would measure larger than expected for the patient's dates. Breech presentation does not cause the uterus to be larger than expected for the gestational age. Since this patient has had two prior ultrasound examinations, hydrocephaly, fibroids, and twins would have previously been diagnosed. In this uncontrolled diabetic, the most likely cause for the excessive fundal height is polyhydramnios, which is a sign of poor glucose control.

86. The answer is a. The decrease in fundal height between visits can be most easily explained by engagement of the fetal head, which is verified on vaginal examination with determination of the presenting part at 0 station. Engagement of the fetal head commonly occurs before labor in nulliparous patients. Therefore, it is appropriate for the patient to return for another scheduled visit in 1 week. IUGR is unlikely because there will usually be a greater discrepancy (> 3 cm) between fundal height and gestational age.

Therefore, the patient does not need to be induced. Since the patient has been reporting good fetal movement and is not post-term, there is no indication to do antepartum testing such as an NST. A fern test is not indicated since the patient has not reported leakage of fluid. An assessment of amniotic fluid to detect oligohydramnios is not indicated since the fundal height is appropriate for the patient's gestational age.

87. The answer is d. Vaginal ultrasound can detect fetal cardiac activity as early as 5 weeks after a missed period. With a traditional stethoscope, fetal heart tones can be heard starting between 17 and 19 weeks' gestation. Doppler stethoscope can detect fetal heart tones by 10 weeks' gestational age in nonobese women.

88. The answer is d. According to ACOG, breech presentation occurs in 3% to 4% of term pregnancies. The patient who has a fetus with a breech presentation has the option of scheduling an ECV, an elective cesarean delivery at or after 39 weeks, or a vaginal breech delivery if certain conditions are met. It is not appropriate to electively deliver any patient prior to 39 weeks without documentation of fetal lung maturity due to the risk of neonatal RDS. An elective cesarean should be scheduled at or after 39 weeks' gestational age to avoid RDS. If a patient would like to avoid a cesarean, but does not want to undergo a vaginal breech delivery, or this is not an option in her medical community, then an ECV is an appropriate management plan. ECV is a procedure where the breech fetus is manipulated through the abdominal wall to change the presentation to vertex. The goal is to increase the proportion of vertex presentations among fetuses formerly in the breech presentation near term, which increases the chances for a successful vaginal delivery. Studies indicate that if an ECV is not performed, 80% of breech presentations will persist at term, versus only 30% if a successful version is performed. ECV has an average success rate of about 60%; it is most successful in parous women with an unengaged breech and a normal amount of amniotic fluid (all conditions that exist in the patient described). A trial of labor for a pregnant woman with a fetus in the breech presentation may be appropriate if the fetus is frank breech, has a flexed head, has a normal amount of amniotic fluid, has an estimated weight between 2500 and 3800 g, and if there are experienced personnel available to counsel the patient about risks and benefits and perform the delivery. In addition, the pelvis should be adequate, usually as assessed by noting a history of delivery of a previous baby of larger size. A fetus with a hyperextended, or "stargazer," head has a higher risk of spinal cord injury during vaginal breech delivery; therefore, delivery should be by cesarean. The best course of management in this case is ECV.

89. The answer is d. According to ACOG, postterm pregnancy refers to a pregnancy that has reached beyond 42 0/7 weeks of gestation from the last menstrual period (LMP). Late-term pregnancy is defined as one that has reached between 41 0/7 weeks and 41 6/7 weeks of gestation. The overall incidence of postterm pregnancy is approximately 5%. Accurate determination of gestational age is essential, and this patient has appropriate dating criteria with an early ultrasound. This patient is currently 40 weeks' gestation, which is considered term, and therefore does not necessarily require immediate plans for delivery. Her cervical examination is unfavorable as determined by Bishop score. If she had a favorable cervix, it would be reasonable to offer her induction at 40 weeks, because the chance of having a successful vaginal delivery is very high. In this situation, it is most appropriate to ask her to return in 1 week to reassess her situation.

90. The answer is b. Late-term and post-term pregnancies are associated with an increased risk of maternal and neonatal morbidity. Due to these risks, at 41 weeks, one must undertake a careful assessment of the options for delivery versus continued pregnancy. Membrane stripping (or sweeping) involves digital separation of the membranes from the lower uterine segment, and has an approximately 50% chance of resulting in labor.

If a patient has a favorable cervix at 41 weeks, it is reasonable to offer induction of labor, because the chance of a successful vaginal delivery is very high. Alternatively, a patient can be induced at 41 weeks with an unfavorable cervix if cervical ripening agents are used. If a patient waits until 42 weeks and still has an unfavorable cervix, then admission with administration of cervical ripening agents prior to Pitocin induction is recommended to improve the likelihood of a successful vaginal delivery.

Table: Bishop Score

BISHOP SCORE					
Points	Dilation	Effacement	Station	Consistency	Position
0	Closed	0%-30%	−3	Firm	Posterior
1	1-2 cm	40%-50%	−2	Medium	Midposition
2	3-4 cm	60%-70%	−1, 0	Soft	Anterior
3	≥ 5 cm	≥ 80%	+1, +2	—	—

The Bishop score is a method to document the favorability of the cervix for induction. The elements of the Bishop score include effacement, dilation, station, consistency, and position of the cervix (Table). Points are assigned for each element, and then totaled to give the Bishop score. Induction to active labor is usually successful with a Bishop score of 8 or greater. In the scenario described here, the patient has a Bishop score of 10, which is favorable for induction. Therefore, it is reasonable to schedule induction of labor at this point. It is not recommended to perform an elective cesarean without a trial of labor because of the risks of major surgery, and the high likelihood of vaginal delivery with a favorable cervix.

91. The answer is b. Patients with oligohydramnios at term should be delivered. If there is no contraindication to vaginal delivery, the patient should be induced. The patient with an unfavorable cervix may undergo cervical ripening after assessment of fetal well-being. If fetal testing is reassuring, the unfavorable cervix can be ripened with a variety of mechanical and pharmacologic agents prior to initiating Pitocin. Pharmacologic agents include PGE 2 preparations available as a vaginal/cervical gel (Prepidil) or vaginal insert (Cervidil). Misoprostol, a synthetic PGE 1 analogue, has been used off-label for preinduction cervical ripening and labor induction. It can be administered via the oral or vaginal route. Mechanical ripening of the cervix can be achieved with laminaria, which is a hygroscopic dilator that is placed in the cervical canal and absorbs water from the surrounding cervical tissue. The cervix can also be mechanically dilated with a balloon catheter. Pitocin is not considered a cervical ripening agent, but a labor-inducing agent. In patients with oligohydramnios, cervical ripening should be performed in the hospital under continuous fetal monitoring, and therefore it is not appropriate to provide a ripening agent and send her home.

92. The answer is d. Diagnostic ultrasound studies of the fetus are generally considered safe in pregnancy. The World Health Organization performed a systematic review of the literature that did not show a close association between ultrasound and adverse pregnancy outcomes. However, there were limitations to this study, and there is no firm evidence demonstrating safety. "Keepsake fetal videos" are considered by the FDA to be an unapproved use of a medical device. Prenatal ultrasound should only be used when clinically indicated, and it is not appropriate to perform an ultrasound at every visit in order to reassure the patient.

93. The answer is e. Maternal perception of decreased fetal movement may precede fetal death in utero. Therefore, kick counts have been employed as a method of antepartum assessment. The optimal number of fetal movements that should be perceived per hour has not been determined. However, studies indicate that the perception of 10 distinct movements in a period of up to 2 hours is reassuring. Since this patient is experiencing only one movement per hour, and this movement is decreased from her previous baseline, further antepartum testing is indicated. A NST is the preferred modality. A contraction stress test involves provoking uterine contractions and evaluating the response of the fetal heart rate tracing to contractions. As this patient is preterm, provoking contractions should be avoided. Delivery is not indicated until nonreassuring fetal status can be documented.

94. The answer is b. The BPP consists of five components, which include a NST and four observations made by real-time ultrasound. These observations are as follows:

(i) Fetal breathing movements—one or more episodes of fetal breathing movements of 30 seconds or more within 30 minutes
(ii) Fetal movement—three or more discrete body or limb movements within 30 minutes
(iii) Fetal tone—one or more episodes of extension of a fetal extremity with return to flexion, or opening or closing of a hand
(iv) Determination of amniotic fluid volume—a single vertical pocket of amniotic fluid exceeding 2 cm

Each of these components is assigned a score of 2 (normal) or 0 (abnormal or absent). In the modified BPP, only the NST and determination of amniotic fluid volume are assessed. Amniotic fluid volume reflects fetal urine production, and can be used to evaluate placental function. The modified BPP combines the NST, as a short-term indicator of fetal acid-base status, with an amniotic fluid volume assessment, as an indicator of long-term placental function. The results of a modified BPP are considered normal if the NST is reactive and there is a 2 cm deep pocket of amniotic fluid. The results are considered abnormal if either the NST is nonreactive, or there is not a 2 cm deep pocket of amniotic fluid present (indicating oligohydramnios).

95. The answer is c. A BPP score of 8 or 10 is normal. A score of 6 is equivocal and requires repeat testing and usually delivery if persistent. A score of 4 or less is abnormal and often requires delivery.

96. The answer is b. The expected date of delivery can be estimated by using Naegele rule. To do this, count back 3 months and then add 7 days to the date of the first day of the last normal menstrual period.

97. The answer is e. At 11 weeks of gestation, the uterus is still within the pelvis and should not be palpable above the symphysis pubis. A uterus that is palpable midway between the symphysis pubis and the umbilicus is 14 to 16 weeks in size. The fetal heart tones are audible in most patients at 10 to 12 weeks. If no fetal heart tones are audible by Doppler auscultation and the patient is 12 weeks or more, an ultrasound of the pregnancy should be ordered. Molar pregnancy, twin gestation, incorrect dates, and uterine fibroids are all possible diagnoses when the uterus is large for dates; therefore, ultrasonography is the first step in the evaluation of size/date discrepancy. Although molar pregnancy is an indication for dilation and curettage, the procedure is not indicated before evaluation of the patient with ultrasonography. This patient is of advanced maternal age (> 35 years of age at the time of delivery); however, genetic amniocentesis should not be performed without first knowing the gestational age and viability of the pregnancy.

98. The answer is e. The desire for sterilization is not an indication for an elective repeat cesarean delivery. The morbidity of repeat cesarean is greater than that of vaginal birth with postpartum tubal ligation. The risk of uterine rupture in a woman who undergoes a trial of labor and has had one prior cesarean section is approximately 0.6%. With a history of two prior cesareans, the risk of uterine rupture is about 1.8%. The risk of uterine rupture in someone who has had a classical or T-shaped uterine incision is 4% to 6%. The success rate for a trial of labor is generally about 60% to 80% depending on the indication for the cesarean delivery. Success rates are higher when the original cesarean was performed for breech or a nonreassuring fetal heart rate tracing (ie, potentially nonrecurring), rather than labor dystocia. Induction of labor should not be performed without an obstetrical indication (eg, preeclampsia) at less than 39 weeks.

99. The answer is e. Preeclampsia is diagnosed by noting new onset hypertension and either proteinuria or end-organ dysfunction after 20 weeks. In 2013, ACOG eliminated dependence on the diagnosis on proteinuria. In the absence of proteinuria, preeclampsia is diagnosed as hypertension in association with thrombocytopenia, impaired liver function, new onset impaired renal function, pulmonary edema, or new onset cerebral or visual disturbances.

Gestational hypertension is diagnosed if the patient develops hypertension without proteinuria or the aforementioned systemic findings after 20 weeks' gestation. Chronic hypertension is hypertension that predates pregnancy, and superimposed preeclampsia is chronic hypertension in association with preeclampsia. The treatment for gestational hypertension and preeclampsia at term is delivery. Select preterm patients may be managed conservatively at home or in the hospital depending on the severity of the hypertension. BPP testing is useful when following the patient conservatively. Although bed rest may transiently improve elevated blood pressure, a patient at full term should be delivered. Based on the severity of this patient's blood pressure, she has preeclampsia with severe features, and she should be delivered. Since this patient's fetus is breech, cesarean delivery rather than induction of labor is the next best step in her management. Diuretics should not be used in the management of preeclampsia, as they deplete the maternal intravascular volume and may compromise placental perfusion.

100. The answer is b. Lower back pain is a common complaint that is reported by about 50% of pregnant women. It is caused by stress placed on the lower spine and associated muscles and ligaments by the gravid uterus, especially in late pregnancy. The pain can be exacerbated with excessive bending and lifting. In addition, obesity predisposes the patient to lower back pain in pregnancy. Treatment options include heat, massage, and analgesia. This patient has no evidence of labor, since she is lacking regular uterine contractions and cervical change. Without any urinary symptoms or a urinalysis suggestive of infection, a urinary tract infection is unlikely. The diagnosis of chorioamnionitis does not fit since the patient has intact membranes, no fever, and a nontender uterus. Round ligament pain is typically characterized by sharp groin pain.

101 to 105. The answers are 101-a, 102-e, 103-b, 104-d, 105-c. Fetal heart rate tracings are obtained in most pregnancies in the United States through the use of electronic fetal monitoring equipment. Accurate interpretation of these tracings with resultant action to expedite delivery in fetuses threatened by hypoxia has improved neonatal outcome. Electronic fetal monitoring has had very little effect on the overall incidence of cerebral palsy, which seems most often to have its etiology remote from the time of labor. Tracing (a) shows a classic hyperstimulation pattern, with a tonic contraction lasting several minutes with distinctly raised intrauterine pressure and a consequent fall in fetal heart rate. Despite the increased uterine pressure, there remains good beat-to-beat variability, which suggests that the fetus is withstanding the stress. Tracing (b) shows fetal heart rate accelerations occurring spontaneously both before and after contractions, with good beat-to-beat variability, and is representative of a healthy fetus. Tracing (c) shows late decelerations following two consecutive contractions. The baseline variability is significantly reduced. This pattern is caused by utero-placental insufficiency. Tracing (d) shows variable decelerations in which the classic V-shaped picture of a variable deceleration is maintained. Such decelerations are a normal, reflex response to umbilical cord compression.

Suggested Readings

AIUM practice guideline for the performance of obstetric ultrasound examinations. American Institute of Ultrasound in Medicine. *J Ultrasound Med.* 2013 Jun;32(6):1083-1101.

American College of Obstetricians and Gynecologists. *Antepartum Fetal Surveillance.* Practice Bulletin Number 145, July 2014.

American College of Obstetricians and Gynecologists. *External Cephalic Version.* Practice Bulletin Number 13, February 2000, Reaffirmed 2014.

American College of Obstetricians and Gynecologists. *Gestational Diabetes Mellitus.* Practice Bulletin Number 137, August 2013.

American College of Obstetricians and Gynecologists. Report on task force on hypertension in pregnancy. *Obstet Gynecol.* 2013;122(5):1122.

American College of Obstetricians and Gynecologists. *Management of Late-Term and Postterm Pregnancies.* Practice Bulletin Number 146, August 2014.

American College of Obstetricians and Gynecologists. *Vaginal Birth After Previous Cesarean Delivery.* Practice Bulletin Number 115, August 2010, Reaffirmed 2013.

Cunningham FG, Leveno KJ, Bloom SL, et al. eds. *Williams Obstetrics.* 23rd ed. New York, NY: McGraw-Hill; 2010. Chapter 2: Pregnancy: overview, organization, and diagnosis, Chapter 3: Anatomy of the reproductive tract, Chapter 19: Dystocia, Chapter 39: Diseases and injuries of the fetus and newborn, Chapter 40: Antepartum assessment.

Torloni MR, Vedmedovska N, Merialdi M, et al. Safety of ultrasonography in pregnancy: WHO systematic review of the literature and meta-analysis. *Ultrasound Obstet Gynecol.* 2009;33(5):599.

Obstetrical Complications of Pregnancy

Questions

106. A 32-year-old G2P1 at 28 weeks' gestation presents to labor and delivery with a chief complaint of vaginal bleeding. Her vital signs are— blood pressure 115/67 mm Hg, pulse 87 beats per minute, temperature 37.0°C, respiratory rate 18 breaths per minute. She reports no contraction and states that the baby is moving normally. On ultrasound, the placenta is located on the anterior wall of the uterus, and completely covers the internal cervical os. Which of the following would most increase her risk for hysterectomy?

a. Desire for sterilization
b. Development of disseminated intravascular coagulopathy (DIC)
c. Placenta accreta
d. Prior vaginal delivery
e. Smoking

107. A patient at 17 weeks' gestation is diagnosed with an intrauterine fetal demise. She desires expectant management. She returns to your office 5 weeks later, and her vital signs are—blood pressure 110/72 mm Hg, pulse 93 beats per minute, temperature 36.38°C, respiratory rate 16 breaths per minute. She has not had a miscarriage, although she has had some occasional spotting. Her cervix is closed on examination. This patient is at increased risk for which of the following?

a. Septic abortion
b. Recurrent abortion
c. Consumptive coagulopathy
d. Future infertility
e. Ectopic pregnancies

Questions 108 and 109

A 24-year-old G1P0 presents at 30 weeks' gestation for a new OB visit. She provides you with the official report of a dating ultrasound performed at 12 weeks; however, shortly thereafter, she moved out of state and has not had prenatal care. She has no medical problems, and has a normal BMI. She reports some abdominal cramping and shortness of breath. During her visit, you examine her cervix and it is closed. You measure her fundal height at 50 cm.

108. What is the next best step in management?

a. Order an ultrasound
b. Tell the patient that she is most likely having twins
c. Teach her how to do fetal kick counts, and instruct her to return in 1 week
d. Tell her that her baby will be very large and recommend a caesarean delivery
e. Order a glucose tolerance test

109. An ultrasound is performed, and demonstrates a singleton fetus with an estimated fetal weight (EFW) in the 53 percentile. The amniotic fluid index is 30 cm, consistent with a diagnosis of polyhydramnios. How should you counsel this patient?

a. She does not require any further evaluation.
b. The incidence of associated malformations is approximately 3%.
c. Maternal edema, especially of the lower extremities and vulva, is rare.
d. Esophageal atresia is accompanied by polyhydramnios in nearly 10% of cases.
e. Potential complications include placental abruption, uterine dysfunction, and postpartum hemorrhage.

110. During routine ultrasound surveillance of a twin pregnancy, twin A weighs 1200 g and twin B weighs 750 g. Polyhydramnios is noted around twin A, while twin B has oligohydramnios. Which of the following statements correctly describes this syndrome?

a. The donor twin develops polyhydramnios more often than the recipient twin.
b. Gross differences may be observed between donor and recipient placentas.
c. The donor twin usually suffers from a hemolytic anemia.
d. The donor twin is more likely to develop widespread thromboses.
e. The donor twin often develops polycythemia.

111. A 32-year-old G5P1 presents for her first prenatal visit. A complete obstetrical, gynecological, and medical history and physical examination is performed. Which of the following would be an indication for elective cerclage placement?

a. Three spontaneous first-trimester abortions
b. Twin pregnancy
c. Three second-trimester pregnancy losses without evidence of labor or abruption
d. History of loop electrosurgical excision procedure for cervical dysplasia
e. Cervical length of 35 mm by ultrasound at 18 weeks

Questions 112 to 116

Match each description with the correct type of abortion. Each lettered option may be used once, more than once, or not at all.

a. Complete abortion
b. Incomplete abortion
c. Threatened abortion
d. Missed abortion
e. Inevitable abortion

112. Uterine bleeding at 12 weeks' gestation accompanied by cervical dilation without passage of tissue.

113. Passage of some but not all placental tissue through the cervix at 9 weeks' gestation.

114. Fetal death at 15 weeks' gestation without expulsion of any fetal or maternal tissue for at least 8 weeks.

115. Uterine bleeding at 7 weeks' gestation without any cervical dilation.

116. Expulsion of all fetal and placental tissue from the uterine cavity at 10 weeks' gestation.

Questions 117 to 119

A 19-year-old P0 presents for her first prenatal visit. She is 12 weeks' pregnant by sure last menstrual period. She reports vaginal bleeding, and on physical examination, you appreciate a 16-week size uterus. You are unable to detect fetal heart tone with a Doppler. The ultrasound shown is obtained.

117. Which of the following best describes the patient's diagnosis?

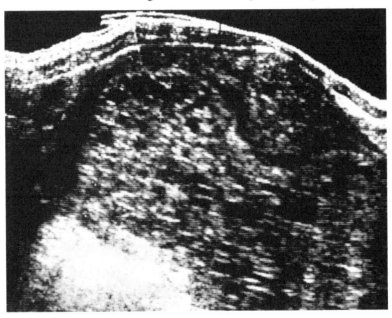

a. The most common chromosomal makeup of a partial (or incomplete) mole is 46, XX, of paternal origin.
b. Older maternal age is not a risk factor for hydatidiform mole.
c. Partial (or incomplete) hydatidiform mole has a higher risk of developing into choriocarcinoma than complete mole.
d. Vaginal bleeding is a common symptom of hydatidiform mole.
e. Hysterectomy is contraindicated as primary therapy for molar pregnancy in women who have completed childbearing.

118. The patient undergoes suction dilation and curettage (D&C) for management of the suspected molar pregnancy. The pathology report reveals trophoblastic proliferation and hydropic degeneration with the absence of vasculature; no fetal tissue is identified. A chest x-ray is negative for any evidence of metastatic disease. Which of the following is the best next step in her management?

a. Weekly human chorionic gonadotropin (hCG) titers
b. Hysterectomy
c. Single-agent chemotherapy
d. Combination chemotherapy
e. Radiation therapy

119. Which of the following would be an indication to start single-agent chemotherapy?

a. A rise in hCG titers
b. A plateau of hCG titers for 1 week
c. Return of hCG titer to normal at 6 weeks after evacuation
d. Appearance of liver metastasis
e. Appearance of brain metastasis

120. A 32-year-old woman presents to the emergency department with abdominal pain and vaginal bleeding. Her last menstrual period (LMP) was 8 weeks ago, and her pregnancy test is positive. Her blood pressure is 85/65 mm Hg and her pulse is 110 beats per minute. On examination, her abdomen is distended and tender. A bedside abdominal ultrasound shows free fluid within the abdominal cavity. The decision is made to take the patient to the operating room for emergency exploratory laparotomy. Which of the following is the most likely diagnosis?

a. Ruptured ectopic pregnancy
b. Hydatidiform mole
c. Incomplete abortion
d. Missed abortion
e. Torsed ovarian corpus luteal cyst

Questions 121 to 123

An 18-year-old G1P0 presents to the emergency department with a 1-day history of abdominal pain and vaginal bleeding. Her LMP was 7 weeks ago. On examination she is afebrile with a normal blood pressure and pulse. Abdominal examination demonstrates left lower quadrant tenderness with voluntary guarding. Laboratory tests reveal a normal white count, hemoglobin of 10.5 g/dL, and a quantitative β-hCG of 2342 mIU/ml. Ultrasound reveals a 10 × 5 × 6 cm uterus with a normal-appearing 1-cm stripe and no gestation sac or fetal pole. A 2.8-cm complex adnexal mass is noted on the left.

121. In the treatment of this patient, laparoscopy has what advantage over laparotomy?

a. Decreased hospital stays
b. Lower fertility rate
c. Lower repeat ectopic pregnancy rate
d. Comparable persistent ectopic tissue rate
e. Greater scar formation

122. At the time of laparoscopy, she is noted to have an approximately 3 cm mass in the ampulla of the left fallopian tube, consistent with an unruptured ectopic pregnancy. There is no blood in the cul de sac. What is the best next step in management?

a. Perform a laparoscopic salpingectomy
b. Perform a laparoscopic salpingostomy
c. Now that you have confirmed the diagnosis, you should leave the fallopian tube alone, and recommend treatment with methotrexate
d. Perform a laparoscopic salpingectomy and recommend postoperative treatment with methotrexate
e. Convert to a laparotomy to remove her fallopian tube

123. Which of the following events would be most likely to predispose this patient to ectopic pregnancy?

a. Previous cervical conization
b. Pelvic inflammatory disease (PID)
c. Use of a contraceptive uterine device (IUD)
d. Induction of ovulation
e. Exposure in utero to diethylstilbestrol (DES)

124. An 18-year-old G1P0 at 8 weeks' gestation presents to your office for her first prenatal visit. She reports daily nausea and vomiting over the past week. Which of the following signs or symptoms would indicate a more serious diagnosis of hyperemesis gravidarum?

a. Hypothyroidism
b. Hypokalemia
c. Weight gain
d. Proteinuria
e. Diarrhea

125. A 32-year-old G2P0101 presents to labor and delivery at 34 weeks' gestation with a chief complaint of regular uterine contractions every 5 minutes for the past several hours associated with the passage of clear fluid from her vagina. The external fetal monitor demonstrates a reactive fetal heart rate tracing, with contractions occurring every 3 to 4 minutes. Sterile speculum examination demonstrates a closed cervix with a pool of clear fluid in the vagina. A sample of this fluid is fern and nitrazine-positive. The patient has a temperature of 38.8°C, pulse 102 beats per minute, blood pressure 100/60 mm Hg, and her fundus is tender to palpation. Her admission blood work shows a WBC of 19,000 mcL. The patient is very concerned because she previously delivered a baby at 35 weeks who developed respiratory distress syndrome (RDS). You perform a bedside ultrasound, which shows oligohydramnios, and a fetus whose size is appropriate for gestational age and in cephalic presentation. Which of the following is the most appropriate next step in the management of this patient?

a. Administer betamethasone
b. Administer tocolytics
c. Place a cervical cerclage
d. Administer antibiotics
e. Perform emergent cesarean section

126. A 30-year-old G1P0 at 25 weeks presents to labor and delivery complaining of irregular uterine contractions and back pain. She reports no leakage of fluid from her vagina, but says that earlier in the day she had some very light vaginal bleeding, which has now resolved. She has had no prenatal care. She is dated by a sure LMP. On arrival to labor and delivery, she is placed on an external fetal monitor, which demonstrates uterine contractions every 2 to 4 minutes. She is afebrile and her vital signs are all normal. Her gravid uterus is nontender and measures 25 cm, consistent with her gestational age by LMP. The nurse calls you to evaluate the patient. Which of the following is the most appropriate first step in the evaluation of vaginal bleeding in this patient?

a. Vaginal examination to determine cervical dilation
b. Ultrasound to assess the placental location
c. Urine culture to evaluate for urinary tract infection
d. Laboratory tests to evaluate for disseminated intravascular coagulopathy
e. Apt test to determine if the blood is from the fetus

127. A 30-year-old G1P0 at 28 weeks' gestation is being evaluated for vaginal bleeding and uterine contractions. A bedside ultrasound demonstrates a cephalic fetus with an anterior placenta and no evidence of placenta previa. The fetal heart rate tracing is reactive, and uterine contractions are seen every 2 to 3 minutes. A sterile speculum examination is negative for ruptured membranes. A digital examination indicates that the cervix is 3 cm dilated and 50% effaced, and the presenting part is at −3 station. Tocolysis with magnesium sulfate is initiated and intravenous antibiotics are started for group B streptococcus prophylaxis. Which of the following statements correctly describes the benefits of betamethasone in the treatment of preterm labor?

a. Betamethasone enhances the tocolytic effect of magnesium sulfate and decreases the risk of preterm delivery.
b. Betamethasone has been shown to decrease intraamniotic infections.
c. Betamethasone promotes fetal lung maturity and decreases the risk of respiratory distress syndrome.
d. The anti-inflammatory effect of betamethasone decreases the risk of GBS sepsis in the newborn.
e. Betamethasone is the only corticosteroid proven to cross the placenta.

Questions 128 and 129

A 30-year-old G1 at 28 weeks' gestation is admitted to the hospital for preterm labor with painful contractions every 2 minutes. She is 3 cm dilated with membranes intact and a small amount of bloody show. Her pregnancy has been complicated by chronic hypertension, which has been well controlled on oral antihypertensive therapy. Ultrasound demonstrates a cephalic fetus with appropriate growth for gestational age and oligohydramnios.

128. Which of the following statements correctly describes the potential benefits of tocolysis?

a. Tocolysis provides fetal neuroprotection.
b. Tocolysis allows the pregnancy to progress to term.
c. The incidence of preterm delivery is decreased with tocolysis.
d. Tocolysis can provide short-term pregnancy prolongation in order to administer steroids and transfer to a tertiary care center.
e. Tocolysis decreases the risk of necrotizing enterocolitis.

129. Which of the following is a contraindication to the use of indomethacin as a tocolytic in this patient?

a. Intact membranes
b. Gestational age greater than 26 weeks
c. Vaginal bleeding
d. Oligohydramnios
e. Fetal growth restriction

130. A healthy 32-year-old G2P1001 presents to labor and delivery at 30 weeks' gestation reporting a small amount of bright red blood per vagina which occurred shortly after intercourse. It started off as spotting and then progressed to a light bleeding. By the time the patient arrived at labor and delivery, the bleeding had completely resolved. She reports no contractions, but admits to occasional abdominal cramping. She was dated by an 18-week ultrasound, and her pregnancy has been uncomplicated. Her obstetric history is significant for a previous low transverse cesarean at term. Vital signs are normal. Tocodynomometer shows contractions every 10 to 15 minutes, and the fetal heart rate tracing is reactive. Which of the following diagnoses may be excluded as the most likely cause for her vaginal bleeding?

a. Cervicitis
b. Preterm labor
c. Placental abruption
d. Placenta previa
e. Vasa previa

Questions 131 to 133

A 34-year-old G4P3003 at 31 weeks' gestation with a known placenta previa presents to the hospital with vaginal bleeding. On assessment, she has normal vital signs, a reactive fetal heart tracing, and no uterine contractions. Heavy vaginal bleeding is noted.

131. Which of the following is a risk factor for placenta previa?

a. Multiparity
b. Nulliparity
c. History of D&C
d. Uterine fibroids
e. Age younger than 25 years

132. Which of the following is the best next step in the management of this patient?

a. Administer intramuscular terbutaline
b. Administer methylergonovine
c. Admit and stabilize the patient
d. Perform cesarean delivery
e. Induce labor

133. The patient continues to bleed heavily and you observe persistent late decelerations on the fetal heart tracing. Her blood pressure and pulse are normal. You explain to the patient that she needs to be delivered, and she is delivered by cesarean under general anesthesia. The baby and placenta are easily delivered, but the uterus is noted to be boggy and atonic despite intravenous infusion of Pitocin. Which of the following is contraindicated in this patient for the treatment of uterine atony?

a. Methylergonovine (methergine) administered intramuscularly
b. Prostaglandin $F_2\alpha$ (hemabate) suppositories
c. Misoprostol (cytotec) suppositories
d. Terbutaline administered intravenously
e. Prostaglandin E_2 suppositories

134. A 25yo P0 at 25 weeks' gestation presents to the emergency department, where she was a restrained passenger in a motor vehicle accident. She reports she was rear-ended while idling at a stop light. She was wearing her seatbelt, and the impact was significant enough that her airbags were deployed. On examination, her vitals are normal. Her fundus is nontender, but she has bruising on her abdomen from the seatbelt. The fetal heart tracing is reactive and she has no contractions on the tocometer. She reports light vaginal bleeding, which is confirmed on sterile speculum examination. Her blood type is A negative. What is best test to determine whether there has been fetal-to-maternal hemorrhage?

a. Type and screen
b. Apt test
c. Kleihauer Betke (K-B) test
d. Complete blood count (CBC)
e. Hemoglobin electrophoresis

135. A 39-year-old G2P1001 presents for a routine OB visit at 30 weeks' gestation. Her obstetric history is significant for a vaginal delivery 10 years ago. That pregnancy was uncomplicated, and she delivered a 6 lb baby at 40 weeks. Her current pregnancy has also been uncomplicated. She has no significant medical history, and she does not use tobacco, alcohol, or other drugs. She weighed 95 lb prior to pregnancy, and she has gained 20 lb to date. Her 20-week anatomy ultrasound was normal, and her first trimester screen did not show an increased risk of chromosomal aneuploidies. Her blood pressure range has been 100 to 120/60 mm Hg to 70 mm Hg. During her examination, you note that her fundal height measures only 26 cm. Which of the following is a most likely explanation for this patient's decreased fundal height?

a. Autosomal trisomy
b. Constitutionally small mother
c. Poor weight gain
d. Lifestyle factors
e. Uteroplacental insufficiency

Questions 136 and 137

A 38-year-old G4P3 at 33 weeks' gestation presents for a routine OB visit, and is noted to have a fundal height of 29 cm. An ultrasound is performed, and demonstrates an EFW in the 5 percentile for the gestational age. The biparietal diameter and abdominal circumference are concordant in size.

136. Which of the following is associated with symmetric growth restriction?

a. Nutritional deficiencies
b. Chromosome abnormalities
c. Hypertension
d. Uteroplacental insufficiency
e. Gestational diabetes

137. Which of the following factors would indicate that this fetus needs to be delivered?

a. A biophysical profile (BPP) of 8/10
b. Estimated fetal weight (EFW) in the 5 percentile
c. Normal umbilical artery dopplers
d. Absence of interval growth on a repeat ultrasound in 2 weeks
e. Amniocentesis demonstrating fetal trisomy 21

138. A 26-year-old G1 at 37 weeks presents to the hospital in active labor. She has no medical problems and has a normal prenatal course except for fetal growth restriction. She undergoes an uncomplicated vaginal delivery of a female infant weighing 1950 g. The infant is at risk for which of the following complications?

a. Hyperglycemia
b. Fever
c. Hypertension
d. Anemia
e. Hypoxia

139. A 38-year-old G2P1 comes to see you for her first prenatal visit at 10 weeks' gestation. She had a previous term vaginal delivery without any complications. You detect fetal heart tones at this visit, and her uterine size is consistent with dates. You also order routine prenatal laboratory tests, which return showing that her blood type is A−, and she has a positive antibody screen, with an anti-D antibody titer of 1:4. Which of the following is the most appropriate next step in the management of this patient?

a. Schedule an amniocentesis for amniotic fluid bilirubin at 16 weeks
b. Repeat the titer in 4 weeks
c. Repeat the titer at 28 weeks
d. Schedule percutaneous umbilical blood sampling (PUBS) to determine fetal hematocrit at 20 weeks
e. Schedule PUBS as soon as possible to determine fetal blood type

140. A 23-year-old G3P1011 at 6 weeks presents for routine prenatal care. She had a cesarean delivery 3 years ago for breech presentation after a failed external cephalic version. Her daughter is Rh-negative. She also had an elective termination of pregnancy 1 year ago. She is Rh-negative and is found to have a positive anti-D titer of 1:8 on routine prenatal laboratory findings. Failure to administer RhoGAM at which time is the most likely cause of her sensitization?

a. After elective termination
b. At the time of cesarean delivery
c. At the time of external cephalic version
d. Within 3 days of delivering an Rh-negative fetus
e. At 28 weeks in the pregnancy for which she had a cesarean delivery

141. A 27-year-old G2P1 at 29 weeks' gestation who is being followed for Rh isoimmunization presents for her OB visit. The fundal height is noted to be 33 cm. An ultrasound reveals fetal ascites and a pericardial effusion. Which of the following can be another finding in fetal hydrops?

a. Oligohydramnios
b. Hydrocephalus
c. Hydronephrosis
d. Subcutaneous edema
e. Over-distended fetal bladder

Questions 142 to 145

A 39-year-old G2P1001 at 39 weeks' gestational age is sent to labor and delivery from her obstetrician's office because of a blood pressure reading of 150/100 mm Hg obtained during a routine OB visit. Her baseline blood pressures during the pregnancy were 100 to 120/60 mm Hg to 70 mm Hg. On arrival to labor and delivery, the patient reports no headache, visual changes, nausea, vomiting, or abdominal pain. The heart rate strip is reactive and the tocodynamometer shows irregular uterine contractions. The patient's cervix is 3 cm dilated. Her repeat blood pressure is 160/90 mm Hg. Hematocrit is 34.0%, platelets are 90,000 mL, SGOT is 22 units per liter, SGPT is 15 units per liter, and urinalysis is negative for protein.

142. Which of the following is the most correct diagnosis?

a. Preeclampsia
b. Preeclampsia with severe features
c. Chronic hypertension with superimposed preeclampsia
d. Eclampsia
e. Gestational hypertension

143. While being evaluated in triage, she is noted to have tonic-clonic seizure. Which of the following is the next step in the management of this patient?

a. Low-dose aspirin
b. Dilantin (phenytoin)
c. Antihypertensive therapy
d. Magnesium sulfate
e. Cesarean delivery

144. The decision is made to deliver the patient promptly. Which factors will help you determine the best mode of delivery?

a. The patient has advanced maternal age, and therefore must be delivered by cesarean immediately.

b. The patient's cervix is 3 cm dilated, and therefore must undergo induction of labor.

c. The patient has low platelets, so she must undergo induction of labor because surgery could cause significant hemorrhage.

d. The patient had a seizure, and therefore must be delivered immediate by cesarean.

e. The patient is a candidate for labor induction or cesarean delivery if the fetal and maternal status are reassuring after her seizure.

145. The patient is successfully inducted and undergoes vaginal delivery. Postpartum, she is on magnesium sulfate for seizure prophylaxis. Her vital signs are—blood pressure 154/98 mm Hg, pulse 93 beats per minute, respiratory rate 24 breaths per minute, and temperature 37.3°C. She has adequate urine output at greater than 40 cc/h. On examination, she is oriented to time and place, but she is somnolent and her speech is slurred. She has good movement and strength of her extremities, but her deep tendon reflexes are absent. Which of the following is the most likely cause of her symptoms?

a. Adverse reaction to hydralazine

b. Hypertensive stroke

c. Magnesium toxicity

d. Sinus venous thrombosis

e. Transient ischemic attack

Obstetrical Complications of Pregnancy

Answers

106. The answer is c. Prior cesarean delivery and placenta previa, especially with an anteriorly located placenta, increase the risk of placenta accreta, increta, and percreta. These are situations where the placenta is abnormally adherent to the uterine wall. In placenta accreta, the placental villi are abnormally attached to the myometrium. In placenta increta, the villi invade into the myometrium, and in placenta percreta, the villi penetrate through the myometrium. Placenta accreta, increta, or percreta typically require treatment with hysterectomy. The incidence of these disorders has increased due to the increased cesarean delivery rate. Placenta accrete may be suspected on ultrasound, but MRI is often required to confirm the diagnosis. Advanced maternal age, multiparity, prior cesarean delivery, and smoking are all risk factors for placenta previa. Painless bleeding is the most common symptom, and is rarely fatal. Vaginal examination to evaluate for placenta previa is contraindicated, unless the woman is in the operating room prepared for immediate cesarean delivery, because even the most gentle examination can cause significant hemorrhage. Vaginal examinations are rarely necessary, because ultrasound is usually readily available to make the diagnosis of placenta previa. Cesarean delivery is necessary in essentially all cases of placenta previa. Because of the poor contractile nature of the lower uterine segment, uncontrollable hemorrhage may follow removal of the placenta. Hysterectomy may be indicated if conservative methods to control hemorrhage fail. Resuscitation with blood products is the treatment for disseminated intravascular coagulopathy, not hysterectomy. Sterilization itself is not an indication for hysterectomy at the time of cesarean delivery, because the complications of surgery are much increased with a cesarean hysterectomy.

107. The answer is c. In women with intrauterine fetal demise, labor usually occurs within 2 weeks. Women are typically offered expectant management versus active management with surgical or medical evacuation of the uterus. If the fetus is retained longer than 1 month, 25% of women can develop coagulopathy, which is manifested by decreased fibrinogen, elevated fibrin degradation products, and decreased platelets. Septic abortions were more frequently seen during the era of illegal abortions, although occasionally sepsis can occur if there is incomplete evacuation of the products of conception in either a therapeutic or spontaneous abortion. However, since her cervix is closed and no tissue has passed, septic abortion is unlikely. Intrauterine fetal demise has no impact on future fertility or association with ectopic pregnancies.

108. The answer is a. This patient has an abnormally large fundal height. A fundal height should typically measure within 3 cm of the patient's gestational age. In this case, the gestational age is known because the patient had an early ultrasound, and was able to produce the report for confirmation. Given this early ultrasound, it is unlikely that the patient is having twins, as this would have been identified at her 12-week ultrasound. Gestational diabetes is sometimes associated with polyhydramnios, and the patient does need a glucose tolerance test as part of her prenatal care, but this is not the next best step. It is possible she will have a large baby, but this alone would not explain the size greater than dates measurement. A fundal height of 50 cm requires further investigation, and the best next step is ultrasound.

109. The answer is e. Polyhydramnios is defined as an excessive quantity of amniotic fluid, and occurs in 1% to 2% of pregnant women. When diagnosed, it requires further evaluation for genetic or anatomic anomalies, diabetes, and infection, although approximately 40% of cases are determined to be idiopathic. The incidence of associated malformations is about 20%, with CNS and GI abnormalities being particularly common, due to their impact on swallowing and absorption of amniotic fluid. Polyhydramnios accompanies about half of cases of anencephaly, and nearly all cases of esophageal atresia. Edema of the lower extremities, vulva, and abdominal wall is common, and results from compression of major venous systems. The most frequent maternal complications are placental abruption, uterine dysfunction, and postpartum hemorrhage.

110. The answer is b. In the twin-to-twin transfusion syndrome (TTTS), the donor twin is always anemic. This is not due to a hemolytic process, but rather to the direct transfer of blood to the recipient twin, who becomes polycythemic. The recipient may suffer thromboses secondary to hyper-transfusion and subsequent hemoconcentration. Although the donor placenta is usually pale and somewhat atrophied, that of the recipient is typically congested and enlarged. Polyhydramnios can develop in either twin, but is more frequent in the recipient twin due to circulatory overload. When polyhydramnios occurs in the donor, it is due to congestive heart failure caused by severe anemia.

111. The answer is c. Cervical insufficiency (or incompetence) describes the inability of the cervix to retain a pregnancy in the absence of contractions (or labor) in the second trimester. It is diagnosed based on a history of painless cervical dilation after the first trimester with delivery usually before 24 weeks, without contractions or other clear pathology (ie, infection, ruptured membranes). Based on current data, a shortened cervical length on ultrasound is associated with an increased risk of preterm birth, but is not sufficient for the diagnosis of cervical incompetence. Cerclage is indicated in a patient with a history of one or more second-trimester losses related to cervical incompetence. Cerclage is not indicated for the prevention of first-trimester losses, nor has it been shown to improve the preterm delivery rate or neonatal outcome in twin gestations. Evidence is currently lacking for the benefit of cerclage solely due to a history of prior loop electrosurgical excision procedure or cone biopsy. Serial transvaginal ultrasound evaluation of cervical length can be considered in women with a history of second and early third-trimester deliveries. A cervical length less than 25 mm or funneling of more than 25% or both is associated with an increased risk of preterm delivery.

112 to 116. The answers are 112-e, 113-b, 114-d, 115-c, 116-a. Bleeding occurs in about 30% to 40% of pregnancies before 20 weeks' gestation, with about half of these pregnancies ending in spontaneous abortion. A threatened abortion describes uterine bleeding that occurs without any cervical dilation or effacement. Inevitable abortion occurs when there is bleeding and cervical dilation, with or without rupture of membranes. Incomplete abortion is when only a portion of the products of conception have been expelled, and the cervix remains dilated. In cases where all fetal and placental tissue have been expelled, the cervix is closed, bleeding is minimal, and uterine cramps have ceased, a diagnosis of complete abortion may be made. A missed abortion is one in which fetal death occurs before 20 weeks' gestation without expulsion of any fetal or maternal tissue for at least 8 weeks thereafter. When a fetus is retained in the uterus beyond 5 weeks after fetal death, consumptive coagulability with hypofibrogenemia may occur. This is uncommon, however, in gestations of less than 14 weeks in duration.

117. The answer is d. The history, clinical picture, and ultrasound of the woman in the question are characteristic of hydatidiform mole, which are usually diagnosed during the first trimester. The most common symptom is vaginal bleeding, often accompanied by an enlarged-for-dates uterus. Other signs and symptoms include absent fetal heart tones, cystic enlargement of the ovaries, hyperemesis gravidarum, hypertension, and abnormally high levels of hCG for gestational age. Ultrasound, such as this one, typically shows a diffuse mixed echogenic pattern, classically referred to a "snowstorm" pattern. The most common chromosomal makeup for partial mole is 69, XXX, or 69, XXY, and for complete mole is 46, XX. Hydatidiform mole is 10 times as common in the Far East as in North America, and it occurs more frequently in women older than 45 years of age. Grossly, these lesions appear as small, clear clusters of grapelike vesicles, the passage of which confirms the diagnosis. Hysterectomy may be considered as primary therapy for molar pregnancy in women who have completed childbearing.

118. The answer is a. Molar pregnancies without evidence of metastatic disease should be followed routinely by hCG titers after uterine evacuation. ACOG guidelines suggest weekly hCG values until nondetectable for 3 weeks, followed by monthly titers for 6 months. After 6 months, the patient may resume trying to get pregnant if she wishes. During this followup period, it is very important that the patient be on reliable contraception, because an elevated hCG may indicate a new pregnancy versus postmolar gestational trophoblastic neoplasia. Most authorities agree that prophylactic chemotherapy should not be routinely employed, because 85% and 90% of affected patients will require no further treatment. For a young woman in whom preservation of reproductive function is important, hysterectomy is not routinely indicated.

119. The answer is a. Single-agent chemotherapy is usually instituted if postmolar gestational trophoblastic neoplasia is diagnosed. Recently, the International Federation of Gynecologists and Obstetricians (FIGO) standardized criteria for the diagnosis of postmolar gestational trophoblastic neoplasia—1– an hCG level plateau of 4 values +/– 10% over 3 weeks; 2– an hCG level increase of greater than 10% of three values over 2 weeks,

3- persistence of detectable hCG for more than 6 months after molar evacuation. New intrauterine pregnancy should always be ruled out. Single-agent chemotherapy (usually with methotrexate or actinomycin-D) should be instituted, provided that the trophoblastic disease has not metastasized to the liver or brain. The presence of such metastases usually requires initiation of multiagent chemotherapy.

120. The answer is a. The most likely diagnosis is ruptured ectopic pregnancy. Molar pregnancy, incomplete abortion, and missed abortion can also be associated with abdominal pain and vaginal bleeding, but would not be associated with free fluid (blood) within the abdominal cavity, hypotension, and tachycardia. A torsed ovarian cyst would present with intermittent abdominal pain. The ultrasound would show a pelvic mass with no doppler flow to the ovary, not free fluid.

121. The answer is a. Laparoscopic treatment of ectopic pregnancy is the preferred surgical treatment if the patient is stable. Studies suggest that the fertility rates and repeat ectopic pregnancy rates are comparable for laparoscopy and laparotomy. Laparoscopy results in shorter hospital stays, and many patients who undergo laparoscopy may be sent home the same day.

122. The answer is b. An unruptured ectopic pregnancy in a patient who desires future fertility could be managed with a laparoscopic salpingostomy. These patients have a higher risk of persistent ectopic tissue, and should be followed with serial hCGs. It is not necessary to perform a laparotomy in this stable patient, nor is removal of the entire fallopian tube (salpingectomy) indicated in this 18-year-old. Methotrexate therapy (without surgery) would also be a reasonable option to manage this stable, unruptured ectopic pregnancy if the patient did not have any contraindications such as immunodeficiency, renal or liver disease, or inability to comply with medical therapy follow up. Better outcomes with methotrexate are also seen with hCG values </= 5,000 mIU/ml, no fetal cardiac activity, and ectopic size less than 4 cm.

123. The answer is b. Any factor delaying transit of the ovum through the fallopian tube may predispose a patient to ectopic pregnancy. The major predisposing factor in the development of ectopic pregnancy is PID, which may cause tubal adhesions. A patient with a history of one episode of salpingitis will have a 9% chance of ectopic pregnancy. Any operative procedure on the fallopian tubes, such as tubal ligation, infertility surgery, or surgical treatment of a previous ectopic, will increase a patient's risk. Tubal sterilization with laparoscopic fulguration has a higher rate of ectopic pregnancy than tubal ligations performed with clips or rings. Prior ectopic pregnancy, history of DES exposure, and use of assisted reproductive technology all increase the risk of ectopic. IUD use decreases the overall pregnancy rate, but if a patient gets pregnant with an IUD (1/500-1/1000), it has a higher chance of being an ectopic pregnancy.

124. The answer is b. Nausea and vomiting of pregnancy is a common condition that affects 70% to 85% of pregnant women. Hyperemesis gravidarum is an extreme version of this that occurs in 0.5% to 2% of pregnancies. The diagnostic criteria include intractable vomiting not related to other causes, a measure of acute starvation (ie, ketonuria), and weight loss (usually at least 5% of body weight). Electrolyte abnormalities such as hypokalemia can also be present due to persistent vomiting. Hyperemesis gravidarum is the most common reason for admission to the hospital during early pregnancy. Patients who have hyperemesis gravidarum are best treated (if the disease is early in its course) with parenteral fluids and electrolytes, sedation, rest, vitamins, and antiemetics if necessary. ACOG recommends antiemetics such as dimenhydrinate, metoclopramide, or promethazine as first line agents, followed by methylprednisolone or ondansetron if this is not effective. Very slow reinstitution of oral feeding is permitted after dehydration and electrolyte disturbances are corrected. The disease usually improves spontaneously as pregnancy progresses.

125. The answer is d. This patient with preterm, premature rupture of membranes (PPROM) has a physical examination consistent with an intrauterine infection or chorioamnionitis. Chorioamnionitis can be diagnosed clinically by the presence of maternal fever, tachycardia, and uterine tenderness. Leukocyte counts are a nonspecific indicator of infection because they can be elevated with labor and the use of corticosteroids. When chorioamnionitis is diagnosed, fetal and maternal morbidity increases and delivery is indicated regardless of the fetus's gestational age. In the case described, antibiotics need to be administered to avoid neonatal sepsis. Ampicillin is the drug of choice to treat group B streptococcal infection. Since the fetal heart rate is reactive, there is no indication for cesarean delivery. Induction or augmentation of labor should be instituted as indicated. There is no role for tocolysis in the setting of chorioamnionitis, since delivery is the goal.

There is also no role for the administration of steroids, since delivery is imminent. Steroids are typically not indicated after 34 weeks' gestation. A cerclage is used to treat an incompetent cervix in the second trimester in the absence of ruptured membranes.

126. The answer is b. The concern with this patient who presents with symptoms of back pain, cramping, and vaginal bleeding is preterm labor. Before performing a digital examination on this patient to determine her cervical status, an ultrasound should be performed to rule out placenta previa in light of her history of vaginal bleeding without a prior ultrasound to document placental location. Intravenous hydration is appropriate in the setting of contractions, because dehydration may cause preterm contractions and uterine irritability. Urinary tract infections can be associated with uterine contractions and preterm labor, and therefore a urinalysis and/or urine culture should be obtained. The type of bleeding described is unlikely to have been caused by coagulopathy. The blood is unlikely to be fetal given the reassuring fetal heart tracing.

127. The answer is c. The patient is in preterm labor, because she has a dilated and effaced cervix in the presence of regular uterine contractions. Therefore, treatment is aimed at delaying delivery to allow continued fetal growth and maturity. The administration of tocolytic therapy to treat the preterm contractions is indicated. In addition, from 24 to 34 weeks, management also includes the administration of steroids, such as betamethasone, to promote fetal lung maturity. These steroids increase fetal surfactant production. RDS is a sequela of preterm neonates and occurs less often in infants given betamethasone in utero, because the surfactant increases pulmonary compliance and decreases surface tension. If delivery seems likely, intravenous antibiotics are administered to prevent possible neonatal sepsis. If the patient's contractions subside and there is no evidence of infection, then the antibiotics can be discontinued. It is advantageous to obtain a neonatology consult on any patient who appears to be in preterm labor so the parents know what to expect if they give birth to preterm infants. There is no need to prepare for a cesarean delivery in this patient at this time. Attempts are made to stop the labor first. If the patient continues to progress, then a vaginal delivery is preferred since the fetus is cephalic.

128. The answer is d. According to ACOG, in the United States, the rate of preterm birth is 12%, and approximately 50% of these births were preceeded by preterm labor. Preterm births account for approximately 70% of neonatal deaths, 36% of infant deaths, and 25% to 50% of cases of long-term neurologic impairment in children. Tocolysis does not provide neuroprotection; however, several studies have shown that predelivery administration of magnesium sulfate reduces the incidence of cerebral palsy when it is given with neuroprotective intent. Tocolysis has not been shown to work longer than 48 hours, and has not been shown to decrease the incidence of preterm birth. There is no evidence that tocolysis has any direct favorable effect on neonatal outcomes, or that any prolongation of pregnancy afforded by tocolytics translates into a statistically significant neonatal benefit.

129. The answer is d. Indomethacin would not be an appropriate tocolytic agent in this patient. Indocin is a prostaglandin synthetase inhibitor that can decrease fetal urine production and cause oligohydramnios. Since this fetus already has oligohydramnios it is best to avoid this therapy. Nifedipine is used for tocolysis and is thought to work by preventing entry of calcium into muscle cells. It can be associated with hypotension, so blood pressure must be followed carefully. Ritodrine and terbutaline are tocolytic agents that are b-adrenergic agents. They work by increasing cAMP in cells, which decreases free calcium. These agents can be associated with tachycardia, hypotension, and pulmonary edema. Magnesium sulfate is a tocolytic agent that works by competing with calcium for entry into cells. At high levels, it can cause respiratory and cardiac depression. Magnesium sulfate is contraindicated in patients with myasthenia gravis.

130. The answer is e. Vasa previa occurs when fetal vessels overlie the cervical os from velamentous insertion of the umbilical cord. They are susceptible to compression and laceration with rupture of membranes. Bleeding from a vasa previa causes fetal exsanguination, and since only a small amount of bleeding is necessary to kill a fetus, death is almost instantaneous if it goes unrecognized. Since the fetal heart tracing is normal, vasa previa is an unlikely diagnosis. Cervical inflammation (cervicitis) can render the cervix friable and prone to bleeding, especially after intercourse. Placental abruption occurs when there is a premature separation of the placenta from the uterine wall. While vaginal bleeding can be observed, the hemorrhage can be completely concealed, with the blood being trapped between the detached placenta and the uterine wall. Labor can be associated with vaginal bleeding caused by cervical dilation. Placenta previa occurs when the placenta is located over or in close proximity to the internal os of the cervix. When the lower uterine segment is formed or cervical dilation occurs in the presence of placenta previa, a certain degree of spontaneous placental separation and hemorrhage from disrupted blood vessels will occur.

131. The answer is a. Placenta previa has been associated with multiparity, especially in women who are para 5 or greater. Prior cesarean delivery provides a two to fivefold increased risk of placenta previa, and this condition is increased twofold in women who smoke. Advancing age is also a risk factor, and some estimates indicate that the incidence is 1/100 for women over age 35. Nulliparity, history of D&C, uterine fibroids, and young age do not increase the incidence of placenta previa.

132. The answer is c. In this patient who is starting to hemorrhage from a placenta previa, steps should be taken to stabilize the patient and prepare for possible emergent cesarean delivery. Patients with placenta previa are typically not candidates for vaginal delivery. The patient is not contracting, therefore there is no role for tocolysis. Terbutaline should never be used in a patient who is actively bleeding, because it is associated with maternal tachycardia and vasodilation. The actively bleeding patient should be resuscitated with intravenous fluids while blood is being cross-matched for possible transfusion. A Foley catheter should be placed because urinary output is a reflection of the patient's volume status. Finally, anesthesia should be notified because the patient may require imminent delivery.

133. The answer is d. Methylergonovine (methergine), prostaglandin $F_2\alpha$ (hemabate), prostaglandin E_1 (misoprostol), and prostaglandin E_2 (dinoprostone) are all uterotonic agents that can be used in situations where there is a postpartum hemorrhage caused by uterine atony. Terbutaline would be contraindicated in this situation because it is a tocolytic that is used to promote uterine relaxation.

134. The answer is c. The K-B test is based on the fact that fetal erythrocytes contain hemoglobin F, which is more resistant to acid elution than hemoglobin A. After exposure to acid, only fetal hemoglobin remains. Fetal red cells can then be identified by uptake of a special stain, and quantified on a peripheral smear. An apt test is usually used to detect the presence or absence (qualitative test, not quantitative) of fetal blood in a vaginal discharge, often to rule out vasa previa in late pregnancy. A type and screen, hemoglobin electrophoresis, or CBC will not provide information about fetomaternal hemorrhage.

135. The answer is b. This fetus is measuring "size less than dates." In a normal singleton pregnancy from about 18 to 36 weeks, the number of weeks of gestation should approximate the fundal height measurement, within 2 cm to 3 cm. The differential for a fundal height measurement that is less than expected includes incorrect dating, oligohydramnios, intrauterine growth restriction, or fetal demise. In this patient, heart tones are present, so the pregnancy is still viable. She had a first trimester ultrasound, so the dates are correct. Fetuses with chromosomal aneuploidies such as trisomy 13, 16, 18, or 21 are associated with growth restriction, but this patient has had a normal first trimester screen and anatomy scan. She has not given a history of leakage of fluid, nor does she have any risk factors for oligohydramnios. She is constitutionally small, and mothers who weigh less than 100 lb prior to pregnancy have a twofold increased risk of having a small-for-gestational age (SGA) infant. While poor maternal weight gain, especially in the second trimester, is associated with fetal growth restriction, the patient has gained 20 lb to date, which is adequate. Habits such as smoking, alcohol, or drug use are also associated with growth restriction, but this patient does not report a history of this. Chronic placenta hypoxia or uteroplacental insufficiency is typically associated with maternal conditions such as vascular disease, chronic renal insufficiency, pregestational diabetes, chronic hypertension, smoking, or pre-eclampsia.

136. The answer is b. Intrauterine growth restriction (IUGR) is diagnosed when the estimated weight of the fetus falls below the 10 percentile for a given age. By the use of ultrasonography, IUGR can be classified as either symmetric or asymmetric. In asymmetric IUGR, the abdominal circumference is low, but the biparietal diameter may be at or near normal. In cases of symmetric IUGR, all fetal structures (including both head and body size) are proportionately diminished in size. Fetal infections, chromosome abnormalities, and congenital anomalies usually result in symmetric IUGR. Asymmetric IUGR is seen in cases where fetal access to nutrients is compromised, such as with severe maternal nutritional deficiencies or hypertension causing utero-placental insufficiency.

137. The answer is d. The timing of deliver depends on many factors, including the underlying etiology of the growth restriction (if known), and the gestational age. Typically, growth restricted fetuses will be monitored with antenatal testing, serial ultrasounds for growth, and Doppler studies. The EFW alone is not necessarily an indication for delivery if other factors are favorable. There is no evidence that early delivery improves outcomes in fetuses with aneuploidy. A BPP of 8/10 and normal umbilical artery dopplers are reassuring. Absence of interval growth would indicate that the fetus should be delivered. Ultrasound measurements for growth should not be performed more frequently than every 2 weeks, because the inherent user error associated with ultrasound measurements can preclude an accurate assessment of interval growth.

138. The answer is e. Fetuses that are growth-restricted often have difficulty transitioning to the extrauterine environment. Therefore, it is critical that neonatologists be involved in such deliveries. Growth-restricted fetuses more commonly pass meconium, and are more likely to develop meconium aspiration syndrome. In addition, growth-restricted fetuses compensate for poor placental oxygen transfer by developing polycythemia, which can then result in multiorgan thrombosis at or after birth. At the time of delivery, growth restricted infants may suffer from hypoxia caused by uteroplacental insufficiency. Infants with IUGR have less subcutaneous fat deposition; therefore, hypothermia and hypoglycemia are a potential concern.

139. The answer is b. During the first prenatal visit, all pregnant women are screened for the ABO blood group and the Rh group, which includes the D antigen. If the woman is Rh-negative, antibody screening is performed. If the antibody D titer is positive, the woman is considered sensitized because she has produced antibodies against the D antigen. Sensitization occurs as a result of exposure to blood from an Rh-positive fetus in a prior pregnancy. A fetus that is Rh-positive possesses red blood cells that express the D antigen. Therefore, the maternal anti-D antibodies can cross the placenta and cause fetal hemolysis. Once the antibody screen is positive for isoimmunization, the titer should be followed at regular intervals (about every 4 weeks). A titer of 1:16 or greater is usually indicative of the possibility of severe hemolytic disease of the fetus. Once this critical titer is reached, further evaluation is done by amniotic fluid assessment or analysis of fetal blood via PUBS. In the presence of fetal hemolysis, the amniotic fluid contains elevated levels of bilirubin that can be determined via spectrophotometric analysis. Cordocentesis, or percutaneous umbilical blood sampling, involves obtaining a blood sample from the umbilical cord under ultrasound guidance. The fetal blood sample can then be analyzed for hematocrit and determination of fetal blood type. Cordocentesis also allows the fetus with anemia to undergo a blood transfusion.

140. The answer is a. To prevent maternal Rh sensitization, pregnant women who are Rh-negative should receive RhoGAM or Rh immune globulin (antibody to the D antigen) in the following situations: after a spontaneous or induced abortion, after an ectopic pregnancy, at the time of an amniocentesis/CVS/PUBS, at 28 weeks' gestation (prophylactically), within 3 days of a delivery of an Rh-positive fetus, at the time of external cephalic version, with second- or third-trimester antenatal bleeding, and in the setting of abdominal trauma.

141. The answer is d. Characteristics of fetal hydrops include abnormal fluid in two or more sites such as the thorax, abdomen, and skin. Fetal hydrops occurs as a result of excessive and prolonged hemolysis which causes anemia. This stimulates erythroid hyperplasia of the bone marrow and extramedullary hematopoiesis in the liver and spleen. The placenta is also markedly erythematous, enlarged, and boggy. Hydrothorax may be so severe that it may restrict lung development and cause pulmonary compromise after delivery. Ascites, hepatomegaly, and splenomegaly may lead to severe dystocia. Hydropic changes are easily seen on fetal ultrasound.

142. The answer is b. In 2013, and the ACOG task force published new evidence based recommendations about hypertension in pregnancy. They recognize four categories of hypertension in pregnancy. These are as follows: (i) preeclampsia-eclampsia, (ii) chronic hypertension, (iii) chronic hypertension with superimposed preeclampsia, and (iv) gestational hypertension. Preeclampsia is defined as blood pressure of 140/90 mm Hg or greater on at least two separate occasions that are 6 hours or more apart after 20 weeks' gestation, in conjunction with proteinuria greater than 300 mg per 24-hour urine collection (or a dipstick reading of +1 if other quantitative methods are not available). In recognition of the syndromic nature of preeclampsia, the task force removed the dependence of the diagnosis on the presence of proteinuria. In the absence of proteinuria, preeclampsia is diagnosed as hypertension in association with thrombocytopenia, impaired liver function, new renal insufficiency, pulmonary edema, or new-onset cerebral or visual disturbances. Gestational hypertension is blood pressure elevation after 20 weeks' gestation without proteinuria or the aforementioned systemic findings. Chronic hypertension is hypertension that predates pregnancy. Superimposed preeclampsia is chronic hypertension in association with preeclampsia. Eclampsia is present when women with preeclampsia develop seizures.

143. The answer is d. Women who have suffered an eclamptic seizure need to be immediately started on magnesium sulfate as a loading dose and then as a continuous infusion to prevent further seizures. This is the most appropriate next step. These women also need to have their blood pressure controlled with antihypertensive medications if the diastolic is increased above 105 mm Hg to 110 mm Hg. The purpose of antihypertensive therapy is to avoid a maternal stroke. Hydralazine, nifedipine, and labetalol are commonly used in acute hypertensive crises. Phenytoin is not indicated for seizure prophylaxis, as magnesium sulfate has been shown to be safer and more effective for prevention of recurrent seizures. Low dose aspirin does not have a role. Eclampsia in a term patient is typically managed with prompt delivery, but does not necessarily require cesarean.

144. The answer is e. The treatment for eclampsia in most situations is prompt delivery; however, this does not preclude a trial of labor. The maternal and fetal status must be considered when determining route of delivery. After the patient is stabilized after her seizure, factors to consider include gestational age, parity, cervical examination, prior delivery history, fetal position, fetal status, and maternal status. Maternal age and a platelet status of 90,000 do not typically contribute to this decision.

145. The answer is c. Magnesium therapy is typically continued for 24 hours postpartum in order to decrease the risk of seizures. This patient is showing signs of magnesium toxicity. The therapeutic range of serum magnesium to prevent seizures is 4 to 7 mg/dL. At levels between 8 mg/dL and 12 mg/dL, patellar reflexes are lost. At 10 mg/dL to 12 mg/dL, somnolence and slurred speech commonly occur. Muscle paralysis and respiratory difficulty occur at 15 mg/dL to 17 mg/dL, and cardiac arrest occurs at levels greater than 30 mg/dL.

Suggested Readings

American College of Obstetricians and Gynecologists. *Cerclage for the Management of Cervical Insufficiency.* Practice Bulletin Number 142, February 2014.

American College of Obstetricians and Gynecologists. *Diagnosis and Treatment of Gestational Trophoblastic Disease.* Practice Bulletin Number 53, June 2004, reaffirmed 2014.

American College of Obstetricians and Gynecologists. *Fetal Growth Restriction.* Practice Bulletin Number 134, May 2013.

American College of Obstetricians and Gynecologists. *Management of Preterm Labor.* Practice Bulletin Number 127, June 2012, reaffirmed 2014.

American College of Obstetricians and Gynecologists. *Medical Management of Ectopic Pregnancy.* Practice Bulletin Number 94, June 2008, reaffirmed 2014.

American College of Obstetricians and Gynecologists. *Nausea and Vomiting of Pregnancy.* Practice Bulletin Number 52, April 2004, reaffirmed 2013.

American College of Obstetricians and Gynecologists. *Premature Rupture of Membranes.* Practice Bulletin Number 139, October 2013.

American College of Obstetricians and Gynecologists. *Prevention of Rh Alloimmunization.* Practice Bulletin Number 4, May 1999, reaffirmed 2013.

American College of Obstetricians and Gynecologists. Task force on hypertension in pregnancy. *Practice Guideline*, 2013.

Cunningham FG, Leveno KJ, Bloom SL, et al. eds. Chapter 25: Obstetrical hemorrhage, Chapter 29: Fetal growth disorders, Chapter 32: Diseases and abnormalities of the placenta, Chapter 33: Abortion, Chapter 39: Diseases and injuries of the fetus and newborn.

Williams Obstetrics. 23rd ed. New York, NY: McGraw-Hill; 2010.

Medical and Surgical Complications of Pregnancy

Questions

146. A 33-year-old G3P2 at 38 weeks' gestation develops flu-like illness and breaks out with a pruritic, vesicular lesions all over her body. Three days later she goes into spontaneous labor and delivers a healthy appearing male infant via vaginal delivery. Her lesions are beginning to heal and she feels well. What is the most appropriate next step in the management of this patient and her baby?

a. Administer intravenous acyclovir to the mother
b. Administer intravenous acyclovir to the baby
c. Administer varicella-zoster immune globulin to the baby
d. Administer varivax (varicella vaccine) to the baby
e. Administer zostavax (herpes zoster vaccine) to the mother

147. A 29-year-old G1 at 9 weeks' gestation presents to your office for a new OB visit. She reports a history of well-controlled hypothyroidism. She takes 88 mcg of levothyroxine daily. How do you expect her thyroid laboratory values to change during pregnancy?

a. The thyroid-stimulating hormone (TSH) and free T4 will not change during pregnancy.
b. The TSH will increase and the free T4 will decrease.
c. The TSH will increase and there will be no change in the free T4.
d. The TSH and the free T4 will increase.
e. The free T4 will not change, and the change in TSH will vary by trimester.

148. A 19-year-old P0 presents for her first OB visit at 10 weeks' gestation. You order routine OB laboratory tests, and it returns showing a positive nucleic acid probe for *Neisseria gonorrhoeae*. One year ago, she was treated with ampicillin for a simple urinary tract infection and developed a severe allergic reaction. Which of the following is the best option for treatment at this time?

a. Tetracycline
b. Doxycycline
c. Azithromycin
d. Ceftriaxone
e. Penicillin

149. A 22-year-old pregnant woman has just been diagnosed with toxoplasmosis. Which of the following risk factors is most likely to have contributed to her diagnosis?

a. Eating raw meat
b. Eating raw fish
c. Owning a dog
d. English nationality
e. Having viral infections in early pregnancy

150. A 17-year-old woman at 22 weeks' gestation presents to the emergency department with a 3-day history of nausea, vomiting, and abdominal pain. The pain started in the middle of the abdomen, and is now located along her mid-to-upper right side. She is noted to have a temperature of 38.4°C (101.1°F). She reports no prior medical problems or surgeries. How does pregnancy alter the diagnosis and treatment of the disease?

a. Owing to anatomical and physiological changes in pregnancy, diagnosis is easier to make.
b. Surgical treatment should be delayed since the patient is pregnant.
c. Fetal outcome is improved with delayed diagnosis.
d. The incidence is unchanged in pregnancy.
e. The incidence is higher in pregnancy.

151. A 24-year-old P1001 presents at 8 weeks' gestation and reports a history of pulmonary embolism 3 years ago during her first pregnancy. She was treated with intravenous heparin followed by several months of oral warfarin (coumadin) and has had no further evidence of thromboembolic disease. How should her current pregnancy be managed?

a. Since she has had no further events or problems for 3 years, her risk of thromboembolism is no longer increased, and she does not require therapy during this pregnancy.
b. Because she has had no problems for 3 years, she may be treated only with a baby aspirin daily.
c. She should be managed with Doppler ultrasonography of the bilateral lower extremities once per trimester to screen for deep vein thrombosis.
d. The patient should be placed on low-dose unfractionated heparin therapy or low molecular weight heparin therapy throughout pregnancy and puerperium.
e. She only requires anticoagulation during the third trimester.

152. A 29-year-old G3P2 black woman in the 33 week of gestation is admitted to the emergency room because of acute abdominal pain that has been increasing during the past 24 hours. The pain is severe and is radiating from the epigastrium to the back. The patient has vomited a few times and has not eaten or had a bowel movement since the pain started. On examination, you observe an acutely ill patient lying on the bed with her knees drawn up. Her blood pressure is 100/70 mm Hg, her pulse is 110 beats per minute, and her temperature is 38.8°C (101.8°F). On palpation, the abdomen is somewhat distended and tender, mainly in the epigastric area, and the uterine fundus reaches 31 cm above the symphysis. Hypotonic bowel sounds are noted. Fetal monitoring reveals a normal pattern of fetal heart rate (FHR) without uterine contractions. On ultrasonography, the fetus is in vertex presentation and appropriate in size for gestational age; fetal breathing and trunk movements are noted, and the volume of amniotic fluid is normal. The placenta is located on the anterior uterine wall and no previa is seen. Laboratory values show mild leukocytosis (12,000 cells per mL); a hematocrit of 43%; mildly elevated serum glutamicoxaloacetic transaminase (SGOT), serum glutamic-pyruvic transaminase (SGPT), and bilirubin; and serum amylase of 180 U/dL. Urinalysis is normal. Which of the following is the most likely diagnosis?

a. Acute degeneration of uterine leiomyoma
b. Acute cholecystitis
c. Acute pancreatitis
d. Acute appendicitis
e. Severe preeclamptic toxemia

153. An 18-year-old G1 is diagnosed with asymptomatic bacteriuria (ASB) at her first prenatal visit at 15 weeks' gestation, based on a urine culture performed as part of her routine new OB laboratory findings. What is the next step in management?

a. Because she is asymptomatic, she does not require treatment.
b. She will only require treatment for ASB if she has sickle cell trait.
c. She only requires treatment if the culture is positive for group B streptococcus.
d. Twenty-five percent of women with ASB subsequently develop an acute symptomatic urinary infection during the same pregnancy, and therefore she should be treated with antibiotics.
e. She does not require treatment because ASB is not associated with adverse pregnancy outcomes.

154. A 20-year-old G1 at 18 weeks of gestation is hospitalized for intravenous antibiotics for the treatment of acute pyelonephritis. She develops shortness of breath and is found to have tachypnea and decreased oxygen saturation. Chest x-ray reveals pulmonary infiltrates consistent with pulmonary edema. What is the most likely cause of this complication?

a. Acute renal failure
b. Allergic reaction
c. Bacteremia
d. Endotoxin release
e. Intravenous hydration

Questions 155 to 157

A 30-year-old G1 at 6 weeks' gestation by last menstrual period presents for prenatal care. Her past medical history is significant for type 1 diabetes, which was diagnosed at the age of 14.

155. What should you tell her about her insulin requirements during pregnancy?

a. Her insulin requirement will not change during pregnancy.
b. She will require less insulin due to increased sensitivity to insulin during pregnancy.
c. She will require less insulin during pregnancy because she will experience decreased insulin resistance.

d. As long as her glycosylated hemoglobin A1c (Hb A1c) is less than 6%, she will not require any changes in her insulin management during pregnancy.

e. She should expect her insulin requirement to increase throughout the pregnancy.

156. Which of the following is the most common birth defect associated with diabetes?

a. Anencephaly
b. Encephalocele
c. Meningomyelocele
d. Sacral agenesis
e. Ventricular septal defect

157. Which of the following diabetic complications is most likely to be permanently worsened by pregnancy?

a. Coronary artery disease (CAD)
b. Gastroparesis
c. Nephropathy
d. Neuropathy
e. Proliferative retinopathy

158. A 33-year-old woman at 10 weeks' gestation presents for her first prenatal visit. Routine laboratory findings are drawn, and her hepatitis B surface antigen is positive. Liver function tests are normal and her hepatitis B core and surface antibody tests are negative. Which of the following is the best way to prevent neonatal infection?

a. Provide immune globulin to the mother
b. Provide hepatitis B vaccine to the mother
c. Perform a cesarean delivery at term
d. Provide hepatitis B vaccine to the neonate
e. Provide immune globulin and the hepatitis B vaccine to the neonate

159. A 38-year-old G1P0 presents to the obstetrician's office at 37 weeks' gestation complaining of a rash on her abdomen that is becoming increasingly pruritic. The rash started on her abdomen, and is starting to spread downward to her thighs. She reports no previous history of any skin disorders or problems, and she reports no malaise or fever. On physical examination, she is afebrile and her physician notes that her abdomen, and most notably her stretch marks, is covered with red papules and plaques. No excoriations or bullae are present. The patient's face, arms, and legs are unaffected by the rash. Which of the following is this patient's most likely diagnosis?

a. Herpes gestationis
b. Pruritic urticarial papules and plaques of pregnancy (PUPPP)
c. Prurigo gravidarum
d. Intrahepatic cholestasis of pregnancy
e. Impetigo herpetiformis

Questions 160 and 161

A 25-year-old G2P0 at 30 weeks' gestation presents with the complaint of intense itching that is worse on the palms and soles of her feet, and is worse at night. Her physical examination does not show any evidence of rash, but she has obvious excoriations from scratching on her abdomen.

160. Which of the following tests would be most likely to confirm your suspected diagnosis?

a. Skin biopsy demonstrating evidence of bile acids in the dermis
b. Elevated serum liver function enzymes
c. Elevated total serum bile acids
d. Liver biopsy demonstrating cholestasis without inflammation
e. Liver ultrasound showing normal liver parenchyma and biliary ducts

161. What is the best next step in treatment for this pregnancy complication?

a. Administration of intramuscular steroids for fetal lung maturity followed by delivery
b. Oral cholestyramine therapy
c. Topical steroids and oral antihistamines
d. Treatment with oral steroids
e. Oral ursodeoxycholic acid therapy

162. A 23-year-old G3P2002 presents for a routine visit at 34 weeks' gestation. She reports a history of genital herpes for 5 years. She says that she has had only two outbreaks during the pregnancy, but is very concerned about the possibility of transmitting this infection to her baby. How should you counsel this patient regarding her management during this pregnancy?

a. There is no risk of neonatal infection during a vaginal delivery if no lesions are present at the time she goes into labor.
b. She should be scheduled for an elective cesarean delivery at 39 weeks' gestation to avoid neonatal infection.
c. Starting at 36 weeks, weekly genital herpes cultures should be performed.
d. The herpes virus is commonly transmitted across the placenta in a patient with a history of herpes.
e. Suppressive antiviral therapy can be started at 36 weeks to help prevent an outbreak from occurring at the time of delivery.

163. A 37-year-old G3P2 presents to your office for her first OB visit at 10 weeks' gestation. She has a history of Graves disease and has been maintained on propylthiouracil (PTU) as treatment for her hyperthyroidism. She is currently euthyroid but asks you if her condition poses any problems for the pregnancy. Which of the following statements should be included in your counseling session with the patient?

a. She may need to discontinue the use of the thionamide drug because it is commonly associated with leukopenia.
b. Infants born to mothers on PTU may develop a goiter and be clinically hypothyroid.
c. PTU does not cross the placenta.
d. Pregnant hyperthyroid women, even when appropriately treated, have an increased risk of developing preeclampsia.
e. Thyroid storm is a common complication in pregnant women with Graves disease.

Questions 164 and 165

A 40-year-old P2002 at 37 weeks presents for her routine OB visit. Her pregnancy has been complicated by obesity and gestational diabetes mellitus (GDM) that has been well controlled with diet. Her blood sugar log shows that her fasting and postprandial values have all been within the normal range. Her fetus has an estimated fetal weight of 6½ lb by Leopold maneuvers.

164. Which of the following is the best next step in her management?

a. Administration of insulin to prevent macrosomia
b. Cesarean delivery at 39 weeks to prevent shoulder dystocia
c. Induction of labor at 38 weeks
d. Kick counts and routine return OB visit in 1 week
e. Weekly biophysical profile

165. This patient asks you if GDM has any long-term implications for her. Which of the following statements should be included in your counseling?

a. GDM resolves following delivery, and she does not need any follow up.
b. She has an increased risk of developing type 2 diabetes later in life.
c. She should have her hemoglobin A1c tested at her postpartum visit, and if elevated, she likely has type 2 diabetes.
d. She should have a fasting glucose tested on postpartum day 1, and if elevated, she likely has type 2 diabetes.
e. She should follow a diabetic diet for the rest of her life.

Questions 166 and 167

A 36-year-old G1P0 at 35 weeks' gestation presents to labor and delivery reporting a several-day history of generalized malaise, anorexia, nausea, and emesis. She reports no headache, vision changes, contractions, vaginal bleeding, or leaking fluid. She reports good fetal movement, and the FHR is in the 150s with good variability and no decelerations. On physical examination, you notice that she is mildly jaundiced and appears to be a little confused. Her vital signs indicate a temperature of 37.7°C (99.9°F), pulse of 70 beats per minute, and blood pressure of 100/62 mm Hg. Laboratory data are as follows—WBC = 25,000, Hct = 42.0%, platelets = 51,000, SGOT/PT = 287/350, glucose = 43 mg/dL, creatinine = 2.0 mg/dL, fibrinogen = 135 g/l, PT/PTT = 16/50 s, serum ammonia level = 90 mmol/L (nl = 11-35). Urinalysis is positive for 3+ protein and large ketones.

166. Which of the following is the most likely diagnosis?

a. Hepatitis B
b. Acute fatty liver of pregnancy
c. Intrahepatic cholestasis of pregnancy
d. Severe preeclampsia
e. Hyperemesis gravidarum

167. Which of the following is the recommended treatment for this patient?

a. Immediate delivery
b. Cholecystectomy
c. Intravenous diphenhydramine
d. MgSO$_4$ therapy
e. Bed rest and supportive measures since this condition is self-limited

168. A 32-year-old G1P0 presents for a routine OB visit at 14 weeks' gestation. Laboratory findings drawn at her first prenatal visit 4 weeks ago showed a platelet count of 60,000/μL. Follow up laboratory findings revealed a normal PT, PTT, and bleeding time. All her other laboratory findings were normal. During the present visit, her blood pressure is 120/70 mm Hg, she has no proteinuria on urine dip, and she reports no complaints. On taking a more in-depth history you learn that, prior to pregnancy, she had a history of occasional nose and gum bleeds, but no serious bleeding episodes. She has considered herself to be a person who just bruises easily. Which of the following is the most likely diagnosis?

a. Alloimmune thrombocytopenia
b. Gestational thrombocytopenia
c. Idiopathic thrombocytopenic purpura
d. HELLP syndrome
e. Pregnancy-induced hypertension

169. A 23-year-old G1P0 presents for a routine OB visit at 28 weeks' gestation. Laboratory findings drawn at her prenatal visit 2 weeks ago reveal a 1-hour glucose test of 128 mg/dL, hemoglobin of 10.8 g/dl, and a platelet count of 80,000/μL. All her other laboratory findings were normal. During the present visit, her blood pressure is 120/70 mm Hg, and her urine dip is negative, and she has no complaints. She has no known medical problems, but does report a history of epistaxis on occasion, but no other bleeding. What is the next step in treatment for her thrombocytopenia?

a. No treatment is necessary
b. Stop prenatal vitamins
c. Oral corticosteroid therapy
d. Intravenous immune globulin
e. Splenectomy

170. A 21-year-old G2P1 at 25 weeks' gestation presents to the emergency room with a chief complaint of shortness of breath. She reports a history of asthma, and states her peak expiratory flow rate (PEFR) with good control is usually around 400 L/min. When speaking, the patient has to stop to catch her breath between words; her PEFR is 210. An arterial blood gas is drawn and oxygen therapy is initiated. She is afebrile, and on physical examination expiratory wheezes are heard in all lung fields. Which of the following is the most appropriate next step in her management?

a. Antibiotics
b. Chest x-ray
c. Inhaled β-agonist
d. Intravenous corticosteroids
e. Theophylline

171. A 28-year-old G1 presents at 25 weeks' gestation complaining of severe left calf pain and swelling. On physical examination, the area of concern is slightly edematous, and the patient demonstrates a positive Homans sign, but no erythema is apparent. Which of the following diagnostic modalities should you order to confirm your suspected diagnosis?

a. MRI
b. Computed tomographic scanning
c. Venography
d. Compression ultrasonography
e. X-ray of lower extremity

Questions 172 to 180

For each clinical scenario presented later, select the most likely causative agent. Each lettered option could be used once, more than once, or not at all.

a. Cytomegalovirus
b. Rubella virus
c. *Treponema pallidum*
d. Parvovirus
e. *Toxoplasmosis gondii*
f. Hepatitis B
g. Herpes simplex virus
h. Varicella zoster
i. Group B streptococcus

172. A 20-year-old G1 patient delivers a live-born infant with cutaneous lesions, limb defects, cerebral cortical atrophy, and chorioretinitis. Her pregnancy was complicated by pneumonia at 18 weeks.

173. A 34-year-old G2 at 36 weeks delivers a growth-restricted infant with cataracts, anemia, patent ductus arteriosus, and sensorineural deafness. She has a history of chronic hypertension, which was well controlled with methyldopa during pregnancy. She had a viral syndrome with rash in early pregnancy.

174. A 25-year-old G3 at 39 weeks delivers a small-for-gestational-age infant with chorioretinitis, intracranial calcifications, jaundice, hepatosplenomegaly, and anemia. The infant displays poor feeding and tone in the nursery. The patient denies eating any raw or undercooked meat and does not have any cats living at home with her. She works as a nurse in the pediatric intensive care unit at the local hospital.

175. A 23-year-old G1 with a history of a flulike illness, fever, myalgias, and lymphadenopathy during her early third trimester delivers a growth-restricted infant with seizures, intracranial calcifications, hepatosplenomegaly, jaundice, and anemia.

176. A 32-year-old G5 delivers a stillborn fetus at 34 weeks. The placenta is noted to be much larger than normal. The fetus appeared hydropic and had petechiae over much of the skin.

177. A 38-year-woman at 39 weeks delivers a 7-lb infant (female) without complications. At 2 weeks of life, the newborn develops fulminant liver failure and dies.

178. A 20-year-old woman who works as a kindergarten teacher presents for her routine visit at 32 weeks. Her fundal height measures 40 cm. An ultrasound reveals polyhydramnios, an appropriately grown fetus with ascites and scalp edema. The patient denies any recent illnesses, but some of the children at her school have been sick recently.

179. A 25-year-old woman in her first pregnancy delivers a 6-lb male neonate at 38 weeks. The newborn develops fever, vesicular rash, poor feeding, and listlessness at 1 week of age.

180. A 22-year-old woman delivers a 7-lb male infant at 40 weeks without any complications. On day 3 of life, the neonate develops respiratory distress, hypotension, tachycardia, listlessness, and oliguria.

Medical and Surgical Complications of Pregnancy

Answers

146. The answer is c. Varicella, or chicken pox, is usually diagnosed based on the clinical findings of a classic pruritic, vesicular rash. Pregnant women should have varicella immunity documented in early pregnancy by a history of previous infection or varicella vaccination. Pregnant women who have no history of chicken pox or have serology demonstrating lack of immunity should avoid varicella infected individuals until their lesions have crusted over and they are no longer infectious. Neonatal mortality rates are close to 25% when maternal varicella develops around the time of delivery, due to the lack of protective maternal antibodies and the relative immaturity of the fetal immune system. Therefore, if a mother has clinical evidence of varicella infection 5 days before or up to 48 hours after delivery, the newborn should receive varicella-zoster immune globulin. Typically, varicella infection in the mother only requires supportive therapy, but pregnant women have a higher and mortality related to development of pneumonia. If pneumonia is diagnosed, intravenous acyclovir should be given. The newborn should be isolated from the mother if she is infective, and if the neonate develops signs or symptoms of varicella infection, then intravenous acyclovir would be administered. Pregnant women should not receive the live-attenuated varicella vaccine.

147. The answer is e. There are considerable changes in maternal thyroid function during pregnancy. Maternal total or bound thyroid hormone levels increase with serum concentration of thyroid-binding globulin. TSH decreases in early pregnancy because of weak stimulation of its receptors by human chorionic gonadotropin (hCG) during the first trimester After the first trimester, TSH levels return to baseline values and progressively increase in the third trimester related to placental growth and production of placental deiodinase. Free T4 remains stable during pregnancy. A high TSH and low free T4 are characteristic of overt hypothyroidism. These physiologic changes should be considered when interpreting thyroid function test results during pregnancy.

148. The answer is c. Patients with a severe allergic reaction to ampicillin should not receive penicillin. Patient with this type of reaction have up to a 20% incidence of reaction to cephalosporins, so ceftriaxone should be avoided as well unless desensitization is undertaken. Spectinomycin used to be the treatment of choice for pregnant women with *Neisseria gonorrhoeae* infections and who were allergic to penicillin; however, the production of this medication was discontinued in the United States in 2006. The use of doxycycline or tetracycline is generally contraindicated in pregnancy. Azithromycin 2 g orally as a single dose may be used as an alternative to treat both gonorrhea and chlamydia.

149. The answer is a. Toxoplasmosis is caused by the intracellular parasite *Toxoplasma gondii*. This infection is usually asymptomatic and self limited, but can present with asymptomatic cervical lymphadenopathy, fever, malaise, night sweats, and myalgias. Symptoms occur in only 10% to 20% of immunocompetent adults. Human infection can result from ingestion of raw or under-cooked meat infected by the organism, or from contact with infected cat feces. The French, because their diet includes raw meat, have a higher incidence (but not the English). The incidence of vertical transmission through the placenta varies by trimester, with the highest risk of transmission in the third trimester. The earlier the fetus is infected, the more severe the disease.

150. The answer is d. The incidence of appendicitis in pregnancy is 1 in 2000, the same as that in the nonpregnant population. The diagnosis can be difficult to make during pregnancy because leukocytosis, nausea, and vomiting are common in pregnancy. In addition, the upward displacement of the appendix by the uterus may cause appendicitis to have a nonclassic presentation. Surgery is necessary even if the diagnosis is not certain. Rupture of the appendix is more likely in pregnant women, likely due to the delay in diagnosis and reluctance to operate on pregnant women.

151. The answer is d. Pregnancy is considered a hypercoaguable state. Patients with a history of thromboembolic disease in pregnancy are at high risk of developing it in subsequent pregnancies, and therefore should be anticoagulated. Baby aspirin is not considered adequate treatment. Pregnant patients with a history of venous thromboembolism should be treated with either low-dose unfractionated heparin therapy or low molecular weight heparin therapy during the pregnancy and through the postpartum period, as this is the time of highest risk of clot formation. Doppler ultrasonography is the most common way to diagnose a deep vein thrombosis, but is not considered a screening test, and should not be ordered each trimester in the absence of clinical symptoms or signs.

152. The answer is c. The most probable diagnosis in this case is acute pancreatitis. The pain caused by a myoma in degeneration is more localized to the uterine wall. Low-grade fever and mild leukocytosis may appear with a degenerating myoma, but liver function tests are usually normal. The other obstetrical causes of epigastric pain, such as preeclampsia may exhibit disturbed liver function (sometimes associated with the hemolysis, elevated liver enzymes, low platelets (HELLP) syndrome), but this patient has only mild elevation of blood pressure and no proteinuria. Acute appendicitis in pregnancy is one of the more common nonobstetric causes of abdominal pain. Symptoms of acute appendicitis in pregnancy are similar to those in nonpregnant patients, but the pain is more vague and poorly localized and the point of maximal tenderness moves to the right upper quadrant with advancing gestation. Liver function tests are normal with acute appendicitis. Acute cholecystitis may cause fever, leukocytosis, and pain of the right upper quadrant with abnormal liver function tests, but amylase levels would be elevated only mildly, if at all, and pain would be less severe than described in this patient. The diagnosis that fits the clinical description and the laboratory findings is acute pancreatitis. This disorder may be more common during pregnancy, with an incidence of 1 in 100 to 1 in 10,000 pregnancies. Cholelithiasis, chronic alcoholism, infection, abdominal trauma, some medications, and pregnancy-induced hypertension are known predisposing factors.

Leukocytosis, hemoconcentration, and abnormal liver function tests are common laboratory findings in acute pancreatitis. However, the most important laboratory finding is an elevation of serum amylase levels, which appears 12 to 24 hours after onset of clinical disease. Values may exceed 200 U/dL (normal values are 50 U/dL to 160 U/dL). Treatment considerations for the pregnant patient with acute pancreatitis are similar to those in nonpregnant patients. Intravenous hydration, nasogastric suction, enteric rest, and correction of electrolyte imbalance and of hyperglycemia are the mainstays of therapy.

153. The answer is d. The term *ASB* is used to indicate persistent, actively multiplying bacteria within the urinary tract without symptoms of a urinary infection. The reported prevalence during pregnancy varies from 2% to 7%. The highest incidence has been reported in black multiparas with sickle cell trait and the lowest incidence among white women of low parity. In women who demonstrate ASB, the bacteriuria is typically present at the time of the first prenatal visit; after an initial negative culture of the urine, fewer than 1% develop a urinary infection. If ASB is not treated during pregnancy, approximately 25% of infected women develop an acute infection. Untreated ASB has been associated with an increase in complications such as low birth weight, preterm birth, and pyelonephritis.

154. The answer is d. Endotoxin release can cause alveolar injury and lead to pulmonary edema and acute respiratory distress. Endotoxin release can also cause renal dysfunction manifested as increase serum creatinine, but this effect is usually reversible with fluid resuscitation. Uterine contractions and hemolytic anemia are also effects of endotoxin release. Bacteremia can be found in up to 20% of women with pyelonephritis, but it is the endotoxin release that leads to alveolar damage. While allergic reactions to antibiotics can cause respiratory symptoms, they do so by causing bronchoconstriction. Intravenous hydration to ensure adequate urinary output (> 50 mL/h) is the mainstay of therapy. Careful monitoring of the input and output of the patient is necessary so that fluid overload will not compound the pulmonary effects of the endotoxin.

155. The answer is e. Pregnancy is characterized by both increased insulin resistance and decreased sensitivity to insulin. The increased insulin resistance is largely due to placental hormones such as human placental lactogen, progesterone, and cortisol. The management of type 1 diabetes in pregnancy focuses on glucose control, maximizing diet, engaging in exercise, and insulin therapy. Insulin requirements will increase during pregnancy, most markedly during the period between 28 and 32 weeks' gestation.

156. The answer is e. Major congenital anomalies are the leading cause of perinatal mortality in pregnancies complicated by type 1 diabetes, occurring in 6% to 12% of infants of women with diabetes. It is believed that the increased risk of congenital anomalies is a consequence of poor glucose control in the preconception and early pregnancy period. Glycosylated hemoglobin (Hgb A_{1c}) level correlates directly with the frequency of anomalies. A HbA1c around 6% is associated with a fetal anomaly rate close to that of the general population (2%-3%), whereas an HbA1c of 10% is associated with a fetal anomaly rate of 20%-25%. The most common single organ system anomalies are complex cardiac (38%), musculoskeletal (15%), and central nervous system (anencephaly and/or spina bifida) (10%). Sacral agenesis is a rare malformation seen in severely diabetic women.

157. The answer is e. Pregnancy has been associated with exacerbation of many diabetes-related complications. The rapid institution of strict glycemic control in women with diabetes during pregnancy has been associated with acute worsening of diabetic proliferative retinopathy, especially in women with coexisting hypertensive disorders. Pregnant women with diabetes should undergo a complete eye examination at the beginning of pregnancy, and should be monitored closely throughout. Most studies have failed to demonstrate permanent worsening in renal function in women with mild to moderate diabetic nephropathy. CAD does not necessarily worsen during pregnancy, but in women with preexisting symptomatic CAD, the pregnancy-associated hemodynamic changes may lead to an increased risk of myocardial infarction and death. Diabetic neuropathy is not very well studied during pregnancy, but may manifest as gastroparesis causing intractable nausea and vomiting.

158. The answer is e. Hepatitis B is transmitted by parenteral and sexual contact. Women with multiple sex partners, those who engage in intravenous drug use, and those who have sexual partners who engage in these risky behaviors are at highest risk to acquire this infection. Infection of the newborn whose mother chronically carries the hepatitis B virus can usually be prevented by the administration of hepatitis B immune globulin very soon after birth, followed promptly by the hepatitis B vaccine.

159. The answer is b. PUPPP is the most common dermatologic condition of pregnancy. It is more common in nulliparous women and occurs most often in the second and third trimesters of pregnancy. PUPPP is characterized by erythematous papules and plaques that are intensely pruritic and appear first on the abdomen. The lesions then commonly spread to the buttocks, thighs, and extremities with sparing of the face.

Herpes gestationis is a blistering skin eruption that occurs more commonly in multiparous patients in the second or third trimester of pregnancy. The presence of vesicles and bullae help differentiate this skin condition from PUPPP. Immunologically, it is indistinguishable from bullous pemphigoid. Prurigo gestationis is a very rare dermatosis of pregnancy that is characterized by small, pruritic excoriated lesions that occur between 25 and 30 weeks. The lesions first appear on the trunk and forearms and can spread throughout the body as well. In cholestasis of pregnancy, bile acids are cleared incompletely and accumulate in the dermis, which causes intense itching. These patients develop pruritus in late pregnancy; there are no characteristic skin changes or rashes except in women who develop excoriations from scratching. Impetigo herpetiformis is a rare pustular eruption that forms along the margins of erythematous patches. This skin condition usually occurs in late pregnancy. The skin lesions usually begin at points of flexure and extend peripherally; mucous membranes are commonly involved. Patients with impetigo herpetiformis usually do not have intense pruritus, but more commonly have systemic symptoms of nausea, vomiting, diarrhea, chills, and fever.

160. The answer is c. The hallmark of intrahepatic cholestasis of pregnancy is elevated serum bile acids. This may be accompanied by elevated liver enzymes, but there are other diseases, such as preeclampsia, that could cause this. Liver biopsy is typically not needed to confirm the diagnosis, but if performed, it would show mild cholestasis with intracellular bile pigments and canalicular bile plugging without necrosis. Liver ultrasound would usually be normal, but may serve to exclude other diagnoses, such as biliary obstruction due to gallstones. Skin biopsy is not used to diagnose cholestasis of pregnancy.

161. The answer is e. Intrahepatic cholestasis of pregnancy is best treated with oral ursodeoxycholic acid therapy, which has been shown to quickly and safely relieve pruritis, lower hepatic enzyme levels, and decrease serum bile acid concentrations. It primarily works by increasing bile flow. Topical steroids and oral antihistamines may be used in conjunction with ursodeoxycholic acid. The data about oral steroids has not shown consistent improvement in symptoms. Cholestyramine may be used, but has been shown to impair fat soluble vitamin absorption, with potential to cause impaired coagulation due to vitamin K deficiency. There is an increased risk of adverse pregnancy outcomes in women who have cholestasis of pregnancy, but this does not require delivery at 30 weeks. Instead, patients should be followed closely with antenatal testing and delivered at 36 to 37 weeks gestation, balancing risks of adverse outcomes such as fetal death with risks of prematurity.

162. The answer is e. A maternal HSV infection can be passed to the fetus via vertical transmission. If a pregnant woman with a history of herpes has no lesions present at the time she goes into labor, vaginal delivery is permitted. If lesions are present at the time of labor, then there is a 3% to 5% risk of transmitting the infection to the fetus, and cesarean delivery is recommended. Viral shedding can occur without the presence of a lesion. It is not recommended that a patient with a history of herpes be scheduled for an elective cesarean section. It is not recommended that weekly genital viral cultures be performed because such cultures do not predict whether a patient will be shedding the virus at the time of delivery. For patients at or beyond 36 weeks' gestation, daily suppressive therapy with an antiviral medication such as acyclovir can be used to try to decrease the risk of viral shedding and outbreaks and the likelihood of a cesarean section.

163. The answer is b. Hyperthyroidism in pregnancy is treated with thionamides, namely, PTU and methimazole. Transient leukopenia occurs in about 10% of patients taking thionamide drugs, but does not necessitate stopping the medication. Agranulocytosis, which is a rare complication, necessitates discontinuation of the drug. Fetal exposure to thionamides, which can cross the placenta, may cause goitrous hypothyroidism. Women who remain hyperthyroid despite therapy have a higher incidence of preeclampsia and heart failure. Thyroid storm occurs only rarely in untreated women with Graves disease. This emergent medical condition involves thyrotoxicosis, which is characterized by fever, tachycardia, altered mental status, vomiting, diarrhea, and cardiac arrhythmia.

164. The answer is d. In general, women with gestational diabetes, who do not require insulin, seldom need early delivery or other interventions. There is no consensus on whether antepartum fetal testing is necessary in women with well-controlled gestational diabetes. Antepartum fetal testing is recommended for women with preexisting diabetes mellitus and those who require insulin therapy, due to an increased risk of fetal demise. There is no good evidence to support routine delivery before 40 weeks when glucose control is good and no other complications supervene. Cesarean delivery may be considered in women with GDM if the estimated fetal weight is 4500 g or more.

165. The answer is b. It has been estimated that 15% to 50% of women who have GDM will develop type 2 diabetes later in life. Women with a history of GDM have a sevenfold increased risk of developing type 2 diabetes compared to women without a history of GDM. Postpartum screening at 6 to 12 weeks is recommended to identify women with type 2 diabetes, impaired fasting glucose levels, or impaired glucose tolerance. A fasting plasma glucose test OR the 2-hour 75-g oral glucose tolerance test may be used to screen. Although the fasting glucose is easier to perform, it would be less likely to detect other forms of impaired glucose metabolism.

166. The answer is b. Acute fatty liver of pregnancy is a rare complication of pregnancy. Estimates of its incidence range from 1 in 7000 to 1 in 15,000 pregnancies. At one time, it was thought to be universally fatal, but early diagnosis and prompt delivery have significantly improved the prognosis. It is thought that recessively inherited mitochondrial abnormalities of fatty acid oxidation predispose a woman to fatty liver in pregnancy. This disorder usually manifests itself late in pregnancy and is more common in nulliparous women. Typically, a patient will present with a several-day or -week history of general malaise, anorexia, nausea, emesis, and jaundice. Liver enzymes are usually not elevated above 500 U/L. Indications of liver failure are present, manifested by elevated PT/PTT, bilirubin, and ammonia levels. In addition, there is marked hypoglycemia. Low fibrinogen and platelet levels occur secondary to a consumptive coagulopathy. In cases of viral hepatitis, serum transaminase levels are usually much higher and marked hypoglycemia or elevated serum ammonia levels would not be seen. Sometimes the HELLP syndrome can initially be difficult to differentiate from acute fatty liver, but in this case the patient has a normal blood pressure. In addition, hepatic failure is not characteristic of severe preeclampsia. Hyperemesis gravidarum is characterized by nausea and vomiting unresponsive to simple therapy. It usually occurs early in the first trimester and resolves by about 16 weeks. In some cases, there can be a transient hepatic dysfunction. Intrahepatic cholestasis of pregnancy is characterized by pruritus and/or icterus. Some women develop cholestasis in the third trimester secondary to estrogen-induced changes. There is an accumulation of serum bile salts, which causes pruritus. Liver enzymes are seldom elevated above 250 U/L.

167. The answer is a. Acute fatty liver resolves spontaneously after delivery. Delayed diagnosis and movement toward delivery can result in risk of coma and death from severe hepatic failure. In addition, procrastination can result in severe hemorrhage and renal failure. Bed rest and supportive therapy would be the treatment for viral hepatitis. Benadryl treatment would apply to therapy for cholestasis of pregnancy. $MgSO_4$ therapy would be applicable to cases of the HELLP syndrome.

168. The answer is c. ITP typically occurs in the second or third decade of life and is more common in women than in men. The diagnosis of ITP is one of exclusion, because there are no pathognomonic signs, symptoms, or diagnostic tests. Traditionally, ITP is associated with a persistent platelet count of less than 100,000/μL in the absence of splenomegaly. Most women have a history of easy bruising and nose and gum bleeds that precede pregnancy. If the platelet count is maintained above 20,000/μL, hemorrhagic episodes rarely occur. In cases of ITP, the patient produces IgG antiplatelet antibodies that increase platelet consumption in the spleen and other sites. Gestational thrombocytopenia occurs in up to 8% of pregnancies. Affected women are usually asymptomatic, have no prior history of bleeding, and usually maintain platelet counts above 70,000/μL. Platelet counts usually return to normal in about 3 months. The cause of gestational thrombocytopenia has not been clearly elucidated. HELLP syndrome is associated with thrombocytopenia, but this condition typically occurs in the third trimester and is associated with hypertension (preeclampsia). In neonatal alloimmune thrombocytopenia, there is a maternal alloimmunization to fetal platelet antigens. The mother is healthy and has a normal platelet count, but produces antibodies that cross the placenta and destroy fetal/neonatal platelets.

169. The answer is a. This patient is most likely to have gestational thrombocytopenia. Asymptomatic pregnant women with platelet counts above 50,000/μL do not need to be treated, because the platelet count is sufficient to prevent bleeding complications. For severely low platelet counts, therapy can include prednisone, intravenous immune globulin, and splenectomy. These therapies are typically not required to treat gestational thrombocytopenia.

170. The answer is c. Inhaled β-agonists are the primary treatment for an acute asthma exacerbation. Intravenous steroids should be given if the exacerbation is severe, if the patient is currently taking oral steroids, or if the response to bronchodilator therapy is incomplete or poor. Antibiotics are used for patients with fever, leukocytosis, or evidence of infection. A febrile patient should have a chest x-ray to rule out pneumonia. Methylxanthines are not used for acute asthma exacerbations.

171. The answer is d. The patient's presentation is concerning for deep vein thrombosis (DVT). Noninvasive modalities are the preferred tests for diagnosing venous thromboemboli. Historically, venography has been considered the gold standard for diagnosis; however, it is not commonly used, because it is cumbersome to perform, expensive, and has potentially serious complications. Compression ultrasonography is the procedure of choice to detect proximal DVT. MRI may be used in cases when ultrasound findings are equivocal.

172. The answer is h. Maternal infection with viruses and bacteria during pregnancy can cause an array of fetal effects from none to congenital malformations and death. Maternal infection with varicella zoster during the first half of pregnancy can cause malformations such as cutaneous and bony defects, chorioretinitis, cerebral cortical atrophy, and hydronephrosis. Adults with varicella infection fare much worse than children; about 10% will develop a pneumonitis, and some of these will require ventilatory support.

173. The answer is b. Rubella is one of the most teratogenic agents known. Fetal manifestations of infection correlate with time of maternal infection and fetal organ development. If infection occurs in the first 12 weeks, 80% of fetuses manifest congenital rubella syndrome, while only 25% develop this syndrome if infection occurs at the end of the second trimester. Congenital rubella syndrome includes one or more of the following—eye lesions, cardiac disease, sensorineural deafness, CNS defects, growth restriction, thrombocytopenia, anemia, liver dysfunction, interstitial pneumonitis, and osseous changes.

174. The answer is a. Cytomegalovirus in the mother is usually asymptomatic, but 15% of adults will have a mononucleosis-like syndrome. Maternal immunity does not prevent recurrence or congenital infection. Congenital infection includes low birth weight, microcephaly, intracranial calcifications, chorioretinitis, mental and motor retardation, sensorineural deficits, hepatosplenomegaly, jaundice, anemia, and thrombocytopenic purpura. The virus is shed in the secretions of affected individuals. Cytomegalovirus is common in day care centers and by age 2 or 3 children usually acquire the infection from one another and transmit it to their parents.

175. The answer is e. *T gondii* is transmitted by eating infected raw or undercooked meat, and by contact with infected cat feces. Maternal immunity appears to protect against fetal infection, and up to one-third of American women are immune prior to pregnancy. Acute infection in the mother is often subclinical, but symptoms can include fatigue, lymphadenopathy, and myalgias. Fetal infection is more common when the disease is acquired later in pregnancy (60% in third trimester vs 10% in first trimester). Congenital disease consists of low birth weight, hepatosplenomegaly, jaundice, anemia, neurological disease with seizures, intracranial calcifications, and mental retardation.

176. The answer is c. Transplacental infection can occur with any stage of syphilis, but the highest incidence of congenital infection occurs in women with primary or secondary disease. The fetal and neonatal effects include hepatosplenomegaly, edema, ascites, hydrops, petechiae or purpuric skin lesions, osteochondritis, lymphadenopathy, rhinitis, pneumonia, myocarditis, and nephrosis. The placenta is enlarged, sometimes weighing as much as the fetus.

177. The answer is f. Transplacental transfer of hepatitis B from the mother to fetus occurs with acute hepatitis, not chronic seropositivity. Acute infection in first trimester infects 10% of fetuses, and in third trimester 80% to 90% are affected. Perinatal transmission occurs by ingestion of infected material during delivery or exposure subsequent to birth in mothers who are chronic carriers. Some infected infants may be asymptomatic, and others develop fulminant hepatic disease. Administration of hepatitis B immune globulin after birth, followed by the vaccine, can prevent disease in infants born to mothers who are chronic carriers.

178. The answer is d. Parvovirus can cause fetal anemia. Maternal infection can lead to fetal hydrops, abortion, or stillbirth. In susceptible adults, 20% to 30% will acquire disease during school outbreaks. If a pregnant woman has this diagnosis confirmed with IgM antibodies, ultrasound is done for fetal surveillance. If hydrops is diagnosed, fetal transfusion can be offered. One-third of fetuses will have spontaneous resolution of hydrops, and 85% of fetuses who receive transfusion will survive.

179. The answer is g. Neonatal herpes infection has three forms—disseminated with involvement of major organs; localized, with involvement confined to the central nervous system; and asymptomatic. A 50% risk of neonatal infection occurs with primary maternal infection, but only 4% to 5% risk with recurrent outbreaks. Postnatal infection can occur through contact with oral and skin lesions. Neonatal infection presentation is nonspecific, with signs and symptoms such as irritability, lethargy, fever, and poor feeding. Less than 50% of infants do not have skin lesions.

180. The answer is i. Early onset group B Streptococcus disease occurs within 1 week of birth. Signs of the disease include respiratory distress, apnea, and shock. Late-onset disease usually occurs after 7 days and manifests as meningitis.

Suggested Readings

American College of Obstetricians and Gynecologists. *Cytomegalovirus, Parvovirus B19, Varicella Zoster, and Toxoplasmosis in Pregnancy.* Practice Bulletin Number 151. June 2015.

American College of Obstetricians and Gynecologists. *Gestational Diabetes Mellitus.* Practice Bulletin Number 137. August 2013.

American College of Obstetricians and Gynecologists. *Pregestational Diabetes Mellitus.* Practice Bulletin Number 60. March 2005, reaffirmed 2014.

American College of Obstetricians and Gynecologists. *Thromboembolism in Pregnancy.* Practice Bulletin Number 123. August 2011, reaffirmed 2014.

American College of Obstetricians and Gynecologists. *Thyroid Disease in Pregnancy.* Practice Bulletin Number 148. April 2015.

Cunningham FG, Leveno KJ, Bloom SL, et al. eds. Chapter 46: Pulmonary disorders; Chapter 47: Renal and urinary tract disorders; Chapter 48: Gastrointestinal disorders; Chapter 49: Hematological disorders; Chapter 54: Dermatological disorders; Chapter 56: Infections; Chapter 57: Sexually transmitted diseases. *Williams Obstetrics.* 23rd ed. New York, NY: McGraw-Hill; 2010.

Normal and Abnormal Labor and Delivery

Questions

Questions 181 to 185

For each description of labor, select the most appropriate next step in management. Each option may be used once, more than once, or not at all.

a. Initiate Pitocin augmentation
b. Place an intrauterine pressure catheter (IUPC)
c. Perform a cesarean delivery
d. Place a fetal scalp electrode
e. No intervention; labor is progressing normally
f. Perform amniotomy

181. A 20-year-old G1 at 38 weeks' gestation presents with regular painful contractions every 3 to 4 minutes lasting 60 seconds. On pelvic examination, she is 3-cm dilated and 90% effaced; an amniotomy is performed and clear fluid is noted. The patient receives epidural analgesia for pain management. The fetal heart rate (FHR) tracing is reactive. One hour later on repeat examination, her cervix is 5-cm dilated and 100% effaced.

182. A 30-year-old G2P0 at 39 weeks is admitted in labor with spontaneous rupture of membranes occurring 2 hours prior to admission and regular uterine contractions. On examination, her cervix is 4-cm dilated and completely effaced. The fetal head is at 0 station and the fetal heart tracing is reactive. Two hours later, on repeat examination, her cervix is 5-cm dilated and the fetal head is at +1 station. Early decelerations are noted on the fetal heart tracing.

183. You are following a 38-year-old G2P1 at 39 weeks in labor. She has had one prior vaginal delivery of a 3800-g infant. One week ago, the estimated fetal weight was 3200 g by ultrasound. Over the past 3 hours her cervical examination remains unchanged at 6 cm. The FHR tracing is reactive. An IUPC reveals two contractions in 10 minutes with amplitude of 40 mm Hg each.

184. You are following a 22-year-old G2P1 at 39 weeks in labor. At 4-cm dilated she is given an epidural for pain management. Three hours later, her cervical examination is unchanged. Her contractions are now every 2 to 3 minutes, lasting 60 seconds. The FHR tracing is 120 beats per minute with accelerations and early decelerations.

185. A 25-year-old G3P2 at 39 weeks is admitted in labor at 5-cm dilated. The fetal heart tracing is reactive. Two hours later, she is reexamined and her cervix is unchanged at 5-cm dilated. An IUPC is placed and the patient is noted to have 280 Montevideo units (MVUs) by the IUPC. After an additional 2 hours of labor, the patient is noted to still be 5-cm dilated. The FHR tracing remains reactive.

186. A 27-year-old G2P1 at 38 weeks' gestation is admitted in active labor. She has had one prior uncomplicated vaginal delivery and has no medical problems. She reports an allergy to penicillin, and says she had a rash. Her vital signs are normal, and the fetal heart tracing is category I. Her prenatal record indicates that her group B Streptococcus (GBS) culture at 36 weeks was positive. What is the best choice for antibiotic prophylaxis during labor?

a. Cefazolin
b. Clindamycin
c. Erythromycin
d. Desensitization then treatment with penicillin
e. Vancomycin

187. A 38-year-old G6P4 undergoes a primary cesarean delivery under regional analgesia for malpresentation of twins at 37 weeks. Immediately after the delivery of the placenta, the anesthesiologist notes maternal seizure activity with profound hypoxia and hypotension. The patient is intubated and provided with circulatory support with vasopressors. Massive hemorrhage from the surgical site ensues, and the patient is given uterotonic agents and blood products. What is the most likely cause of her hemorrhage?

a. Amniotic fluid embolism
b. Halogenated anesthetic agent
c. Placenta accreta
d. Severe preeclampsia with HELLP syndrome
e. Uterine atony from overdistended uterus

188. A 23-year-old G1 at 38 weeks' gestation presents in active labor at 6-cm dilated with ruptured membranes. On cervical examination the fetal nose, eyes, and lips can be palpated. The fetal heart tracing is 140 beats per minute with accelerations and no decelerations. Which of the following is the most appropriate next step in management for this patient?

a. Perform immediate cesarean delivery
b. Allow spontaneous labor with vaginal delivery
c. Perform forceps rotation in the second stage of labor to convert mentum posterior to mentum anterior and to allow vaginal delivery
d. Allow the patient to labor spontaneously until complete cervical dilation is achieved and then perform an internal podalic version with breech extraction
e. Attempt manual conversion of the face to vertex in the second stage of labor

189. A 32-year-old G3P2 at 39 weeks' gestation presented to labor delivery with ruptured membranes. On examination, she was contracting regularly, and her cervix was 4-cm dilated. Her history was significant for two prior vaginal deliveries, with her largest child weighing 3800 g. Over the next 2 hours she progressed to 7-cm dilation. Four hours later, she remained 7-cm dilated. She had regular contractions and IUPC showed MVUs of 220. The estimated fetal weight by ultrasound was 3200 g. Which of the following labor abnormalities best describes this patient?

a. Prolonged latent phase
b. Protracted active phase
c. Hypertonic dysfunction
d. Secondary arrest of dilation
e. Second stage arrest

190. A 29-year-old P0 at 41 weeks' gestation presents in labor. At the time of delivery, a shoulder dystocia is encountered. An episiotomy is cut to assist with dystocia maneuvers. Compared with a midline episiotomy, which of the following is an advantage of mediolateral episiotomy?

a. Ease of repair
b. Fewer breakdowns
c. Less blood loss
d. Lower incidence of dyspareunia
e. Less chance of extension of the incision

Questions 191 to 193

For each clinical description, select the most appropriate procedure. Each lettered option may be used once, more than once, or not at all.

a. External cephalic version
b. Internal podalic version
c. Low transverse cesarean
d. Classical cesarean

191. A 24-year-old P0 at 25 weeks' gestation presents in active preterm labor in breech presentation. She changes from 4 cm to 6 cm dilation and is contracting regularly.

192. A 34-year-old P2002 with no prenatal care presents in labor. She is completely dilated and effaced. She progresses within minutes to vaginal delivery of a 2500 g infant. Because the uterus still feels large, you do a vaginal examination. A second set of membranes is bulging through a fully dilated cervix, and you feel a small part presenting in the sac. A fetal heart is auscultated at 60 beats per minute.

193. A 24-year-old woman (G3P2) is at 37 weeks' gestation. The fetal presentation is a transverse lie by ultrasound.

Questions 194 to 196

Select the most appropriate diagnosis for each clinical situation described. Each lettered option may be used once, more than once, or not at all.

a. First stage arrest
b. Second stage arrest

c. Failed induction of labor
d. Protracted first stage
e. Protracted second stage

194. No progress in descent for 4 hours or more in nulliparous women with an epidural or 3 hours or more in multiparous women with an epidural.

195. No cervical change for 4 hours or more with adequate uterine contractions and 6 cm or greater dilation with membrane rupture, or 6 hours or more with inadequate contractions.

196. Failure to generate regular contractions and cervical change after at least 24 hours of oxytocin, and with amniotomy if feasible.

Questions 197 to 200

Match each description with the most appropriate type of obstetric anesthesia. Each lettered option may be used once, more than once, or not at all.

a. Intravenous meperidine
b. Pudendal block
c. Spinal analgesia
d. Epidural analgesia

197. Appears to lengthen the second stage of labor

198. Is associated with fetal sedation

199. May be complicated by profound hypotension

200. May be associated with increased need for augmentation of labor with oxytocin and for instrument-assisted delivery

201. A 23-year-old G1 at 39 weeks' gestation presents to triage with a chief complaint of uterine contractions. They began 2 hours ago, are painful, and occur every 4 to 8 minutes. She reports good fetal movement, and no bleeding or leaking fluid. The external tocometer shows contractions every 5 to 15 minutes. The fetal monitor shows a category 1 tracing. On examination, her cervix is 1-cm dilated, 60% effaced, and the fetal vertex is at −1 station. The patient had the same cervical examination in your office last week. What is the most appropriate next step in management?

a. Send her home
b. Admit her for an epidural for pain control
c. Perform an amniotomy
d. Administer terbutaline
e. Augment her labor with Pitocin

202. A 19-year-old P0 at 41 weeks presents in spontaneous labor. Her membranes rupture spontaneously after she is admitted to labor and delivery, demonstrating meconium-stained amniotic fluid. What is the best management strategy for this patient and fetus at the time of delivery?

a. No special measures need to be taken, and this infant can be managed per the normal routine.
b. The obstetrician should suction the oropharynx and nasopharynx on the perineum after delivery of the head but before the delivery of the shoulders (intrapartum suctioning).
c. A pediatrician should be called to the delivery in order to perform intubation of the neonate.
d. A pediatrician should be called to perform routine tracheal suctioning.
e. A pediatrician should be called, and if the newborn is depressed, they should intubate the trachea and suction meconium or other aspirated material from beneath the glottis.

203. A 38-year-old G3P2 at 40 weeks' gestation presents to labor and delivery with gross rupture of membranes occurring 1 hour prior to arrival. The patient is having contraction every 3 to 4 minutes on the external tocometer, and each contraction lasts 60 seconds. The FHR tracing is 120 beats per minute with accelerations and no decelerations. The patient has a history of rapid vaginal deliveries, and her largest baby was 3200 g. On cervical examination she is 5-cm dilated and completely effaced, with the vertex at −2 station. The estimated fetal weight is 3300 g. The patient is in a lot of pain and requesting medication. Which of the following is the most appropriate method of pain control for this patient?

a. Intramuscular meperidine
b. Pudendal block
c. Perineal block
d. Epidural analgesia
e. General anesthesia

Questions 204 and 205

A 35-year-old G2P1 at 39 weeks' gestation presents to labor and delivery in active labor. Her cervix is 5-cm dilated and 80% effaced, and the vertex is at 0 station. The tocometer shows that she is having contractions every 3 minutes. The fetal heart tracing shows a baseline rate of 140 beats per minute, moderate variability, with accelerations and no decelerations.

204. This FHR tracing may best be interpreted as which of the following?

a. Category I
b. Category II
c. Category III
d. Category IV
e. Category V

205. One hour after she is admitted, her membranes rupture spontaneously. Shortly thereafter, she develops recurrent variable decelerations. What is the best next step in management?

a. Continue to monitor, as variable decelerations do not require intervention
b. Initiate an amnioinfusion
c. Since she is remote from delivery, perform a cesarean
d. Administer oxygen by nasal cannula
e. Administer terbutaline

206. A 29-year-old G2P1 at 40 weeks is in active labor. Her cervix is 5-cm dilated, completely effaced, and the vertex is at 0 station. She is on oxytocin to augment her labor, and she has just received an epidural for pain management. The nurse calls you to the room because the FHR has been in the 70s for the past 3 minutes. The contraction pattern is noted to be every 3 minutes, each lasting 60 seconds, with return to normal tone in between contractions. The patient's vital signs are: blood pressure 90/40 mm Hg, pulse 105 beats per minute, respiratory rate 18 breaths per minute, and temperature 36.1°C (97.6°F). On repeat cervical examination, the vertex is well applied to the cervix and the patient remains 5-cm dilated and at 0 station, and no vaginal bleeding is noted. Which of the following is the most likely cause for the deceleration?

a. Cord prolapse
b. Epidural analgesia
c. Pitocin
d. Placental abruption
e. Tachysystole

Questions 207 and 208

You are delivering a 26-year-old G3P2002 at 40 weeks' gestation. She has a history of two previous uncomplicated vaginal deliveries, and has had no problems during this pregnancy. After 15 minutes of pushing, the baby's head delivers spontaneously, but then retracts back against the perineum. As you apply gentle downward traction to the head, the baby's anterior shoulder fails to deliver.

207. Which of the following is the best next step in the management of this patient?

a. Call for help
b. Cut a symphysiotomy
c. Instruct the nurse to apply fundal pressure
d. Perform a Zavanelli maneuver
e. Push the baby's head back into the pelvis

208. After performing the appropriate maneuvers, the baby finally delivers. The pediatricians note that the right arm is hanging limply to the baby's side with the forearm extended and internally rotated. Which of the following is the baby's most likely diagnosis?

a. Erb palsy
b. Klumpke paralysis
c. Humeral fracture
d. Clavicular fracture
e. Paralysis from intraventricular bleed

209. A 41-year-old G1P0 at 39 weeks, who has been completely dilated and pushing for 4 hours, has an epidural in place and remains undelivered. She is exhausted and crying and tells you that she can no longer push. Her temperature is 38.3°C (101°F). The FHR is in the 190s with decreased variability. The patient's membranes have been ruptured for over 24 hours, and she has been receiving intravenous penicillin for a history of colonization with group B streptococcus. The fetal head is in the direct OA position and is visible at the introitus between pushes. Extensive caput is noted, but the fetal bones are at the +3 station. Which of the following is the most appropriate next step in the management of this patient?

a. Perform a cesarean delivery
b. Encourage the patient to continue to push after a short rest
c. Attempt operative vaginal delivery
d. Rebolus the patient's epidural
e. Cut an episiotomy

210. A 28-year-old G1 at 38 weeks had a normal progression of her labor. She has an epidural and has been pushing for 2 hours. The fetal head is direct occiput anterior at +3 station. The FHR tracing is 150 beats per minute with recurrent variable decelerations. With the patient's last push, the FHR had a prolonged deceleration to the 80s for 3 minutes. You recommend operative vaginal delivery due to the nonreassuring FHR tracing. Compared to the use of the vacuum extractor, forceps are associated with an increased risk of which of the following neonatal complications?

a. Cephalohematoma
b. Retinal hemorrhage
c. Jaundice
d. Intracranial hemorrhage
e. Corneal abrasions

211. You performed a forceps-assisted vaginal delivery on a 20-year-old G1 at 40 weeks for maternal exhaustion. The patient had pushed for 3.5 hours with an epidural for pain management. A second-degree episiotomy was cut to facilitate delivery. Eight hours after delivery, you are called to see the patient because she is unable to void and complains of severe pain. On examination you note a large fluctuant purple mass inside the vagina. What is the best management for this patient?

a. Apply an ice pack to the perineum
b. Embolize the internal iliac artery
c. Incise and evacuate the hematoma
d. Perform dilation and curettage to remove retained placenta
e. Place a vaginal pack for 24 hours

212. A 20-year-old G1 at 41 weeks has been pushing for 2½ hours. The fetal head is at the introitus and beginning to crown. It is necessary to cut an episiotomy. The tear extends through the sphincter of the rectum, but the rectal mucosa is intact. How should you classify this type of episiotomy?

a. First-degree
b. Second-degree
c. Third-degree
d. Fourth-degree
e. Mediolateral episiotomy

213. A 16-year-old G1P0 at 38 weeks' gestation presents to labor and delivery for the second time during the same weekend that you are on call. She initially presented at 2:00 PM Saturday afternoon complaining of regular uterine contractions. Her cervix was 1-cm dilated, 50% effaced with the vertex at −1 station, and she was sent home after walking for 2 hours in the hospital without any cervical change. It is now Sunday night at 8:00 PM, and the patient returns to labor and delivery with increasing pain. She is exhausted because she did not sleep the night before because her contractions kept waking her up. The patient is placed on the external fetal monitor. Her contractions are occurring every 2 to 3 minutes. You reexamine the patient and determine that her cervix is unchanged. Which of the following is the best next step in the management of this patient?

a. Perform artificial rupture of membranes to initiate labor
b. Administer an epidural
c. Administer Pitocin to augment labor
d. Achieve cervical ripening with prostaglandin gel
e. Administer 10 mg intramuscular morphine

Questions 214 and 215

A 25-year-old G1P0 patient at 37 weeks presents to labor and delivery reporting gross rupture of membranes and painful uterine contractions. The tocometer shows contractions every 2 to 3 minutes, and the fetal heart tracing is category I. On cervical examination, she is 4-cm dilated and completely effaced with the presenting part at −3 station. The presenting part is soft and felt to be the fetal buttock. A bedside ultrasound reveals a breech presentation with both hips flexed and knees extended. The estimated weight of the fetus is approximately 6 lb.

214. Which of the following is the best method to achieve delivery?
a. Deliver the fetus vaginally by breech extraction
b. Deliver the baby vaginally after external cephalic version
c. Perform an emergent cesarean delivery
d. Perform an internal podalic version
e. Perform a forceps-assisted vaginal breech delivery

215. What type of breech presentation is described?
a. Frank
b. Incomplete, single footling
c. Complete
d. Double footling

Normal and Abnormal Labor and Delivery

Answers

181. The answer is e. Patient has normal labor; no intervention is needed at this time.

182. The answer is a. The patient has a protracted active phase of labor (cervical dilation < 1.2 cm/h). Either expectant management or Pitocin augmentation may be used for treatment.

183. The answer is a. The best evidence available indicates that this labor is hypotonic and that the contractions are inadequate. Two contractions of 40 mm Hg intensity during a 10-minute period equates to 80 MVUs. About 200 MVUs are needed to consider contractions to be adequate to affect delivery. Since the ultrasound indicates a fetus without obvious abnormalities and smaller than her first infant, we assume the absence of cephalopelvic disproportion (CPD). Oxytocin is the treatment of choice in this situation.

184. The answer is b. Arrest of labor cannot be diagnosed during the first stage of labor until the cervix has reached 4-cm dilation and until adequate uterine contractions (both in frequency and intensity) have been documented. The actual pressure within the uterus cannot be measured via an external tocodynamometer; an IUPC needs to be placed. It is generally accepted that 200 MVUs (number of contractions in 10 minutes × average contraction intensity in mm Hg) are required for normal labor progress.

185. The answer is c. The patient is having adequate uterine contractions as determined by the IUPC. Therefore, augmentation with Pitocin is not indicated. The patient's diagnosis is secondary arrest of labor, which requires cesarean delivery. In the active phase of labor, a multiparous patient should undergo dilation of the cervix at a rate of at least 1.5 cm/h if uterine contractions are adequate.

186. The answer is a. GBS is an important cause of perinatal morbidity and mortality. Implementation of national guidelines for intrapartum antibiotic prophylaxis since the 1990s has resulted in an 80% reduction in the incidence of early onset neonatal sepsis due to GBS. The Gram-positive organism can colonize the lower gastrointestinal tract, and secondary spread to the genitourinary tract is common. Between 10% and 30% of pregnant women are colonized with GBS in the vagina or rectum. Universal prenatal screening is recommended between 35 and 37 weeks. Penicillin G (5 million units IV initially, then 2.5-3 million units/4 hours until delivery) remains the agent of choice for intrapartum prophylaxis, although ampicillin is an acceptable alternative. Data show that GBS isolates are increasingly resistant to second-line therapies. Up to 32% of isolates are resistant to erythromycin, and therefore, this is no longer recommended. Clindamycin is only recommended if the isolate is susceptible to both clindamycin and erythromycin. A patient with a penicillin or cephalosporin allergy should be asked about her specific symptoms. If she has had anaphylaxis, angioedema, respiratory distress, or urticarial, she should receive vancomycin 1g IV every 12 hours until delivery or clindamycin as described earlier. If she has not had these symptoms, and perhaps just had a mild rash, she should receive cefazolin 2 g IV as an initial dose, then 1 g IV every 8 hours until delivery.

187. The answer is a. Amnionic fluid embolism is a complex disorder characterized by abrupt onset of maternal hypoxia, hypotension, and disseminated intravascular coagulopathy. Amnionic fluid enters the maternal circulation from a breach in the normal maternal-fetal physiological barriers. This typically happens with labor and delivery, and cesarean delivery offers ample opportunity. The typical clinical presentation is dramatic. Patients may gasp for air, develop seizures from hypoxia, and have cardiopulmonary collapse, followed by massive hemorrhage from consumptive coagulopathy. It unfortunately often results in death given the quickness of events. Immediate support with oxygenation through intubation and circulatory support and blood products is vital. Profound neurological impairment is common in survivors. While halogenated anesthetic agents and multiple gestations can cause uterine atony leading to hemorrhage and while placenta accreta can also be a cause of hemorrhage, these are not the culprits in this drastic presentation.

188. The answer is b. With face presentation, the fetal head is hyperextended so the occiput is in contact with the fetal back, and the chin (mentum) is presenting. In the event of a face presentation, successful vaginal delivery will occur the majority of the time with an adequate pelvis. Spontaneous internal rotation during labor is required to bring the chin to the anterior position, which allows the neck to pass beneath the pubis. Therefore, the patient is allowed to labor spontaneously; a cesarean delivery is employed for labor abnormality or for fetal distress. Manual conversion to vertex, forceps rotation, and internal version are not used to deliver the face presentation because of undue trauma to both the mother and the fetus.

189. The answer is d. The labor portrayed is characteristic of a secondary arrest of dilation. The woman has entered the active phase of labor, as she previously progressed from 4 cm to 7 cm in less than 2 hours and then remains 7 cm over an additional 4 hours. New criteria for first stage arrest include 6 cm or more dilation with membrane rupture and no cervical change for 4 or more hours with adequate contractions, or 6 or more hours with inadequate contractions. New data suggests that historical criteria defining normal labor progress (cervical change of 1.2 cm/h for nulliparous women and 1.5cm/h for multiparous women) are no longer valid.

190. The answer is e. Midline episiotomies are easier to repair, and have a lower incidence of surgical breakdown, involve less pain, and lower blood loss. However, the incidence of extensions of the incision to include the rectum is higher for midline episiotomies compared with mediolateral episiotomies. Mediolateral episiotomies lead to more pain, blood loss, and dyspareunia. Regardless of technique, attention to hemostasis and anatomic restoration is the key element of a technically appropriate repair.

191. The answer is d. Cesarean delivery is indicated in this extremely preterm breech fetus. At 25 weeks, the lower uterine segment is likely to be poorly developed, and therefore classical uterine incision is indicated.

192. The answer is b. Twins are typically diagnosed during pregnancy with the use of routine ultrasound. Therefore, it is rare these days to diagnose twins at the time of delivery.

Delivery of the second twin is probably the only remaining situation where internal podalic version is indicated. Some obstetricians might perform a cesarean delivery for a noncephalic second twin; however, in this case, fetal bradycardia dictates that immediate delivery be undertaken, and internal podalic version is the quickest procedure.

193. The answer is a. A transverse lie is undeliverable vaginally. At 37 weeks, one treatment option is to do nothing and hope that the lie will be longitudinal by the time labor commences. However, in order to try to increase the chance of cephalic presentation at the time of labor, the next best step is to offer the patient an external cephalic version. This maneuver should be done in the hospital, with monitoring of the fetal heart rate.

194 to 196. The answers are 194-b, 195-a, 196-c. The diagnosis of arrest and protraction disorders is based on deviation from norms that have recently been reevaluated by the American College of Obstetricians and Gynecologists, the Society for Maternal-Fetal Medicine, and the National Institute of Child Health and Human Development. For many years, Friedman curves were used to assess whether labor was progressing normally. However, more recent data indicates that labor in nulliparous women takes longer than expected based on Friedman curves, and that the active phase of labor does not start for most women until they are at least 6 cm dilated. This has changed how patients are managed in labor and has resulted in new definitions, which are the basis for these three questions.

197 to 200. The answers are 197-d, 198-a, 199-c, 200-d. Parenteral narcotics are commonly used for labor pain. Meperidine is the most common opioid used for labor pain relief. It has a depressant effect on the fetus and can cause neonatal sedation. Pudendal block may provide adequate temporary pain relief for outlet operative vaginal deliveries in women not using regional analgesia. The success of a pudendal block depends on a clear understanding of the anatomy of the pudendal nerve and its surroundings. Complications (intravascular injection, hematoma, infection or abscess) are quite rare. Single-shot spinal analgesia provides prompt and adequate relief for procedures of limited duration such as cesarean delivery, rapidly progressing labor, or postpartum tubal ligation. The long-acting local anesthetic (with or without an opioid agonist) is injected at the level of the L4 to L5 interspace. Because of the inability to extend the duration of action, single-shot spinal analgesia is of limited use for management of labor. Epidural analgesia provides the most effective form of pain relief for the first and second stages of labor and for delivery. A catheter is placed in the epidural space, allowing for continuous infusion of local anesthetic agents or narcotics. The advantage of this method is that it can be titrated over time, and can be used for cesarean deliveries or postpartum tubal ligations. The most common side effect of regional analgesia is hypotension, which occurs in 25% to 67% of women undergoing spinal analgesia. Epidurals appear to lengthen the second stage of labor, and are associated with both an increased need for augmentation of labor with oxytocin and for instrument-assisted delivery.

201. The answer is a. This patient is most likely experiencing false labor, or Braxton-Hicks contractions. False labor is characterized by contractions that are irregular in timing and duration, and do not result in any cervical dilation. The intensity of Braxton-Hicks contractions does not change, the discomfort is mainly felt in the lower abdomen, and the pain is usually relieved by sedation. In the case of true labor, the uterine contractions occur at regular intervals, tend to become increasingly more intense over time, and results in progressive dilation and effacement of the cervix. Sedation does not stop the discomfort. There are three stages of labor. The first stage of labor is the interval between the onset of labor and full cervical dilation. The first stage consists of a latent phase (with gradual cervical change), and an active phase (characterized by rapid cervical change). The second stage of labor begins with complete cervical dilation and ends with the delivery of the fetus. The third stage of labor is the time from delivery of the fetus to expulsion of the placenta. Since this patient is not in true labor, the best plan of management is to send her home and await spontaneous labor.

202. The answer is e. In 2006, the American Academy of Pediatrics and the American Heart Association published new guidelines on neonatal resuscitation, which the American College of Obstetricians and Gynecologists adopted as well. Infants with meconium-stained amniotic fluid should no longer receive routine intrapartum suctioning, which used to be the standard of care. Current evidence no longer supports this practice, because routine intrapartum suctioning has not been shown to prevent or alter the course of meconium aspiration syndrome. If the newborn is depressed, tracheal suctioning should be undertaken. Attempted intubation of a vigorous newborn may potentially result in more injuries to the vocal cords.

203. The answer is d. The most appropriate modality for pain control in this patient is administration of an epidural analgesia. An epidural block provides relief from the pain of uterine contractions and delivery. It is accomplished by injecting a local anesthetic agent into the epidural space at the level of the lumbar intervertebral space. An indwelling catheter can be left in place to provide continuous infusion of an anesthetic agent throughout labor and delivery via a volumetric pump. In this patient, intramuscular narcotics such as meperidine or morphine would not be preferred because these agents can cause respiratory depression in the newborn if delivery is imminent. A pudendal block involves local infiltration of the pudendal nerve, which provides anesthesia to the perineum for delivery but no pain relief for uterine contractions. A local perineal block refers to infusing a local anesthetic to the area of an episiotomy. The inhalation of anesthetic gases (general anesthesia) is reserved primarily for situations involving emergent cesarean deliveries and difficult deliveries. All anesthetic agents that depress the maternal CNS cross the placenta and affect the fetus. In addition, a major complication of general anesthesia is maternal aspiration, which can result in aspiration pneumonitis.

204. The answer is a. In 2008, a workshop sponsored by the American College of Obstetricians and Gynecologists, the National Institute of Child Health and Human Development, and the Society for Maternal-Fetal Medicine convened to update fetal heart tracing nomenclature and interpretation. A normal baseline FHR is 110 beats per minute to 160 beats per minute. Moderate (normal) variability is an amplitude range of 6 beats per minute to 25 beats per minute. An acceleration is an abrupt increase in the FHR, with onset to peak in less than 30 seconds. If an acceleration lasts 10 minutes or longer, it is a baseline change. The committee adopted a three-tiered FHR interpretation system. Category I tracings include: baseline FHR 110 beats per minute to 160 beats per minute, moderate variability, no decelerations, and either presence or absence of accelerations. A category II tracing includes all tracings not categorized as category I or III. These tracings require evaluation, increased surveillance, initiation of corrective measures where appropriate, and reevaluation. They may include tachycardia, minimal variability, absence of induced accelerations after fetal stimulation, or episodic decelerations. Category III tracings include either absent variability with recurrent late decelerations, recurrent variable decelerations, or bradycardia, or a sinusoidal pattern. Category III tracings are abnormal and indicate an increased risk for fetal academia. If unresolved, these tracings usually require prompt delivery.

205. The answer is b. Intermittent variable decelerations by definition occur with fewer than 50% of contractions. They are the most common FHR abnormality that occurs during labor, and typically do not require treatment. Recurrent variable decelerations by definition occur with greater than or equal to 50% of contractions and may be more indicative of impending fetal academia. Management of recurrent variables should include relieving umbilical cord compression. Changing the maternal position is a reasonable first step. Amnioinfusion has been shown to decrease both recurrent variables and the cesarean delivery rate. Terbutaline and oxygen are not indicated for treatment of recurrent variable decelerations.

206. The answer is b. A prolonged FHR deceleration is a decrease in the FHR that is 15 beats per minute or more, lasting 2 minutes or longer, but less than 10 minutes from onset to return to baseline. Epidural analgesia is a common cause of FHR decelerations because it can be associated with maternal hypotension and decreased placental perfusion. Therefore, maternal blood pressure should always be noted in cases of FHR decelerations. If maternal blood pressure is abnormally low, ephedrine can be given to correct the hypotension. Because an umbilical cord prolapse can be associated with decelerations, the patient should undergo a cervical examination to evaluate for a prolapsed cord. In addition, the Pitocin infusion should be discontinued to reduce uterine contraction frequency. The patient should be turned to the left lateral position to decrease uterine pressure on the great vessels and enhance uteroplacental flow. Supplemental oxygen should be given to the patient in an attempt to increase oxygen to the fetus. A cesarean delivery may be performed if the FHR does not respond to these resuscitative measures.

207. The answer is a. In this clinical scenario, a shoulder dystocia is encountered. A shoulder dystocia occurs when the fetal shoulders fail to spontaneously deliver secondary to impaction of the anterior shoulder against the pubic bone after delivery of the head has occurred. Shoulder dystocia is an obstetric emergency; the first step should always be to call for help when such a situation is encountered. An episiotomy may be necessary to allow the obstetrician to have adequate room to perform a number of manipulations to try to relieve the dystocia. Such maneuvers include the following—suprapubic pressure, McRoberts maneuver (flexing maternal legs upon the abdomen), Wood's corkscrew maneuver (rotating the posterior shoulder), Rubin maneuver (rotate accessible shoulder toward anterior surface of the chest), and delivery of the posterior shoulder (sweeping the posterior arm across the chest). There is no role for fundal pressure, because this action further impacts the shoulder against the pubic bone and makes the situation worse. A Zavanelli maneuver is replacement of the fetal head into the pelvis so that cesarean delivery can be performed. It should only be attempted when all other methods have failed. A symphysiotomy involves cutting the pubic symphysis and has a high morbidity for the mother.

208. The answer is a. Shoulder dystocias can be associated with significant fetal morbidity including brachial plexus injuries, clavicular fractures, and humeral fractures. Fractures of the clavicle and humerus usually heal rapidly and do not have any long-term orthopedic or neurologic consequences. Brachial plexus injury usually results from downward traction on the brachial plexus during delivery of the anterior shoulder. Injury to the brachial plexus may be localized to the upper or lower roots. In Erb palsy, the upper roots of the brachial plexus are injured (C5-C6), resulting in paralysis of the shoulder and arm muscles; the arm hangs limply to the side and is extended and internally rotated. In the case of Klumpke paralysis, the lower nerves of the brachial plexus are affected (C7-T1) and the hand is paralyzed.

209. The answer is c. Indications for an operative vaginal delivery with a vacuum extractor or forceps occur in situations where the fetal head is engaged, the cervix is completely dilated, and there is a prolonged second stage. It may also be indicated when there is suspicion of potential fetal compromise, or need to shorten the second stage for maternal benefit. In this clinical scenario, all of these indications for operative delivery apply. This patient has been pushing for 4 hours, which meets criteria for protracted second stage of labor in a nulliparous patient with an epidural, based on contemporary data. In addition, potential maternal and fetal compromise exists since the patient has the clinical picture of chorioamnionitis, and the FHR is nonreassuring. It is best to avoid cesarean delivery if possible, since it would take more time to achieve, and because the patient is infected.

210. The answer is e. Corneal abrasions and ocular trauma are more common with forceps versus the vacuum, unless the vacuum is inadvertently placed over the eye. Vacuum deliveries have a higher rate of neonatal cephalohematomas, scalp lacerations, retinal hemorrhages, intracranial hemorrhages, and jaundice.

211. The answer is c. The described mass is a vaginal hematoma. Following operative vaginal delivery, the symptoms of severe pain and urinary retention should lead to a vaginal examination to evaluate for a fluctuant mass consistent with hematoma. Small vulvar hematomas identified post-partum may be treated expectantly. If severe pain occurs, or if the hema-toma continues to expand, the best treatment is incision and evacuation of the blood clots, with ligation of the bleeding vessels if they can be identified. Often no sites of active bleeding are found, in which case the defect should be closed and the vagina packed for 12 to 24 hours. Laparotomy may be indicated if the hematoma extends into the broad ligament. Embolization of the vaginal branch of the internal pudendal artery, uterine artery, and internal pudendal artery can be performed if bleeding is intractable.

212. The answer is c. A first-degree tear involves the vaginal mucosa or perineal skin, but not the underlying tissue. In a second-degree laceration, the underlying subcutaneous tissue (the fascia and muscles of the perineal body) is also involved, but not the rectal sphincter or rectal mucosa. Third-degree lacerations involve the anal sphincter. A fourth-degree laceration involves a tear that extends into the rectal mucosa to expose the lumen of the rectum.

213. The answer is e. This patient is either experiencing prolonged latent labor or is in false labor. Friedman criteria for the normal progress in labor were established in the 1950s, and until recently, were used for assessment and management of labor. Friedman data indicated that the transition from the latent to the active phase of labor occurred around 4 cm of cervical dilation, and that active phase dilation should proceed at 1.2 cm per hour for nulliparous women, and 1.5 cm per hour for multiparous women. How-ever, contemporary data suggests that changes in obstetric and anesthesia practices have resulted in changes in typical labor, and therefore, criteria for labor progress have been reviewed and revised based on data from the Consortium for Safe Labor (CSL). This data showed that cervical change between 3 cm and 6 cm is much slower than originally thought, and that the active phase of labor is more likely to start around 6 cm dilation. Women who dilate at a rate less than 1 cm per hour before 6 cm are still likely to proceed to spontaneous vaginal delivery. Data needed to establish the nor-mal range for the duration of labor in the latent phase are not readily avail-able because the onset of the latent phase in most women occurs outside the hospital and therefore cannot be accurately determined. One way to manage a protracted latent labor is to administer a strong sedative such as morphine along with intravenous fluids. This is sometimes referred to as "hydration and sedation." This is preferred over augmentation with Pitocin or performing an amniotomy, because 10% of patients will actually have been in false labor. Patients who are not truly in labor will usually stop contracting after administration of morphine and hydration with rest. If a patient truly is in labor, then, after the sedative wears off, she will have undergone cervical change and will have benefited from the rest in terms of having additional energy to proceed with labor. An epidural would not be recommended because the patient may not truly be in labor. There is no role for cervical ripening in this patient, because if she is not in labor, she can go home and wait for natural cervical ripening and spontaneous labor.

214 and 215. **The answers are 214-c, 215-a.** The patient described here has a fetus in frank breech presentation, which occurs when both hips are flexed and both knees are extended so that the feet lie in close proximity to the head and the fetal buttocks is the presenting part. With a complete breech presentation, both hips and knees are flexed. In the case of an incomplete breech presentation, one or both hips are not completely flexed; this may result in single footling or double footling presentations. Due to improved outcomes, it is generally recommended that fetuses with breech presentations undergo cesarean delivery. External cephalic version is a procedure whereby the presentation of the fetus is changed from breech to cephalic by manipulating the fetus externally through the abdominal wall. It is not indicated in this patient because the membranes are ruptured and the risk of cord prolapse is great. In addition, this procedure generally requires that the uterus be soft and relaxed, which is not the case with this patient in labor. Internal podalic version is a procedure used in the delivery of a second twin. It involves turning the fetus by inserting a hand into the uterus, grabbing both feet, and delivering the fetus by breech extraction.

Suggested Readings

American College of Obstetricians and Gynecologists. *Management of Delivery of a Newborn with Meconium-Stained Amniotic Fluid.* Committee Opinion Number 379. September 2007, reaffirmed 2013.
American College of Obstetricians and Gynecologists. *Management of Intrapartum Fetal Heart Rate Tracings.* Practice Bulletin Number 116. November 2010, reaffirmed 2015.

American College of Obstetricians and Gynecologists. *Obstetric Analgesia and Anesthesia.* Practice Bulletin Number 36. July 2002, reaffirmed 2013.

American College of Obstetricians and Gynecologists. *Prevention of Early-Onset Group B Streptococcal Disease in Newborns.* Committee Opinion Number 485. April 2011, reaffirmed 2013.

Cunningham FG, Leveno KJ, Bloom SL, et al. eds. Chapter 13: Conduct of normal labor and delivery, Chapter 14: Intrapartum assessment; Chapter 18: Dystocia: abnormal labor and fetopelvic disproportion; Chapter 19: Dystocia; Chapter 21: Forceps delivery and vacuum extraction; Chapter 25: Obstetrical hemorrhage. *Williams Obstetrics.* 23rd ed. New York, NY: McGraw-Hill; 2010.

Spong CY, Berghella V, Wenstrom KD, Mercer BM, Saade GR. Preventing the first cesarean delivery: summary of a joint Eunice Kennedy Shriver National Institute of Child Health and Human Development, Society for Maternal-Fetal Medicine, and American College of Obstetricians and Gynecologists Workship. *Obstet Gynecol.* 2012;120(5):1181.

Zhang J, Landy JH, Branch DW, et al. Contemporary patterns of spontaneous labor with normal neonatal outcomes. *Obstet Gynecol.* 2010;116(6):1281.

The Puerperium, Lactation, and Immediate Care of the Newborn

Questions

216. A 34-year-old G3P2 delivers a baby by spontaneous vaginal delivery. She had scant prenatal care and no ultrasound, so she is anxious to know the sex of the baby. At first glance you notice female genitalia, but on closer examination the genitalia are ambiguous. Which of the following is the best next step in the evaluation of this neonate?

a. Chromosomal analysis
b. Evaluation at 1 month of age
c. Pelvic ultrasound
d. Thorough physical examination
e. Laparotomy for gonadectomy

217. A 24-year-old primigravid woman, who plans to breastfeed, decides to have a home delivery. Immediately after the birth of a 4.1-kg (9-lb) newborn, the patient experiences massive hemorrhage from extensive vaginal and cervical lacerations. She is brought to the nearest hospital in shock. Over the course of 2 hours, nine units of blood are transfused, and the patient's blood pressure returns to a reasonable level. A hemoglobin value the next day is 7.5 g/dL, and three more units of packed red blood cells are given. The most likely late sequela to consider in this woman is which of the following?

a. Hemochromatosis
b. Stein-Leventhal syndrome
c. Sheehan syndrome
d. Simmonds' syndrome
e. Cushing syndrome

218. A 27-year-old G4P3 at 37 weeks presents to labor and delivery with heavy vaginal bleeding and painful uterine contractions. A bedside ultrasound demonstrates a fundal placenta. The patient's vital signs are: blood pressure 140/92 mm Hg, pulse 118 beats per minute, respiratory rate 20 breaths per minute, and temperature 37°C (98.6°F). The fetal heart rate tracing reveals tachycardia with decreased variability and intermittent late decelerations. She is taken to the OR for an emergency cesarean, and delivers a male infant with Apgar scores of 4 and 9. When the placenta is delivered, a large retroplacental clot is noted. The patient becomes hypotensive, and bleeding is noted from the wound edges and her IV catheter sites. Which of the following blood products will most quickly resolve her cause of hemorrhage?

a. Cryoprecipitate
b. Fresh frozen plasma (FFP)
c. Packed red blood cells
d. Platelets
e. Recombinant factor VII

Questions 219 to 222

A 30-year-old G5P3 has undergone a repeat cesarean delivery. She wants to breastfeed. Her past medical history is significant for hepatitis B infection, hypothyroidism, depression, and breast reduction. She is receiving intravenous antibiotics for endometritis. The baby latches on appropriately and begins to suckle.

219. In the mother, which of the following is a response to newborn suckling?

a. Decrease of oxytocin
b. Increase of prolactin-inhibiting factor (PIF)
c. Increase of hypothalamic dopamine
d. Increase of hypothalamic prolactin
e. Increase of luteinizing hormone—releasing factor

220. Which of the following aspects of her history might prevent this patient from breastfeeding?

a. Maternal reduction mammoplasty with transplantation of the nipples
b. Maternal treatment with ampicillin
c. Maternal treatment with fluoxetine
d. Maternal treatment with levothyroxine
e. Past hepatitis B infection

221. The patient asks you about the pros and cons of breastfeeding. Which of the following is an accurate statement regarding breastfeeding?

a. Breastfeeding decreases the time to return of normal menstrual cycles.
b. Breastfeeding is associated with a decreased incidence of sudden infant death syndrome.
c. Breastfeeding is a poor source of nutrients for required infant growth.
d. Breastfeeding is associated with an increased incidence of childhood obesity.
e. Breastfeeding is associated with a decreased incidence of childhood attention deficit disorder.

222. The patient returns to see you in 6 weeks for a routine postpartum visit. She has been nursing her baby without any major problems, and wants to continue to do so for at least 9 months. She is ready to resume sexual activity and wants to know what her options are for contraception. She is a nonsmoker, and her only other medication is a prenatal vitamin. Which of the following methods may decrease her milk supply?

a. Intrauterine device (IUD)
b. Progestin only pill
c. Depo-Provera
d. Combination oral contraceptive
e. Condoms and spermicide

223. On postpartum day 2 after a vaginal delivery, a 32-year-old G2P2 develops acute shortness of breath and chest pain. Her vital signs are: blood pressure 120/80 mm Hg, pulse 130 beats per minute, respiratory rate 32 breaths per minute, and temperature 37.6°C (99.8°F). She has new onset of cough. She appears to be in mild distress. Lung examination reveals clear bases with no rales or rhonchi. The chest pain is reproducible with deep inspiration. Cardiac examination reveals tachycardia with 2/6 systolic ejection murmur. Pulse oximetry shows an oxygen saturation of 88% on room air, and oxygen supplementation is initiated. Which of the following is the best diagnostic tool to confirm the diagnosis?

a. Arterial blood gas
b. Chest x-ray
c. CT angiography
d. Lower extremity Dopplers
e. Ventilation-perfusion scan

224. A 26-year-old G1P1 is now postoperative day (POD) 6 after a low-transverse cesarean delivery for arrest of active phase. On POD 2, the patient developed a fever of 39°C (102.2°F) and was noted to have uterine tenderness and foul-smelling lochia. She was started on broad-spectrum antibiotic coverage for endometritis. The patient states she feels fine now and wants to go home, but continues to spike fevers each evening. Her lung, breast, and cardiac examinations are normal. Her abdomen is nontender with a firm, nontender uterus below the umbilicus. On pelvic examination, her uterus is appropriately enlarged, but nontender. The adnexa are non-tender without masses. Her lochia is normal. Her white blood cell count is 12 with a normal differential. Blood, sputum, and urine cultures are all negative for growth after 3 days. Her chest x-ray is negative. Which of the following statements accurately describes this patient's condition?

a. It usually involves both the iliofemoral and ovarian veins.
b. Antimicrobial therapy is usually ineffective.
c. Fever spikes are rare.
d. Heparin therapy is always needed for resolution of fever.
e. Vena caval thrombosis may accompany either ovarian or iliofemoral thrombophlebitis.

Questions 225 and 226

A 24-year-old who delivered her first baby 5 weeks ago calls your office and asks to speak to you. She states that she is feeling very overwhelmed and anxious about taking care of her newborn son. She feels she cannot do anything right, and feels sad throughout the day. She tells you that she cries on most days, and is having difficulty sleeping at night. She also states she doesn't feel like eating or doing any of her normal activities. She reports no suicidal or homicidal ideation.

225. Which of the following is the most likely diagnosis?

a. Postpartum depression
b. Maternity blues
c. Postpartum psychosis
d. Bipolar disorder
e. Postpartum blues

226. Which of the following accurately describes this patient's condition?

a. A history of depression is not a risk factor for developing postpartum depression.
b. Prenatal preventive intervention for patients at high risk for postpartum depression is best managed alone by a mental health professional.

c. Young, multiparous patients are at highest risk.

d. Postpartum depression is a self-limiting process that lasts for a maximum of 3 months.

e. Women should be screened for depression at least once during the perinatal period using a standard, validated assessment tool.

227. A 35-year-old G3P3 presents to your office 3 weeks after an uncomplicated vaginal delivery. She has been successfully breastfeeding. She reports chills and a fever up to 38.3°C (101°F) at home. She states that she feels like she has flu, but has not had any sick contacts. She has no medical problems, prior surgeries, or allergies to medications. On examination, she has a temperature of 38°C (100.4°F) and generally appears in no distress. Head, ear, throat, lung, cardiac, abdominal, and pelvic examinations are all normal. A triangular area of erythema and tenderness is noted in the upper outer quadrant of the left breast. No masses or axillary lymphadenopathy are noted. Which of the following is the best option for treatment of this patient?

a. Admission to the hospital for intravenous antibiotics

b. Bromocriptine to suppress breast milk production

c. Incision and drainage

d. Oral dicloxacillin for 10 to 14 days

e. Oral erythromycin for 7 to 10 days

228. A 22-year-old G1 at 34 weeks is tested for tuberculosis because her father, with whom she lives, was recently diagnosed with tuberculosis. Her skin test is positive and her chest x-ray demonstrates a granuloma in the upper left lobe. Which of the following is true concerning infants born to mothers with active tuberculosis?

a. The risk of active disease during the first year of life may approach 90% without prophylaxis.

b. Bacille Calmette-Guérin (BCG) vaccination of the newborn infant without evidence of active disease is not appropriate.

c. Future ability for tuberculin skin testing is lost after BCG administration to the newborn.

d. Neonatal infection is most likely acquired by aspiration of infected amniotic fluid.

e. Congenital infection is common despite therapy.

229. A 23-year-old G2P1 develops chorioamnionitis during labor and is started on ampicillin and gentamicin. She requires a cesarean delivery for arrest of active phase labor. What is the most optimal way to reduce her chance of developing postoperative endometritis?

a. Add 2 g of cefazolin to her antibiotic regimen
b. Add clindamycin 900 mg IV to her antibiotic regimen
c. Continue her antibiotics for 1 week following delivery
d. She only needs to add a third antibiotic agent if she develops a fever postpartum
e. Add vancomycin 1 g IV to her antibiotic regimen

230. A 21-year-old G2P2 calls her physician 7 days postpartum because she is concerned that she is still experiencing vaginal bleeding. She describes the bleeding as light pink to bright red, and less heavy than the first few days postdelivery. She reports no fever or pain. On examination, she is afebrile and has an appropriately sized, nontender uterus. The vagina contains about 10 cc of old, dark blood. The cervix is closed. Which of the following is the most appropriate treatment?

a. Antibiotics for endometritis
b. High-dose oral estrogen for placental subinvolution
c. Oxytocin for uterine atony
d. Suction dilation and curettage for retained placenta
e. Reassurance

231. A 28-year-old G2P2 presents to the hospital 2 weeks after vaginal delivery with a chief complaint of sudden onset heavy vaginal bleeding that soaks a sanitary napkin every hour. Her pregnancy was complicated by preterm labor, and she delivered precipitously at 26 weeks' gestation. Her pulse is 89 beats per minute, blood pressure 120/76 mm Hg, and temperature 37.1°C (98.9°F). Her abdomen is nontender and her fundus is located above the symphysis pubis. On physical examination, you note active bleeding from the uterus, and you estimate a blood loss of 500 cc during the examination. Her uterus is about 12 to 14 weeks size and nontender. Her cervix is closed. An ultrasound reveals an irregularly thickened endometrial stripe. Her hemoglobin is 10.9 g/dL, unchanged from the one at her vaginal delivery. β-HCG is negative. Which of the following is the most appropriate treatment for the cause of her vaginal bleeding?

a. Methylergonovine maleate (methergine)
b. Oxytocin injection (Pitocin)
c. Ergonovine maleate (ergotrate)
d. Prostaglandins
e. Dilation and curettage

232. A 22-year-old G1P0 has just undergone a spontaneous vaginal delivery. As the placenta is being delivered, a red fleshy mass is noted to be protruding out from behind the placenta. Which of the following is the best next step in management of this patient?

a. Begin intravenous oxytocin infusion
b. Call for immediate assistance from other medical personnel
c. Continue to remove the placenta manually
d. Have the anesthesiologist administer magnesium sulfate
e. Push the placenta back into the uterus

Questions 233 to 235

Three days ago you delivered a 40-year-old G1P1 by cesarean following arrest of descent after 2 hours of pushing. Labor was also significant for prolonged rupture of membranes. The patient had an epidural, which was removed the day following delivery. The nurse calls you to come to see the patient on the postpartum floor because she has a fever of 38.8°C (102°F) and is experiencing shaking chills. Her blood pressure is 120/70 mm Hg and her pulse is 120 beats per minute. She has been eating a regular diet without difficulty and had a normal bowel movement this morning. She is attempting to breastfeed, but says her milk has not come in yet. On physical examination, her breasts are mildly engorged and tender bilaterally. Her lungs are clear. Her abdomen is tender over the fundus, but no rebound is present. Her incision has some serous drainage at the right apex, but no erythema is noted.

233. Which of the following is the most likely diagnosis?

a. Pelvic abscess
b. Septic pelvic thrombophlebitis (SPT)
c. Wound infection
d. Endometritis
e. Atelectasis

234. Which of the following is the most appropriate antibiotic to treat this patient with initially?

a. Oral bactrim
b. Oral dicloxacillin
c. Oral ciprofloxacin
d. Intravenous ampicillin
e. Intravenous gentamicin and clindamycin

235. After 48 hours of treatment, the patient remains febrile. What is the most appropriate next step in management?

a. Begin intravenous heparin
b. Add intravenous ampicillin to the current antibiotic regimen
c. Order a CT scan to evaluate her pelvis
d. Continue her current treatment for another 24 hours to see if the fever resolves
e. Discontinue her current antibiotic regimen, and begin intravenous vancomycin

236. A 22-year-old G1P1 is brought to the emergency department by EMS after having a seizure at home. She is 2 weeks' postpartum after an uncomplicated spontaneous vaginal delivery. She has no medical problems, and her pregnancy, labor, and immediate postpartum period were unremarkable. On arrival, her vitals were: blood pressure 165/95 mm HG, pulse 82 beats per minute, respiratory rate 20 breaths per minute. What is the most appropriate next step in management?

a. Begin magnesium sulfate therapy
b. Request a neurology consult
c. Order a head CT
d. Start phenytoin therapy
e. Order a toxicology screen

237. You are doing postpartum rounds on a 23-year-old G1P1 who is postpartum day 2 after an uncomplicated vaginal delivery. As you walk into the room, you note that she is crying. She states she can't seem to help it. She says she does not feel sad or anxious. She has not been sleeping well because she is getting up every 2 to 3 hours to breastfeed her new baby. Her past medical history is unremarkable. Which of the following is the most appropriate treatment recommendation?

a. Time and reassurance, because this condition is self-limited
b. Referral to psychiatry for counseling and antidepressant therapy
c. Referral to psychiatry for admission to a psychiatry ward and therapy with Haldol
d. A sleep aid
e. Referral to a psychiatrist who can administer electroconvulsive therapy

Questions 238 and 239

A 20-year-old G1P1 is postpartum day 2 after an uncomplicated vaginal delivery of a 6-lb 10-oz baby boy. She is trying to decide whether to have you perform a circumcision on her newborn. The boy is in the well-baby nursery and is doing very well.

238. In counseling this patient, you tell her which of the following recommendations from the American Pediatric Association?

a. Circumcisions should be performed routinely because they decrease the incidence of male urinary tract infections.
b. Circumcisions should be performed routinely because they decrease the incidence of penile cancer.
c. Circumcisions should be performed routinely because they decrease the incidence of sexually transmitted diseases.
d. Circumcisions should not be performed routinely because of insufficient data regarding risks and benefits.
e. Circumcisions should not be performed routinely because it is a risky procedure and complications such as bleeding and infection are common.

239. The parents ask if you will use analgesia during the circumcision. What do you tell them regarding the recommendations for administering pain medicine for circumcisions?

a. Analgesia is not recommended because there is no evidence that newborns undergoing circumcision experience pain.
b. Analgesia is not recommended because it is unsafe in newborns.
c. Analgesia in the form of oral tylenol is the pain medicine of choice recommended for circumcisions.
d. Analgesia in the form of a penile block is recommended.
e. The administration of sugar orally during the procedure will keep the neonate preoccupied and happy.

240. A 33-year-old G1P0 was induced for being postterm at 42½ weeks' gestation. Immediately following the delivery, you examine the baby with the pediatricians and note the following on physical examination: a small amount of cartilage in the earlobe, occasional creases over the anterior two-thirds of the soles of the feet, 4-mm breast nodule diameter, fine and fuzzy scalp hair, and a scrotum with some but not extensive rugae. Based on this physical examination, what is the approximate gestational age of this male infant?

a. 28 weeks
b. 33 weeks
c. 36 weeks
d. 38 weeks
e. 42 weeks

241. A 40-year-old G4P5 at 39 weeks' gestation has progressed rapidly in labor with a reassuring fetal heart rate pattern. She has had an uncomplicated pregnancy with normal prenatal laboratory tests, including an amniocentesis for advanced maternal age. The patient begins the second stage of labor, and after 15 minutes of pushing, starts to demonstrate recurrent variable heart rate accelerations. You suspect that she may have a fetus with a nuchal cord. You expediently deliver the baby by low-outlet forceps, and hand the baby over to the neonatologists called to attend the delivery. As soon as the baby is handed off to the pediatric team, it lets out a strong spontaneous cry. The infant is pink with slightly blue extremities that are actively moving and kicking. The heart rate is noted to be 110 beats per minute on auscultation. What Apgar score should the pediatricians assign to this baby at 1 minute of life?

a. 10
b. 9
c. 8
d. 7
e. 6

242. A 32-year-old G2P1 at 41 weeks' gestation is undergoing an induction of labor for oligohydramnios. During the course of her labor, the fetal heart rate tracing demonstrates recurrent variable decelerations that do not respond to oxygen, intravenous fluid, or amnioinfusion. The patient's cervix is dilated to 4 cm. A low-transverse cesarean delivery is performed for a nonreassuring fetal heart tracing remote from delivery. After delivery of the fetus, you send a cord gas, which comes back with the following arterial blood values: pH 7.29, Pco_2 50 mm Hg, and Po_2 20 mm Hg. What condition does the cord blood gas indicate?

a. Normal fetal status
b. Fetal acidemia
c. Fetal hypoxia
d. Fetal asphyxia
e. Fetal metabolic acidosis

243. You are asked to assist in the well-born nursery with neonatal care. Which of the following is a part of routine care in a healthy infant?

a. Administration of ceftriaxone cream to the eyes for prophylaxis for gonorrhea and chlamydia
b. Administration of vitamin A to prevent bleeding problems
c. Administration of hepatitis B vaccination for routine immunization
d. Cool-water bath to remove vernix
e. Placement of a computer chip in left buttock for identification purposes

Questions 244 to 246

A 35-year-old G2P2 presents for her routine postpartum visit. Her pregnancy was complicated by gestational diabetes, which was diagnosed in the second trimester during routine screening. She has no other medical problems, and she has no family history of diabetes. She gained 25 pounds during her pregnancy, and her gestational diabetes was managed with diet modification.

244. She asks whether she is at an increased risk for diabetes later in life. How should you counsel her?

a. She is not at an increased risk for development of diabetes.
b. She has an increased risk of type 1 diabetes later in life.
c. She has an increased risk of type 2 diabetes later in life.
d. If she loses all of the weight she gained during her pregnancy, she will not be at an increased risk for development of diabetes later in life.
e. She has an increased risk of diabetes only if she has a family history of diabetes in a first degree relative.

245. The patient asks if the fact that she had gestational diabetes might have any long-term effects on her baby. How should you counsel her?

a. Offspring of mothers with gestational diabetes are at an increased risk for obesity later in life.
b. Her baby has an increased risk of developing type 1 diabetes.
c. As long as her baby maintains a normal weight during childhood and adolescence, there is no increased risk for development of diabetes later in life.
d. Her baby has an increased risk of neurodevelopmental complications.
e. Offspring of mothers with gestational diabetes do not have any increased risks compared to offspring of mothers without gestational diabetes.

246. How should this patient be managed postpartum?

a. She should have a fasting glucose on postpartum day 1, and if normal, no other evaluation is needed.
b. She should have a glucose tolerance test performed on postpartum day 1.
c. She should have a glucose tolerance test performed 6 to 12 weeks' postpartum.
d. She should be referred back to her primary care provider for further evaluation.
e. She does not need any further evaluation.

247. A 30-year-old G3P3, who is 8 weeks' postpartum and regularly breastfeeding calls you and is very concerned because she is having pain with intercourse secondary to vaginal dryness. Which of the following should you recommend to help her with this problem?

a. Instruct her to stop breastfeeding
b. Apply hydrocortisone cream to the perineum
c. Apply testosterone cream to the vulva and vagina
d. Apply estrogen cream to the vagina and vulva
e. Apply petroleum jelly to the perineum

248. A 34-year-old G1P1 comes to see you 6 weeks after an uncomplicated vaginal delivery for a routine postpartum examination. She reports no problems, and has been breastfeeding her newborn without any difficulties since leaving the hospital. During the bimanual examination, you note that her uterus is irregular, firm, nontender, and about a 15-week size. Which of the following is the most likely etiology for this enlarged uterus?

a. Subinvolution of the uterus
b. The uterus is appropriate size for 6 weeks' postpartum
c. Fibroid uterus
d. Adenomyosis
e. Endometritis

Questions 249 and 250

A 39-year-old G3P3 comes to see you on day 5 after a repeat cesarean delivery. During the surgery she received two units of packed red blood cells for a hemorrhage related to uterine atony. Her past medical history is significant for type 2 diabetes mellitus and chronic hypertension. She weighs 110 kg. She is concerned because her incision has become very red and tender, and pus started draining from a small opening in the incision this morning. She has been experiencing general malaise and reports a fever of 38.8°C (102°F). Her vital signs are: temperature 37.8°C (100.1°F), pulse 69 beats per minute, respiratory rate 18 breaths per minute, and blood pressure is 143/92 mm Hg. Physical examination shows erythema around the incision, and a 1-cm defect at the left corner of the skin incision, which is draining a small amount of purulent liquid. There is tenderness along the wound edges.

249. Which of the following is the best next step in the management of this patient?
a. Apply Steri-Strips to close the wound
b. Administer local antibiotic ointment
c. Probe the fascia
d. Take the patient to the OR for debridement and closure of the skin
e. Reapproximate the wound edge under local analgesia

250. Which of the following is her greatest risk factor for her complication?
a. Anemia
b. Corticosteroid therapy
c. Diabetes
d. Hypertension
e. Obesity

The Puerperium, Lactation, and Immediate Care of the Newborn

Answers

216. The answer is d. Ambiguous genitalia at birth is a medical emergency, not only for psychological reasons for the parents, but also because hirsute female infants with congenital adrenal hyperplasia (CAH) may die if undiagnosed. CAH is an autosomally inherited disease of adrenal failure that causes hyponatremia and hyperkalemia due to lack of mineralo-corticoids. A thorough physical examination is the best initial evaluation. While it will not provide the definitive diagnosis of the gender, it can provide clues. Examination should include inspection and palpation of the genitalia, palpation for gonads in the inguinal canal or labioscrotal folds, evaluation for fused labia, evaluation for presence of a vagina or pouch, and assessment for other nongenital dysmorphic features. The newborn should also be quickly evaluated for presence of hyper- or hypotension, or signs of dehydration. Karyotype, electrolyte analysis, blood or urine assays for progesterone, 17α-hydroxyprogesterone, and serum androgens such as dehydroepiandrosterone sulfate are essential to the workup as well. Pelvic ultrasound or MRI can detect ovaries or undescended testes, but that is not the first step in management. Laparotomy or laparoscopy is sometimes necessary for ectopic gonadectomy after puberty has occurred.

217. The answer is c. A disadvantage of home delivery is the lack of facilities to control postpartum hemorrhage. The woman described in the question delivered a large baby, suffered multiple soft tissue injuries, and went into shock, needing nine units of blood by the time she reached the hospital. Sheehan syndrome seems a likely possibility in this woman. This syndrome of anterior pituitary necrosis related to obstetric hemorrhage can be diagnosed by 1-week postpartum, as lactation fails to commence normally. Other symptoms of Sheehan syndrome include amenorrhea, atrophy of the breasts, and loss of thyroid and adrenal function. The other presented choices for late sequelae are less likely. Hemochromatosis would not be expected to occur in this healthy young woman, especially since she did not receive prolonged transfusions. Cushing, Simmonds, and Stein-Leventhal syndromes are not known to be related to postpartum hemorrhage. It is important to note that home delivery is not a predisposing factor to postpartum hemorrhage.

218. The answer is b. This patient has a large placental abruption, which is the most common cause of consumptive coagulopathy in pregnancy. The bleeding described signifies that the patient has a significant coagulopathy with hypofibrinogenemia. Prompt and vigorous transfusion is needed. Packed red blood cells will restore blood volume and increase oxygen carrying capacity. FFP contains about 600 mg to 700 mg of fibrinogen and will promote clotting, and is the best choice to quickly resolve her cause of hemorrhage. Cryoprecipitate contains clotting factors and fibrinogen, but in a much lower amount (200 mg) than FFP, and has no advantage over the use of FFP in this bleeding patient. Recombinant factor VII can be used for the treatment of severe obstetrical hemorrhage but will not be effective if fibrinogen is low. Platelet transfusion is considered in bleeding patients with platelets less than 50,000.

219. The answer is d. The normal sequence of events triggered by suckling is as follows: through a response of the central nervous system, dopamine is decreased in the hypothalamus. Dopamine suppression decreases production of PIF, which normally travels through a portal system to the pituitary gland; because PIF production is decreased, production of prolactin by the pituitary is increased. At this time, the pituitary also releases oxytocin, which causes milk to be expressed from the alveoli into the lactiferous ducts. Suckling suppresses the production of luteinizing hormone—releasing factor and, as a result, acts as a mild (but not reliable) contraceptive (because the mid-cycle surge of luteinizing hormone does not occur).

220. The answer is a. There are very few contraindications to breastfeeding. Most medications taken by the mother enter into breast milk to some degree. Breastfeeding is inadvisable when the mother is being treated with antimitotic drugs, tetracyclines, diagnostic or therapeutic radioactive substances, or lithium carbonate. Acute puerperal mastitis may be managed quite successfully while the mother continues to breastfeed. Reduction mammoplasty with autotransplantation of the nipple makes breastfeeding impossible.

However, there are reduction mammoplasty techniques that do potentially allow for some amount of breastfeeding; this would be most likely in patients who underwent a surgery where the areola and nipple were not completely severed. Ampicillin or levothyroxine can be safely used by breastfeeding mothers. A past history of hepatitis B is not a contraindication to breastfeeding. With some acute viral infections such as hepatitis B, there is the possibility of transmitting the virus in milk.

221. The answer is b. According to the American Academy of Pediatrics, some of the benefits of nursing include a decrease in infant diarrhea, urinary tract infections, ear infections, and death from sudden infant death syndrome. Human milk is the ideal food for neonates. It provides species- and age-specific nutrients for the baby. It has immunological factors and antibacterial properties, and contains factors that act as biological signals to promote cellular growth. Breastfeeding can delay the resumption of ovulation and menses but should not be considered contraception.

222. The answer is d. The use of an IUD, barrier methods, and hormonal contraceptive agents containing only progestins are all appropriate methods of birth control for breastfeeding women. It is best for nursing mothers to avoid estrogen-containing contraceptives because estrogen preparations can inhibit lactation or decrease milk supply.

223. The answer is c. The patient most likely has a pulmonary embolism (PE). All three components of Virchow's triad are present during pregnancy and the postpartum period: venous stasis, endothelial injury, and a hypercoaguable state. The reported incidence of venous thromboembolism during pregnancy is 1 in 500 to 1 in 2000. PE is the seventh leading cause of maternal mortality, responsible for 9% of maternal deaths, and therefore, rapid diagnosis and treatment are critical. The classic triad—hemoptysis, pleuritic chest pain, and dyspnea—appears in only 20% of cases. The most common sign on physical examination is tachypnea (> 16 breaths/min). Ventilation-perfusion scans with large perfusion defects and ventilation mismatches support the putative diagnosis of PE, but this finding can also be seen with atelectasis or other disorders of lung aeration. Conversely, a normal ventilation-perfusion scan suggests that massive PE is not the etiology of the clinical symptoms. To confirm the diagnosis, a CT pulmonary angiography is the best diagnostic tool in this setting, and has high sensitivity and specificity for the diagnosis of PE. An arterial blood gas will confirm hypoxia, but not confirm PE as the cause. A chest x-ray could be done to rule out other causes such as pulmonary edema or pneumonia, but will not make the diagnosis of PE.

224. The answer is e. The patient described has SPT. SPT may involve the ovarian vein, or other deep pelvic veins. The clinical presentation is usually that of pain and fever; therefore, it is usually diagnosed as endometritis, and antibiotic therapy is started. Following antimicrobial therapy, clinical symptoms usually resolve, but fever spikes persist. Patients typically do not appear clinically ill between fevers. The diagnosis of ovarian vein thrombosis is made by computerized tomography (CT) or magnetic resonance imaging (MRI). Deep septic pelvic thrombophlebitis that does not involve the ovarian vein is usually a diagnosis of exclusion, and should be suspected in patients with persistent postpartum fever despite antibiotics, with normal imaging. The treatment of choice is anticoagulation. There are no studies documenting the optimal time for anticoagulation, but most institutions recommend 6 weeks.

225. The answer is a. This patient is exhibiting classic symptoms of postpartum depression. Postpartum depression develops in about 8% to 15% of women, and generally is characterized by an onset about 2 weeks to 12 months postdelivery, with an average duration of 3 to 14 months. Perinatal depression includes major and minor depressive episodes that occur during pregnancy or in the first 12 months after delivery, and is one of the most common medical complications during pregnancy or the postpartum period. It often goes unrecognized, because changes in sleep, appetite, and libido may be attributed to normal pregnancy and postpartum changes. Women with postpartum depression may display irritability, labile mood, difficulty sleeping, phobias, and anxiety. About 50% of women experience postpartum blues within 3 to 6 days after delivering. This mood disturbance is thought to be precipitated by progesterone withdrawal following delivery, and usually resolves in 10 to 14 days. Postpartum blues is characterized by mild insomnia, tearfulness, fatigue, irritability, poor concentration, and depressed effect. Postpartum psychosis usually has its onset within a few days of delivery and is characterized by confusion, disorientation, and loss of touch with reality. Postpartum psychosis is very rare and occurs in only 1 to 4 in 1000 births. Bipolar disorder or manic-depressive illness is a psychiatric disorder characterized by episodes of depression followed by mania.

226. The answer is e. Patients at high risk for postpartum depression often have a history of depression or postpartum depression. They are more likely to be primiparous or older; they may have had a long interval between pregnancies or an unplanned pregnancy or be without a supportive partner. Other risk factors include experiencing a stressful life event during pregnancy or early postpartum period, a traumatic birth experience, having a baby in the neonatal intensive care unit, or breastfeeding problems. ACOG recommends that all women be screened during the perinatal period with a validated, standardized assessment tool such as the Edinburgh Postnatal Depression Scale. Recent evidence suggests that collaborative care models improve long-term patient outcomes; this may involve medical therapy, social work, psychotherapy, and support under the supervision of a mental health specialist. Prenatal intervention must include the obstetric team, with family or peer support when possible. Postpartum depression is variable in duration, but occasionally will not resolve without intervention such as therapy, medication, or in rare cases, hospitalization.

227. The answer is d. Puerperal mastitis may be subacute, but is often characterized by chills, fever, and breast tenderness. If undiagnosed, it may progress to suppurative mastitis with abscess formation that requires drainage. The most common causative organism is *Staphylococcus aureus*, which is probably transmitted from the infant's nose and throat. Initial antibiotic therapy should be directed at this organism, and should consist of either dicloxacillin 500 mg orally four times a day, or cephalexin 500 mg orally four times a day, for a total of 10 to 14 days. In penicillin-allergic patients, clindamycin 300 mg orally three times a day is recommended. If a mass is palpable, an abscess should be suspected. Incision and drainage is recommended for a breast abscess. Milk production should not be suppressed, and the patient should continue to breastfeed or pump on the affected breast. Symptomatic relief with ibuprofen and ice packs may also be of benefit.

228. The answer is c. The goal of management in the infant born to a mother with active tuberculosis is prevention of early neonatal infection. Congenital infection, acquired either by a hematogenous route or by aspiration of infected amniotic fluid, is rare. Most neonatal infections are acquired by postpartum maternal contact. The risk of active disease during the first year of life may approach 50% if prophylaxis is not instituted. BCG vaccination and daily isonicotinic acid hydrazide (isoniazid, INH) therapy are both acceptable means of therapy. BCG vaccination may be easier because it requires only one injection; however, the ability to perform future tuberculin skin testing is lost.

229. The answer is b. Postpartum endometritis is much more common after cesarean delivery, and the infection is commonly polymicrobial. Fever is the most common criteria for the diagnosis. The addition of anaerobic coverage to the primary antibiotic regimen of ampicillin and gentamicin has reduced the rates of postcesarean endometritis. Ideally, this should be given preincision as part of antibiotic prophylaxis for cesarean delivery, and should consist of either clindamycin 900 mg IV or metronidazole 500 mg IV. There is not conclusive evidence regarding the optimal duration of therapy postpartum; however, based on limited studies, it is reasonable to continue antibiotics for one more postpartum dose following delivery.

230. The answer is e. The bleeding this patient describes is normal. Bloody lochia can persist for up to 2 weeks without indicating an underlying pathology; however, if heavy bleeding continues beyond 2 weeks, it may indicate placental site subinvolution, retention of small placental fragments, or both. At that point, appropriate diagnostic and therapeutic measures should be initiated. The physician should first estimate the blood loss and then perform a pelvic examination in search of uterine subinvolution or tenderness. Excessive bleeding or tenderness should lead the physician to suspect retained placental fragments or endometritis. A larger than expected but otherwise asymptomatic uterus supports the diagnosis of subinvolution.

231. The answer is e. Uterine hemorrhage after the first postpartum week is most often the result of retained placental fragments or subinvolution of the placental site. Risk factors for retained placenta include extreme prematurity, precipitous delivery, succenturiate lobe of the placenta, placenta accreta, and manual extraction of the placenta. Ultrasound can aid in the diagnosis, and when retained products of conception are present, the endometrial stripe may appear thickened and/or irregular. In some cases, if the cervix is open, this tissue may spontaneously expel. Surgery is required if the cervix is closed. The standard of treatment is dilation and curettage.

232. The answer is b. This patient has a uterine inversion. The most important first step is to summon assistance immediately, including an anesthesiologist. Next, discontinue any uterotonic agents, and ensure that the patient has adequate IV access and blood available if needed. The placenta should not be removed, as this may cause profound hemorrhage. Instead, attempts should be made to manually replace the inverted uterus into its normal position. Uterine relaxants such as nitroglycerine, terbutaline, or inhaled anesthetic agents may need to be given in order to aid attempts at manual replacement. Once the uterus is restored to its normal configuration, the placenta may be removed by waiting for spontaneous separation or by manual removal if indicated. After the placenta delivers, uterotonic agents should be given to enhance myometrial contraction and decrease the risk of uterine atony.

233. The answer is d. Endometritis, or infection of the uterus, is the most common infection that occurs after a cesarean delivery. A long labor and prolonged rupture of membranes are predisposing factors for endometritis. Other risk factors include chorioamnionitis, group b streptococcus colonization, manual removal of the placenta, and diabetes mellitus. In the presence of a pelvic abscess, usually signs of peritoneal irritation such as rebound tenderness, ileus, and decreased bowel sounds are present. Wound infections occur with an incidence of about 6% following cesarean deliveries. Fever usually begins on the fourth or fifth POD, and erythema around the incision along with purulent drainage is often present. Atelectasis can be a cause of postoperative fever, but the fever occurs generally in the first 24 hours. In addition, on physical examination, atelectasis is generally accompanied by decreased breath sounds at the lung bases on auscultation. It more commonly occurs in women who have had general anesthesia, not an epidural like the patient described here. SPT occurs uncommonly as a sequela of pelvic infection. Venous stasis occurs in dilated pelvic veins; in the presence of bacteria, it can lead to septic thromboses. Diagnosis is usually made when persistent fever spikes occur after treatment for endometritis. The patient usually has no uterine tenderness, and bowel function tends to be normal.

234. The answer is e. The etiology of endometritis, like that of all pelvic infections, is polymicrobial. Therefore, the antibiotic coverage selected should treat aerobic and anaerobic organisms. Common aerobes associated with metritis are staphylococci, streptococci, enterococci, *Escherichia coli, Proteus*, and *Klebsiella*. The anaerobic organisms associated with pelvic infections are most commonly *Bacteroides, Peptococcus, Peptostreptococcus*, and *Clostridium*. Generally, endometritis should be treated with intravenous broad-spectrum antibiotic coverage. Intravenous clindamycin (900 mg/8 h) plus gentamicin (1.5 mg/kg/8 h OR 5 mg/kg/24 h) is a commonly used effective therapy. The antibiotic therapy is generally continued until the patient has been afebrile for at least 24 hours. Oral therapy is not as effective as intravenous therapy, and is therefore not the most appropriate choice for treatment. Bactrim is a sulfa drug that is commonly given orally to treat uncomplicated urinary tract infections. Dicloxacillin is commonly used orally to treat women with mastitis because it has good coverage against *S aureus*, which is the most common organism responsible for this infection. Ciprofloxacin, a quinolone, is useful in the treatment of complicated urinary tract infections. This medication is not recommended for pregnant or lactating women because animal studies show an association of fluoroquinolones with cartilage damage and/or arthropathy.

235. The answer is b. Most patients should respond to intravenous antibiotic treatment for endometritis within 48 hours. If no improvement is noted, further investigation is warranted. Approximately 20% of treatment failures are due to resistant organisms such as enterococcus. Therefore, a reasonable next step in management is to add ampicillin to extend her antibiotic coverage. If she continues to remain febrile after adding ampicillin, it may be appropriate to evaluate for SPT ore pelvic abscess with CT or MRI.

236. The answer is a. This patient is most likely to have postpartum preeclampsia. This may present up to 6 weeks after delivery, and in greater than 50% of cases, follows a pregnancy and labor that were not complicated by hypertension. Although the differential diagnosis may include new onset seizure disorder, illicit drugs, and brain tumor, she is most likely to have postpartum preeclampsia, especially given her hypertension on arrival, and should be initially managed as such. The most appropriate first step is to begin magnesium therapy for seizure prophylaxis. The rest of the treatment is aimed at managing her blood pressure.

237. The answer is a. Women experiencing postpartum blues usually do fine with reassurance alone, because this condition usually resolves spontaneously in a short period of time. Women with postpartum depression may need a referral to a psychiatrist who can administer psychotherapy and prescribe antidepressants. Haldol is an antipsychotic that might be administered in the treatment of postpartum psychosis. Sleep aids are not recommended. Electroconvulsive therapy would be used to treat depression only if a patient were unresponsive to pharmacologic therapy.

238. The answer is d. According to the American Academy of Pediatrics, current evidence indicates that health benefits of newborn male circumcision outweigh the risks, and that the procedure's benefits justify access to this procedure for families who choose it. The American College of Obstetricians and Gynecologists has also adopted this statement. Specific health benefits include a decreased incidence of urinary tract infections, penile cancer, and some sexually transmitted infections, including HIV.

When performed by an experienced person on a healthy, stable infant, circumcisions are generally safe procedures, although potential complications include infection and bleeding. Although the health benefits are not great enough to recommend routine circumcision for all newborns, it is important for clinicians to counsel patients about the benefits and risks in an unbiased and accurate manner.

239. The answer is d. Analgesia should always be provided to a newborn undergoing a circumcision procedure, because much evidence suggests that infants who undergo this procedure without pain medicine experience pain and stress. The administration of oral tylenol or sucrose is not adequate for operative pain relief. Topical lidocaine cream, dorsal penile nerve block, and subcutaneous ring block are all effective and safe modalities to achieve analgesia in newborns undergoing a circumcision procedure.

240. The answer is d. An estimate of the gestational age of a newborn can be made rapidly by a physical examination immediately following delivery. Important physical characteristics that are evaluated are the sole creases, breast nodules, scalp hair, earlobes, and scrotum. In newborns who are 39 weeks' gestational age or greater, the soles of the feet will be covered with creases, the diameter of the breast nodules will be at least 7 mm, the scalp hair will be coarse and silky, the earlobes will be thickened with cartilage, and the scrotum will be full with extensive rugae. In infants that are 36 weeks or less, there will be an anterior transverse sole crease only, the breast nodule diameter will be 2 mm, the scalp hair will be fine and fuzzy, the earlobes will be pliable and lack cartilage, and the scrotum will be small with few rugae. In infants of gestational age between 37 and 38 weeks, the soles of the feet will have occasional creases on the anterior two-thirds of the feet, the breast nodule diameter will be 4 mm, the scalp hair will be fine and fuzzy, the earlobes will have a small amount of cartilage, and the scrotum will have some but not extensive rugae.

241. The answer is b. The Apgar scoring system, applied at 1 minute and again at 5 minutes, was developed as an aid to evaluate infants who require resuscitation. Heart rate, respiratory effort, muscle tone, reflex irritability, and color are the five components of the Apgar score. A score of 0, 1, or 2 is given for each of the five components, and the total is added up to give one score. The following table demonstrates the scoring system.

Table: APGAR score

Sign	0 Points	1 Point	2 Points
Heart rate	Absent	Below 100	More than 100
Respiratory effort	Absent	Slow, irregular	Good, crying
Muscle tone	Flaccid	Some extremity flexion	Active motion
Reflex irritability	No response	Grimace, feeble cry when stimulated	Sneeze/cough/pulls away when stimulated
Color	Blue, pale	Body pink, extremities blue	Completely pink, no cyanosis

The baby described here receives an Apgar score of 9. One point is deducted for the baby not being completely pink and having blue extremities.

242. The answer is a. The blood gas results described in this case are normal. Normal values for umbilical arterial samples are pH 7.25 to 7.3, Pco_2 50 mm Hg, Po_2 20 mm Hg, and bicarbonate 25 mEq. Acidemia is generally defined as a pH less than 7.20. Birth asphyxia generally refers to hypoxic injury so severe that the umbilical artery pH is less than 7.0, a persistent Apgar score is between 0 and 3 for more than 5 minutes, neonatal sequelae exist such as seizures or coma, and there is multiorgan dysfunction.

243. The answer is c. The Centers for Disease Control recommends that all newborns receive routine immunization against hepatitis B prior to being discharged from the hospital. Only if the mother is positive for hepatitis B surface antigen should the neonate also be passively immunized with hepatitis B immune globulin. According to the Centers for Disease Control, all newborns should receive eye prophylaxis against chlamydia and gonorrhea with either silver nitrate, erythromycin ophthalmic ointment, or tetracycline ophthalmic ointment. Vitamin K is routinely administered to prevent hemorrhagic disease of the newborn; breast milk contains only very small amounts of vitamin K. Since the temperature of newborns drops very rapidly after birth, newly delivered infants must be monitored in a warm crib. All neonates must be accurately identified via identification bands.

244-246. 244-c, 245-a, 246-c. It is estimated that 15% to 50% of women with gestational diabetes will develop type 2 diabetes later in life. Postpartum screening at 6 to 12 weeks is recommended to identify women with diabetes, impaired fasting glucose, or impaired glucose tolerance. Women with GDM have a sevenfold increased risk of developing type 2 diabetes when compared to women without GDM. Either a fasting plasma glucose or the 75-g oral glucose tolerance test may be ordered in the postpartum period. Offspring of mothers with gestational diabetes are at an increased risk for obesity later in life. There is some data that development of type 2 diabetes may be impacted by intrauterine exposure to hyperglycemia. Both types 1 and 2 diabetes have a large genetic component.

247. The answer is d. Intercourse can be painful in breastfeeding women because of an increase in vaginal dryness caused by hypoestrogenism. Water-soluble lubricants or estrogen cream applied topically to the vaginal mucosa can be helpful. In addition, the female superior position may be recommended during intercourse so that the woman can control the depth of penile penetration. Testosterone cream is not used for the treatment of vaginal atrophy.

248. The answer is c. The uterus achieves its previous nonpregnant size by about 4 weeks' postpartum. Subinvolution (cessation of the normal involution) of the uterus can occur in cases of retained placenta or uterine infection. In such cases, the uterus is larger and softer than it should be on bimanual examination. In addition, the patient usually experiences prolonged discharge and excessive uterine bleeding. With endometritis, the patient will also have a tender uterus on examination, and will complain of fever and chills. In adenomyosis, portions of the endometrial lining grow into the myometrium, causing menorrhagia and dysmenorrhea. On physical examination, the uterus is usually tender to palpation, boggy, and symmetrically enlarged. The patient described here has a physical examination most consistent with fibroids. Uterine leiomyomas would cause the uterus to be firm, irregular, and enlarged.

249 and 250. The answers are 249-c, 250-e. The incidence of incisional wound infection following cesarean delivery is approximately 6%. Risk factors that predispose to wound infections include obesity, diabetes, corticosteroid therapy, anemia, poor hemostasis, and immunosuppression. Obesity confers the highest risk. The use of preoperative prophylactic antibiotics decreases the incidence of wound infection to about 2%. Usually, incisional abscesses will cause a fever around POD 4, and erythema, induration, and drainage from the incision are also frequently noted. Opening of the incision and surgical drainage are key to curing the infection. Broad-spectrum antimicrobial agents are also administered. In all cases of wound infection, the incision must be probed to rule out a wound dehiscence (separation of the wound involving the fascial layer). As long as the fascial layer is intact, the open wound is kept clean and allowed to heal by secondary intention.

Suggested Readings

American Association of Pediatrics. Policy statement on circumcision. *Pediatrics*. 2012;130(3):e585-586.

American College of Obstetricians and Gynecologists. *Gestational Diabetes Mellitus*. Practice Bulletin Number 137, August 2013.

American College of Obstetricians and Gynecologists. *Screening for Perinatal Depression*. Committee Opinion Number 630, May 2015.

American College of Obstetricians and Gynecologists. *Use of Prophylactic Antibiotics in Labor and Delivery*. Practice Bulletin Number 120, June 2011, reaffirmed 2014.

American College of Obstetricians and Gynecologists. *Use of Psychiatric Medications During Pregnancy and Lactation*. Practice Bulletin Number 92, April 2008, reaffirmed 2014.

Cunningham FG, Leveno KJ, Bloom SL, et al. eds. Chapter 16: The newborn infant; Chapter 17: The puerperium; Chapter 23: Cesarean delivery and postpartum hysterectomy; Chapter 25: Obstetrical hemorrhage; Chapter 26: Pulmonary disorders. *Williams Obstetrics*. 23rd ed. New York, NY: McGraw-Hill; 2010.

Lee PA, Houk CP, Ahmed SF, Hughes IA, International Consensus Conference on Intersex organized by the Lawson Wilkins Pediatric Endocrine Society and the European Society for Paediatric Endocrinology. Consensus statement on management of intersex disorders. International Consensus Conference on Intersex. *Pediatrics*. 2006;118(2):e488.

Mackeen AD, Packard RE, Ota E, Speer L. Antibiotic Regimens for Postpartum Endometritis. *Cochrane Database Sys Rev*. 2015 Feb;2:CD001067.

Marik PE, Plante LA. Venous thromboembolic disease and pregnancy. *N Engl J Med*. 2008;359(19):2025.

Gynecology

Preventive Care and Health Maintenance

Questions

251. A 71-year-old G2P2 presents to your gynecology office for a routine examination. She says she is very healthy and denies taking any medication. She has no history of abnormal Pap smears and has only had one sexual partner in her lifetime. She is a nonsmoker and has an occasional cocktail with her dinner. She does not have any complaints. In addition, she denies any family history of cancer. The patient tells you that she is a widow and lives alone in an apartment in town. Her grown children have families of their own and live far away. She states that she is self-sufficient and spends her time visiting friends and volunteering at a local museum. Her blood pressure is 140/70 mm Hg. Her height is 5 ft 4 in and she weighs 130 lb. Which of the following are the most appropriate screening tests to order for this patient?

a. Pap smear and mammogram
b. Pap smear, mammogram, and colonoscopy
c. Mammogram, colonoscopy, and bone densitometry
d. Mammogram, colonoscopy, bone densitometry, and TB skin test
e. Mammogram, colonoscopy, bone densitometry, TB skin test, and auditory testing

252. A 72-year-old G5P5 presents to your office for well-woman examination. Her last examination was 7 years ago, when she turned 65. She has routine checks and laboratory tests with her internist each year. Her last mammogram was 6 months ago and was normal. She takes a diuretic for hypertension. She is a retired school teacher. Her physical examination is normal. Which of the following is the best vaccination to recommend for this patient?

a. Diphtheria-pertussis
b. Hepatitis B vaccine
c. Influenza vaccine
d. Measles-mumps-rubella
e. Pneumocystis

253. A 65-year-old G3P3 presents to your office for annual checkup. She had her last well-woman examination 20 years ago when she had a hysterectomy for fibroids. She reports no medical problems, except some occasional stiffness in her joints early in the morning. She takes a multivitamin daily. Her family history is significant for cardiac disease in both her parents and breast cancer in a maternal aunt at the age of 42 years. Her physical examination is normal. Which of the following is the most appropriate set of laboratory tests to order for this patient?

a. Lipid profile and fasting blood sugar
b. Lipid profile, fasting blood sugar, and TSH
c. Lipid profile, fasting blood sugar, TSH, and CA-125
d. Lipid profile, fasting blood sugar, TSH, and urinalysis
e. Lipid profile, fasting blood sugar, TSH, urinalysis, and CA-125

254. You are following up on the results of routine testing of a 68-year-old G4P3 for her well-woman examination. Her physical examination was normal for a postmenopausal woman. Her Pap smear revealed parabasal cells, her mammogram and lipid profile was normal, and the urinalysis shows hematuria. Which of the following is the most appropriate next step in the management of this patient?

a. Colposcopy
b. Endometrial biopsy
c. Renal sonogram
d. Urine culture
e. No further treatment or evaluation is necessary if the patient is asymptomatic.

255. A 74-year-old woman presents to your office for well-woman examination. Her last Pap smear and mammogram were 3 years ago. She has hypertension, high cholesterol, and osteoarthritis. She stopped smoking 15 years ago, and does not use alcohol. Based on this history, which of the following medical conditions should be this patient's biggest concern?

a. Alzheimer disease
b. Breast cancer
c. Cerebrovascular disease
d. Heart disease
e. Lung cancer

256. A 21-year-old G0 presents to your office for a routine annual gynecologic examination. She reports that she has previously been sexually active, but currently is not dating anyone. She has had three sexual partners in the past, and says she diligently used condoms. She is a senior in college and is doing well academically and has many friends. She lives at home with her parents and a younger sibling. She reports her 80-year-old grandmother was recently diagnosed with breast cancer. She has no other family history of cancer. She says she is healthy and has no history of medical problems or surgeries. She smokes tobacco and drinks beer occasionally, but denies any illicit drug use. Her menses started at the age of 13 years, and are regular and light without dysmenorrhea. Her blood pressure is 90/60 mm Hg. Her height is 5 ft 6 in and she weighs 130 lb. Based on this patient's history, what would be the most likely cause of death if she were to die at the age of 21 years?

a. Suicide
b. Homicide
c. Motor vehicle accidents
d. Cancer
e. Heart disease

257. A 17-year-old G1P1 presents to your office for her yearly well-woman examination. She had an uncomplicated vaginal delivery the previous year. She has been sexually active for the past 4 years and has had four different sexual partners, but has been monogamous in the previous year with the same partner. Her menses occurs every 28 days and lasts for 4 days. She denies any intermenstrual spotting, postcoital bleeding, or vaginal discharge. She reports no tobacco, alcohol, or illicit drug use. Which of the following are appropriate screening tests for this patient?

a. Gonorrhea and chlamydia screening
b. Gonorrhea, chlamydia, and cervical cancer screening
c. Gonorrhea, chlamydia, and syphilis screening
d. Gonorrhea, chlamydia, hepatitis B, hepatitis C, and syphilis screening
e. Gonorrhea, chlamydia, hepatitis B, hepatitis C, herpes simplex, and syphilis

258. A 15-year-old woman presents to your office for her routine physical examination while she is on summer break from school. She denies any medical problems or prior surgeries. She had chicken pox at the age of 4 years. Her menses started at the age of 12 years and are regular. She has recently become sexually active with her 16-year-old boyfriend. She states that they use condoms for contraception. Her physical examination is normal. Which of the following vaccines is appropriate to administer to this patient?

a. Hepatitis A vaccine
b. Human papilloma virus vaccine
c. Meningococcal vaccine
d. Pneumococcal vaccine
e. Varicella vaccine

259. A 26-year-old woman presents to your office for her well-woman examination. She reports no medical problems or prior surgeries. She states that her cycles are monthly. She is sexually active and uses oral contraceptive pills for birth control. Her physical examination is normal. She reports that her 43-year-old paternal aunt was recently diagnosed with breast cancer and is undergoing treatment. She reports that her paternal grandmother died from ovarian cancer at the age of 75 years. She wants genetic testing (BRCA) for breast and ovarian cancer. Which of the following statements regarding genetic testing for breast and ovarian cancer is true?

a. All female relatives of an individual with breast cancer should undergo genetic testing.
b. Genetic testing detects all germline mutations associated with the *BRCA1* and *BRCA2*.
c. Genetic testing is only recommended for individuals with affected individuals on the maternal side of the family.
d. Most cases of breast cancer are due to germline mutations in *BRCA1* and *BRCA2*.
e. When possible, the genetic testing should begin with the person who has ovarian cancer or early on-set breast cancer.

260. A 21-year-old woman presents to your office for well-women examination and screening for sexually transmitted infections. Her menses started at the age of 13 years and are regular. She is currently sexually active with her 20-year-old boyfriend and has had three sexual partners in her lifetime. She uses Depo-Provera and condoms for contraception. She has a history of asthma, for which she uses an inhaler as needed. She reports no prior surgeries. Her family history is significant for hypertension, high cholesterol and heart disease in her father, aged 48. She weighs 125 lb and is normotensive. Besides screening for cervical cancer and sexually transmitted infections, what other routine screening should be done for her at this visit?

a. Bone mineral density
b. Hemoglobin A_{1c}
c. Lipid profile
d. Thyroid stimulating hormone
e. Urinalysis

261. A married 41-year-old G5P3114 presents to your office for a routine examination. She reports being healthy except for a history of migraine headaches. All her Pap smears have been normal. She developed gestational diabetes in her last pregnancy. She drinks alcohol socially, and admits to smoking occasionally. Her grandmother was diagnosed with ovarian cancer when she was in her fifties. Her blood pressure is 140/90 mm Hg, height is 5 ft 5 in, and weight is 150 lb. Which of the following is the most common cause of death in women of this patient's age?

a. HIV
b. Cardiac disease
c. Accidents
d. Suicide
e. Cancer

262. A 44-year-old G2P2 presents for her well-women examination. She reports no prior medical problems or surgeries. She does not use tobacco, but reports that she drinks two glasses of wine on the weekends and occasionally smokes marijuana. She works as a secretary. She is recently divorced and has become sexually active with a new partner. She has not had STD testing since her divorce. She asks whether she should be tested for HIV. How should you counsel her?

a. She should be tested for HIV because she uses illicit drugs.
b. She should be tested for HIV because she has a new partner.
c. She should be tested only if her new partner uses intravenous drugs.
d. She does not need to have testing for HIV.
e. She does not need testing since she has only had one partner since her last HIV test.

263. A 40-year-old G3P2012 presents for her well-woman examination. Her last Pap smear and visit to a doctor was 5 years ago. She has had two vaginal deliveries and her largest baby weighed 4000 g. She has no current medical problems, but had a history of gestational diabetes in her last pregnancy. She had a postpartum bilateral tubal ligation. Her menstrual cycles occur every 28 days and last 5 days. She is sexually active in a monogamous relationship with her husband of 16 years. She reports that she occasionally leaks urine when she coughs; otherwise she has no complaints. On physical examination, she weighs 198 lbs and her blood pressure is 132/81 mm Hg. Her breast and pelvic examinations are normal. What are the most appropriate screening tests for this patient?

a. Pap smear, gonorrhea, chlamydia testing
b. Pap smear, fasting glucose, lipid profile
c. Pap smear, fasting glucose, lipid profile, urinalysis
d. Pap smear, fasting glucose, lipid profile, TSH, urinalysis
e. Pap smear, fasting glucose, lipid profile, mammogram, urinalysis

264. A 36-year-old G2P2 presents for her well-woman examination. She has had two spontaneous vaginal deliveries without complications. Her largest child weighed 3500 g at birth. She uses oral contraceptive pills and has never had an abnormal Pap smear. She does not smoke, but drinks about four times per week. Her weight is 70 kg. Her vital signs are normal. After placement of the speculum, you note a clear cyst approximately 2.5 cm in size on the lateral wall of the vagina on the right side. The cyst is nontender and does not cause the patient any dyspareunia or discomfort. Which of the following is the most likely diagnosis of this mass?

a. Bartholin duct cyst
b. Gartner duct cyst
c. Lipoma
d. Hematoma
e. Inclusion cyst

265. A 50-year-old G4P4 presents for her well-woman examination. She had one cesarean delivery followed by three vaginal deliveries. Her menses stopped 1 year ago and she occasionally still has a hot flash. She tells you that about 10 years ago she was treated with a loop electro-excision procedure (LEEP) for cervical intraepithelial neoplasia (CIN) III. Since that time, all of her Pap tests have been normal. What recommendation should you make regarding how frequently she should undergo Pap smear testing?

a. She needs an annual Pap smear for 20 years following her LEEP.
b. She needs an annual Pap smear for the rest of her life since she had CIN III.
c. She should undergo routine age-based screening.
d. She should have HPV co-testing, and if negative, can discontinue Pap smears.
e. You should recommend a hysterectomy so she can stop having Pap smears.

266. A 45-year-old G3P3 presents for her yearly examination. She last saw a doctor 7 years ago after she had her last child. She had three vaginal deliveries, the last of which was complicated by gestational diabetes and pre-eclampsia. She has not been sexually active in the past year. She once had an abnormal Pap smear for which she underwent cryotherapy. Her cycles are every 35 days and last for 7 days. She describes the flow as heavy for the first 2 days and occasionally passes blood clots the size of quarters. She reports no medical problems. Her family history is significant for coronary artery disease in her dad at the age of 65 years and a maternal aunt who developed ovarian cancer at the age of 67 years. She is normotensive, and her breast and pelvic examinations are normal. Along with a Pap smear, mammogram, fasting glucose, and lipid profile, what other screening test is recommended for this patient?

a. CA-125
b. Hemoglobin level
c. Hepatitis C
d. Thyroid stimulating hormone
e. Urinalysis

267. A 30-year-woman presents to your office because she is afraid of developing ovarian cancer. Her 70-year-old grandmother recently died from ovarian cancer, and she is upset and tearful. You discuss with her the risk factors and prevention strategies for ovarian cancer. Which of the following can decrease a woman's risk of ovarian cancer?

a. Use of combination oral contraceptive therapy
b. Menopause after the age of 55 years
c. Nonsteroidal anti-inflammatory drugs
d. Nulliparity
e. Ovulation induction medications

268. A 42-year-old G4P3104 presents for her well-woman examination. She has had three vaginal deliveries and one cesarean delivery for breech presentation. She states her cycles are regular and reports no history of sexually transmitted infections. Currently she and her husband use condoms, but they dislike the hassle of a coital-dependent method. She is interested in a more effective contraception because they do not want any more children. She reports occasional migraine headaches, and had a serious allergic reaction to anesthesia as a child when she underwent a tonsillectomy. She drinks and smokes socially. She weighs 78 kg, and her blood pressure is 142/89 mm Hg. During her office visit, you counsel the patient at length regarding birth control methods. Which of the following is the most appropriate contraceptive method for this patient?

a. Intrauterine device
b. Laparoscopic bilateral tubal ligation
c. Combination oral contraceptives
d. Diaphragm
e. Transdermal patch

269. A 55-year-old Caucasian G2P2 presents for her well-woman examination. She had two uneventful vaginal deliveries. Her last menstrual period was 2 years ago. She has occasional night sweats, but they are not bothersome. Her medical history is significant for hypothyroidism, which is well controlled on medication. She does not take any other medicines. She does not use tobacco, alcohol, or drugs. Her family history is significant for stroke, diabetes, and high blood pressure. On examination she is a pleasant female, stands 5 ft 6 in tall, and weighs 115 lbs. Her blood pressure is 130/72 mm Hg, pulse 70 beats per minute, respiratory rate 14 breaths per minute, and temperature 37°C (98.4°F). Her breast, lung, cardiac, abdomen, and pelvic examinations are normal. Which of the following aspects of her history would be an indication to order bone mineral density screening?

a. She has been in menopause for 2 years.
b. She weighs 115 pounds.
c. She is Caucasian.
d. She has a family history of diabetes.
e. She does not meet criteria for bone mineral density screening.

270. A 32-year-old woman presents for her yearly examination. She has been smoking one pack of cigarettes a day for the past 12 years. She wants to stop, and you make some recommendations to her. Which of the following is true regarding smoking cessation in women?

a. Ninety percent of those who stop smoking relapse within 3 months.
b. Nicotine replacement in the form of chewing gum or transdermal patches has not been shown to be effective in smoking cessation programs.
c. Smokers do not benefit from repeated warnings from their doctor to stop smoking.
d. Stopping cold turkey is the only way to successfully achieve smoking cessation.
e. No matter how long one has been smoking, smoking cessation appears to improve the health of the lungs.

Preventive Care and Health Maintenance

Answers

251. The answer is c. In postmenopausal women, routine screening for colon cancer is recommended with a colonoscopy to be performed every 10 years. Alternatively, flexible sigmoidoscopy can be performed every 5 years along with a yearly fecal occult blood test. Mammography should be performed every 1 to 2 years in all women 50 to 74 years of age. Postmenopausal women, who are not on hormone replacement therapy, and all women 65 years or older should be screened for osteoporosis with a DEXA scan to determine bone mineral density. Screening for cervical cancer with Pap smears may be discontinued after the age of 65 years in women with adequate negative prior screening results and no history of CIN II or higher. Adequate prior screening is defined as three consecutive negative Pap smears or two consecutive negative HPV co-test results within the previous 10 years, with the most recent test performed in the last 5 years. Women with a history of CIN II, CIN III, or adenocarcinoma in situ should continue screening for a total of 20 years after treatment. Tuberculosis skin testing need to be performed only in individuals with HIV infection, those who have close contact with individuals suspected of having TB, who are IV drug users, who are residents of nursing homes or long-term-care facilities, or who work in a profession that is health care related. This patient does not have any risk factors that would necessitate TB testing. Auditory testing is not a routine screening test.

252. The answer is c. Women older than 65 years should have all of the following immunizations: tetanus-diphtheria booster every 10 years, influenza virus vaccine annually, and a one-time pneumococcal vaccine. Hepatitis B vaccine would be indicated only in individuals at high risk (ie, international travelers, intravenous drug users, and their sexual contacts, those who have occupational exposure to blood or blood products, persons with chronic liver or renal disease, or residents of institutions for the developmentally disabled, and inmates of correctional institutions). Herpes zoster is indicated for women older than 65 years if not previously immunized.

253. The answer is d. Women older than 65 years should undergo cholesterol testing every 5 years, fasting glucose testing every 3 years, screening for thyroid disease with a TSH every 5 years, and periodic urinalysis is recommended in women older than 65 years. CA-125 testing is not recommended for screening for ovarian cancer. There are many benign conditions which can cause an elevated CA-125, such as pregnancy, endometriosis, fibroids, menses, pelvic inflammatory disease, peritoneal disease, and liver disease.

254. The answer is d. A urinalysis that is positive for blood should be followed up with a urine culture to evaluate for an asymptomatic urinary tract infection before further workup is done or referral to a urologist is made. Parabasal cells on a Pap smear indicate lack of estrogen, and are a normal finding in postmenopausal women. It requires no further evaluation.

255. The answer is d. In order of decreasing incidence, the leading causes of death in women older than 65 years are the following: diseases of the heart, cancer, cerebrovascular diseases, chronic obstructive pulmonary diseases, Alzheimer disease, diabetes, pneumonia and influenza, accidents, renal disease, and septicemia.

256. The answer is c. The leading causes of death in women between the ages of 20 and 24 years, in order of decreasing frequency, are as follows: injuries/accidents, suicide, malignancy, homicide, heart disease, pregnancy complications, birth defects, influenza and pneumonia, stroke, septicemia, and diabetes.

257. The answer is a. Routine screening for sexually transmitted disease is not warranted for all women; however, all sexually active women younger than 25 years of age should be routinely screened for gonorrhea and chlamydia, and older women with risk factors such as new or multiple partners, sex work, or concurrent STD should also be screened. There is no routine screening recommended for hepatitis B virus or herpes simplex virus. Hepatitis C screening should occur in those with risk factors such as intravenous drug use, dialysis, partner with hepatitis C, multiple partners, and received blood products prior to 1990. Syphilis screening should also occur in those with risk factors such as sex work, confinement in an adult correction facility or men having sex with men. Screening for cervical cancer should begin at the age of 21 years.

Cervical Cancer screening	
Age at initiation	21 years regardless of age of onset of sexual activity
Screening intervals for women with average risk	Age 21-29 years: cytology every 3 years ≥ 30 years: cytology and co-testing every 3-5 years if 3 consecutive negative Paps or negative high-risk HPV DNA test
Age to discontinue screening	Age 65 if adequate negative prior screening results. Women with a history of CIN 2 or CIN 3 or adenocarcinoma in situ should continue routine age-based screening for at least 20 years.
Screening after hysterectomy	No screening is necessary if there is no history of CIN 2, CIN 3, or adenocarcinoma in situ in the past 20 years. If supracervical hysterectomy, follow screening guidelines shown earlier. Screening should be continued if history of diethylstilbestrol exposure or cervical cancer.

258. The answer is b. It would be appropriate for this patient to receive a human papilloma vaccination, since it is recommended for all previously unvaccinated women aged 9 to 26 years. She is not a candidate for the varicella vaccine since she has had chicken pox. The hepatitis A vaccine is indicated for international travelers, illegal drug users, and health care workers. The pneumococcal vaccine is indicated in immunocompromised persons, those with chronic illnesses, and individuals older than 65 years. Meningococcal vaccination is recommended for college freshmen living in dorms, asplenia, or travel or residence in countries where meningococcal disease is endemic.

259. The answer is e. Germline mutations in *BRCA1* and *BRCA2* account for the vast majority of families with hereditary breast and ovarian cancer syndrome. Approximately 10% of cases of ovarian cancer and 3% to 5% of cases of breast cancer are due to germline mutations in *BRCA1* and *BRCA2*. In the general population, it is estimated that approximately 1 in 300 to 1 in 800 individuals carry a mutation in *BRCA1* or *BRCA2*. For a woman with a *BRCA1* mutation, the risk of ovarian cancer is 39% to 46%. For a woman with a *BRCA2* mutation, the risk of ovarian cancer is 12% to 20%. The estimated lifetime risk of breast cancer with a *BRCA1* or *BRCA2* mutation is 65% to 74%. Evaluating a patient's risk for hereditary breast and ovarian cancer syndrome should be a routine part of obstetric and gynecologic practice. When evaluating a family history, it is important to remember that breast cancer and ovarian cancer predisposing genes can be transmitted through the father as well as the mother. If possible, genetic testing should begin with a person in the family who has ovarian cancer or early onset breast cancer (affected individual). For obstetrician–gynecologists, certain clinical criteria have been developed to assist in determining which patients would benefit from a genetic risk assessment. The first group of criteria includes those patients with greater than an approximate 20% to 25% chance of having an inherited predisposition to breast cancer and ovarian cancer and for whom genetic risk assessment is recommended. The second group of criteria includes those patients with greater than an approximate 5% to 10% chance of having an inherited predisposition to breast and ovarian cancer and for whom genetic risk assessment may be helpful. Although, in most cases, an inherited predisposition to ovarian cancer is caused by mutations in *BRCA1* or *BRCA2*, current technology does not allow identification of all mutations that must exist in these genes.

260. The answer is c. The National Cholesterol Education Program recommends that all adults 20 years and older have a serum lipoprotein profile every 5 years. Lipid profiles are also recommended if there is a family history of premature cardiovascular disease (age younger than 50 in men and 60 in women). Even though use of Depo-Provera is associated with decreased bone mineral density there is no indication for bone mineral density screening for women using it. Testing for diabetes is indicated for individuals with BMI greater than 25, family history of diabetes, polycystic ovarian syndrome, hypertension, prior history of gestational diabetes. Thyroid testing is reserved for symptoms, strong family history of thyroid disease or autoimmune disease. Urinalysis is indicated for symptoms of infection or yearly screening in diabetics and periodically in women older than 65 years.

261. The answer is e. The leading causes of death in women aged 35 to 44 years, in order of decreasing incidence, are as follows: cancer, accidents, heart disease, suicide, chronic liver disease, stroke, diabetes mellitus, homicide, HIV, influenza, and pneumonia.

262. The answer is b. The CDC and ACOG recommend that females aged 13 to 64 years be tested at least once during their lifetime, and annually thereafter based on risk factors. This patient has a new partner, and therefore should be offered testing. Repeat HIV testing should be offered annually to women who use IV drugs, are sex partners of a person who uses IV drugs, exchanges sex for drugs or money, are sex partners of HIV infected individuals, have sex with men who have sex with men, or have had more than one sex partner since their last HIV test.

263. The answer is e. Pap smear is indicated since it has been over 5 years since her last Pap smear. Given her history of gestational diabetes and the large birth weight of her child, diabetes screening is indicated. Also a lipid profile is indicated every 5 years after the age of 20 years. Her symptoms of urinary incontinence require that urinary tract infection be ruled out as a cause. Most national agencies recommend screening with mammogram for breast cancer beginning at the age of 40 years.

BREAST CANCER SCREENING RECOMMENDATIONS				
	Mammography	Clinical Breast Examination	Breast Self-Examination Instruction	Breast Self-Awareness
American College of Obstetricians and Gynecologists	Age 40 years and older annually	Age 20-39 years every 1-3 years Age 40 years and older annually	Consider for high-risk patients	Recommended
American Cancer Society	Age 40 years and older annually	Age 20-39 years every 1-3 years Age 40 years and older annually	Optional for age 20 years and older	Recommended
National Comprehensive Cancer Network	Age 40 years and older annually	Age 20-39 years every 1-3 years Age 40 years and older annually	Recommended	Recommended
National Cancer Institute	Age 40 years and older every 1-2 years	Recommended	Not Recommended	—
U.S. Preventative Services Task Force	Age 50-74 years biennially	Insufficient Evidence	Not Recommended	____

Source: ACOG Practice Bulletin Number 122, August 2011.

264. The answer is b. Gartner duct cysts arise from embryonic remnants of the mesonephric duct that course along the lateral vaginal wall. These are usually small and asymptomatic and are found incidentally during a pelvic examination. They can be followed conservatively unless the patient becomes symptomatic, at which time excision is recommended. Inclusion cysts are usually seen on the posterior lower vaginal surface. Inclusion cysts are the most common vaginal cysts and result from birth trauma or previous gynecologic surgery. Bartholin duct cysts are the most common large cysts of the vulva. Bartholin ducts open into a groove between the hymen and labia minora on the posterior lateral vaginal opening. Lipomas are benign, encapsulated tumors of fat cells; they are most commonly discovered in the labia majora and are superficial in location. Hematomas of the vulva usually occur as a result of blunt trauma or straddle injury. Spontaneous hematomas can occur as a result of rupture of a varicose vein in pregnancy or the postpartum period.

265. The answer is c. Cervical cancer screening should begin at 21 years of age. Cervical cytology screening is recommended every 3 years for women aged 21 to 29 years. Women aged 30 to 65 years may have cytology and co-testing every 5 years, or cytology alone every 3 years. Women with a history of CIN 2, CIN 3, or adenocarcinoma in situ should continue routine age-based screening for at least 20 years following treatment. Hysterectomy is not indicated. Certain risk factors have been associated with CIN in observational studies; women with any of the following risk factors may require more frequent cervical cytology screening: HIV infection, immunosuppression (such as transplant patients), or women with in-utero diethylstilbestrol exposure. Women older than 65 years may discontinue screening after adequate negative prior screening results. This is defined as three consecutive negative cytology results or two consecutive negative HPV co-test tests results within the past 10 years, with the most recent test performed within the past 5 years.

266. The answer is b. Hemoglobin level assessment is warranted in women with excessive menstruation as described in her history. Mammography is indicated for her age. Measuring CA-125 levels has not been shown to be effective in population-based screening for ovarian cancer. Hepatitis C screening should occur in those with risk factors such as intravenous drug use, dialysis, partner with hepatitis C, multiple partners, and received blood products prior to 1990. She is not diabetic or hypertensive and has no urinary symptoms so urinalysis is not indicated. Thyroid testing is reserved for symptoms, strong family history of thyroid disease or autoimmune disease.

267. The answer is a. Oral contraceptive use, multiparity, breastfeeding, and early menopause are all factors believed to decrease the risk of developing ovarian cancer because they reduce the number of years a woman spends ovulating. The use of combination oral contraceptives decreases the risk of developing ovarian cancer by about 40%. Nulliparity, increasing age, and fertility drugs all increase ovulatory cycles and therefore are risk factors for developing ovarian cancer. In the general population, the risk of developing ovarian cancer is about 1% to 1.5%. This risk increases to about 5% if a woman has one first-degree relative with ovarian cancer and to about 7% if she has two or more first-degree relatives with ovarian cancer.

268. The answer is a. An intrauterine device is a highly effective long-term method for which the patient has no contraindication. A bilateral tubal ligation would be another option; however, the patient had a serious allergic reaction to anesthesia as a child, and general anesthesia is required for female laparoscopic sterilization. The patient's smoking and age contra-indicate the use of combination oral contraceptives. Migraine headaches accompanied by neurologic symptoms such as loss of vision, paresthesias, and numbness are generally considered to be a contraindication to combination oral contraceptive use. Use of a diaphragm is a coital-dependent action and the patient relates that it is not something she desires.

269. The answer is b. The patient meets criteria for screening based on her low body weight. Bone mineral density screening should be started at the age of 65 years in most women. Postmenopausal women with risk factors may require screening earlier if any of these risk factors are present: prior osteoporotic fracture, body weight less than 127 pounds, medications or diseases that cause bone loss, parental medical history of a hip fracture, current smoker, alcoholism, or rheumatoid arthritis.

270. The answer is e. Cigarette smoking has been linked to many pathologic conditions, including coronary artery disease, obstructive pulmonary disease, and lung cancer. There are studies that demonstrate that smoking cessation is of benefit to pulmonary health regardless of how long one has smoked. Doctors should repeatedly counsel their patients to stop smoking, and follow-up visits to achieve these goals are effective. The "5 A's" model is an evidence-based model that may be used successfully to address patient smoking. The 5 A's are as follows: Ask (about tobacco use), Advise patients who smoke to quit, Assess the patient's willingness to try to stop smoking, Assist in the attempt to quit for those who are willing, and Arrange follow up. In addition to counseling, all patients should be offered medication to improve quit success and reduce withdrawal symptoms. Medications include nicotine replacement therapy, prescription antidepressants such as bupropion, and varenicline, which blocks the pleasant effects of smoking from the brain.

Suggested Readings

American College of Obstetricians and Gynecologists. Annual well women's health care: well-woman recommendations. Available at acog.org.

American College of Obstetricians and Gynecologists. *Breast Cancer Screening*. Practice Bulletin Number 122, August 2011, reaffirmed 2014.

American College of Obstetricians and Gynecologists. *Colorectal Cancer Screening Strategies*. Committee Opinion Number 609, October 2014.

American College of Obstetricians and Gynecologists. *Hereditary Breast and Ovarian Cancer Syndrome*. Practice Bulletin Number 103, April 2009, reaffirmed 2015.

American College of Obstetricians and Gynecologists. *Integrating Immunizations into Practice*. Committee Opinion Number 558, April 2013, reaffirmed 2015.

American College of Obstetricians and Gynecologists. *Routine Human Immunodeficiency Virus Screening*. Committee Opinion Number 596, May 2014.

American College of Obstetricians and Gynecologists. *Screening for Cervical Cancer*. Practice Bulletin Number 131, November 2012, reaffirmed 2015.

American College of Obstetricians and Gynecologists. *Tobacco Use and Women's Health*. Committee Opinion Number 503, September 2011, reaffirmed 2013.

American College of Obstetricians and Gynecologists. *Well-Woman Visit*. Committee Opinion Number 534, August 2012, reaffirmed 2014.

Centers for Disease Control. Leading causes of death in females, 2011. Available at CDC.gov, Accessed 2011.

Benign and Malignant Disorders of the Breast and Pelvis

Questions

271. A 21-year-old woman presents with left lower quadrant pain. An anterior 7-cm firm adnexal mass is palpated. Ultrasound confirms a complex left adnexal mass with solid components that appears to contain a tooth. What percentage of these tumors is bilateral?

a. Less than 1
b. 2 to 3
c. 10
d. 50
e. Greater than 75

272. A 54-year-old woman is scheduled for laparotomy due to a pelvic mass. At the time of exploratory laparotomy, a unilateral ovarian neoplasm is discovered that is accompanied by a large omental metastasis. Frozen section diagnosis confirms metastatic serous cystadenocarcinoma. Which of the following is the most appropriate intraoperative course of action?

a. Excision of the omental metastasis and ovarian cystectomy
b. Omentectomy and ovarian cystectomy
c. Excision of the omental metastasis and unilateral oophorectomy
d. Omentectomy and bilateral salpingo-oophorectomy
e. Omentectomy, total abdominal hysterectomy, and bilateral salpingo-oophorectomy

273. A 68-year-old woman is seen for evaluation of a swelling in the right, posterior aspect of her vaginal opening. She has noted pain in this area when walking and during intercourse. At the time of pelvic examination, a mildly tender, firm mass is noted just outside the introitus in the right vulva at approximately 8 o'clock. Which of the following is the most appropriate treatment?

a. Marsupialization
b. Administration of antibiotics
c. Surgical excision
d. Incision and drainage
e. Observation

274. A 51-year-old woman is diagnosed with invasive cervical carcinoma by cone biopsy. Pelvic examination and rectal-vaginal examination reveal the parametrium to be free of disease, but the upper portion of the vagina is involved with tumor. Intravenous pyelography (IVP) and sigmoidoscopy are negative, but a computed tomography (CT) scan of the abdomen and pelvis shows grossly enlarged pelvic and periaortic nodes. This patient is classified at which of the following stages?

a. IIa
b. IIb
c. IIIa
d. IIIb
e. IV

Questions 275 to 278

A 45-year-old G1P1 presents for her routine annual examination. The patient is a healthy smoker who has no medical problems. Her surgical history is significant for a cesarean delivery with bilateral tubal interruption. You perform a Pap smear, which returns showing high grade squamous intraepithelial lesion (HSIL). She undergoes colposcopy, which is inadequate.

275. What is the next step in management?

a. Repeat Pap smear in 6 months.
b. HPV testing.
c. Cone biopsy.
d. Repeat Pap smear with co-testing in 1 year.
e. Repeat the colposcopy in 4 to 6 months.

276. Cone biopsy of the cervix shows squamous cell cancer that has invaded only 2 mm beyond the basement membrane with a lateral spread of 5 mm. There are no confluent tongues of tumor, and there is no evidence of lymphatic or vascular invasion. The margins of the cone biopsy specimen are free of disease. How should you stage this patient's disease?

a. Microinvasive cancer, stage Ia2
b. Carcinoma in situ
c. Microinvasive cancer, stage Ia1
d. Invasive cancer, stage Ib
e. Invasive cancer, stage IIa

277. Which lymph node group would be the first involved in metastatic spread of this disease beyond the cervix and uterus?

a. Common iliac nodes
b. Sacral nodes
c. External iliac nodes
d. Paracervical nodes
e. Para-aortic nodes

278. This patient now asks you for your advice on how to treat her cervical cancer. Your best recommendation is for the patient to undergo which of the following?

a. Treatment with external beam radiation
b. Implantation of radioactive cesium into the cervical canal
c. Extrafascial hysterectomy
d. Radical hysterectomy with pelvic lymphadenectomy
e. Treatment with adjuvant chemoradiation

Questions 279 and 280

279. A woman is found to have a unilateral invasive vulvar carcinoma that is 3 cm in diameter but not associated with evidence of lymph node spread. Initial management should consist of which of the following?

a. Chemotherapy
b. Radiation therapy
c. Simple vulvectomy
d. Radical vulvectomy with bilateral lymphadenectomy
e. Radical local excision and ipsilateral inguinal lymphadenectomy

280. If this woman had multiple medical comorbidities, what would be the best option for management?

a. Chemotherapy.
b. Radiation therapy.
c. She should still undergo the same surgery that would be recommended for a healthy patient.
d. Simple vulvectomy.
e. She should not receive any treatment, and should be referred to hospice.

281. A pregnant 35-year-old patient is at highest risk for the concurrent development of which of the following malignancies?

a. Cervix
b. Ovary
c. Breast
d. Vagina
e. Colon

282. Stage Ia2 microinvasive cervical cancer is diagnosed based on cervical biopsy in a 34-year-old woman who is 12 weeks' pregnant. What is the best next step in management?

a. Recommend pregnancy termination so her cervical cancer can be treated
b. Perform a cone biopsy
c. Treat her with chemotherapy during the pregnancy
d. Wait until after the pregnancy to treat her cervical cancer
e. Treat the cervical cancer with radiation during the pregnancy

283. A 54-year-old woman presents for well-woman examination. On pelvic examination you palpate an enlarged, tender right adnexal mass. You order a pelvic ultrasound as the next step in this patient's evaluation. Which of the following sonographic characteristics of the cyst in this patient would warrant further evaluation for possible ovarian malignancy?

a. Lack of pelvic ascites
b. The presence of a unilocular cyst in one ovary
c. Papillary vegetations within a cystic ovary
d. An ovarian cyst with a diameter of 4 cm
e. Demonstration of arterial and venous flow by Doppler imaging

284. A 70-year-old woman presents for evaluation of a pruritic lesion on the vulva. Examination shows a white, friable lesion on the right labia majorum that is 3 cm in diameter. No other suspicious areas are noted.

Biopsy of the lesion confirms squamous cell carcinoma. In this patient, lymphatic spread of the cancer would be first to which of the following lymph nodes?

a. External iliac lymph nodes
b. Superficial inguinal lymph nodes
c. Deep femoral lymph nodes
d. Periaortic nodes
e. Internal iliac nodes

285. A 17-year-old girl is seen by her primary care physician for the evaluation of left lower quadrant pain. The physician felt a pelvic mass on physical examination and ordered a pelvic ultrasound. You are consulted because an ovarian neoplasm is identified by the ultrasound. Which of the following is the most common ovarian tumor in this type of patient?

a. Germ cell
b. Papillary serous epithelial
c. Fibrosarcoma
d. Brenner tumor
e. Sarcoma botryoides

286. A 41-year-old woman undergoes exploratory laparotomy for a persistent adnexal mass. Frozen section diagnosis is serous carcinoma. What is the likelihood that the contralateral ovary is involved in this malignancy?

a. 5%
b. 15%
c. 33%
d. 50%
e. 75%

287. A postmenopausal woman presents with pruritic white lesions on the vulva. Punch biopsy of a representative area is obtained and is consistent with lichen sclerosus. Which of the following is the most appropriate treatment for this patient?

a. Topical estrogen
b. Wide local excision of the lesion
c. Intralesional injection of corticosteroids
d. Skinning vulvectomy
e. Topical corticosteroids

288. A 22-year-old woman returns to your office for evaluation of an abnormal Pap smear. The Pap smear was reported as HSIL. Colposcopic biopsy confirms the presence of a cervical lesion consistent with severe cervical dysplasia (CIN III). Which of the following human papilloma virus (HPV) types is most often associated with this type of lesion?

a. HPV type 6
b. HPV type 11
c. HPV type 16
d. HPV type 18
e. HPV type 44

289. A 20-year-old woman presents complaining of bumps around her vaginal opening. The bumps have been there for several months and are getting bigger. Her boyfriend has the same type of bumps on his penis. On physical examination, the patient has multiple 2- to 10-mm lesions around her introitus consistent with condyloma. Her cervix has no gross lesions. A Pap smear is performed. One week later, the Pap smear returns showing atypical squamous cells of undetermined significance (ASCUS). Reflex HPV typing showed no high-risk HPV. Which of the following viral types is most likely responsible for the patient's condyloma?

a. HPV type 11
b. HPV type 16
c. HPV type 18
d. HPV type 45
e. HPV type 56

Questions 290 to 295

Select the ovarian tumor from the following list that is most likely to be associated with the clinical picture. Each lettered option may be used once, more than once, or not at all.

a. Granulosa tumor
b. Sertoli-Leydig cell tumor
c. Immature teratoma
d. Gonadoblastoma
e. Krukenberg tumor

290. A 26-year-old G2P1 presents to the gynecologist complaining of increasing hair growth on her face, chest, and abdomen, but the hair on her head is receding in the temporal regions. She also has had problems with acne. On physical examination, the patient has significant amounts of coarse, dark hair on her face, chest, and abdomen. On pelvic examination she has an enlarged clitoris. She has a 7-cm left adnexal mass.

291. A 56-year-old postmenopausal woman presents complaining of vaginal bleeding. Her uterus is slightly enlarged and she has a 6-cm right adnexal mass. Endometrial biopsy shows adenocarcinoma of the endometrium.

292. A 67-year-old woman is found to have bilateral adnexal masses while undergoing evaluation of her recently diagnosed colon cancer.

293. A 17-year-old woman is referred by her primary care physician for the evaluation of primary amenorrhea. On physical examination, the patient has evidence of virilization. She also has a pelvic mass. During the workup of the patient, she is found to have sex chromosome mosaicism (45, X/46, XY).

294. A 19-year-old woman is undergoing diagnostic laparoscopy for a 9-cm right ovarian mass. The final pathology report shows evidence of glial tissue and immature cerebellar and cortical tissue.

295. A 51-year-old menopausal woman is undergoing exploratory laparotomy for bilateral adnexal masses. A frozen section is performed on the excised ovaries and shows significant numbers of signet cells.

Questions 296 to 301

Match the chemotherapeutic agents with the most common side effects. Each lettered option may be used once, more than once, or not at all.

a. Hemorrhagic cystitis
b. Renal failure
c. Tympanic membrane fibrosis
d. Necrotizing enterocolitis
e. Pulmonary fibrosis
f. Pancreatic failure
g. Ocular degeneration
h. Cardiac toxicity
i. Peripheral neuropathy
j. Bone marrow depression

296. Cyclophosphamide

297. Cisplatin

298. Paclitaxel

299. Bleomycin

300. Doxorubicin

301. Vincristine

Questions 302 to 308

Match each figure with the correct description. Each lettered option may be used once, more than once, or not at all.

a. Well-differentiated adenocarcinoma of the endometrium
b. Proliferative endometrium
c. Choriocarcinoma
d. Late secretory endometrium
e. Uterine carcinosarcoma
f. Mature cystic teratoma
g. Clear cell cancer of the endometrium

302.

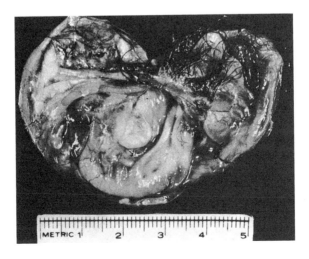

303.

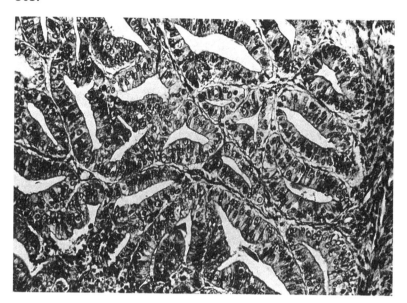

304.

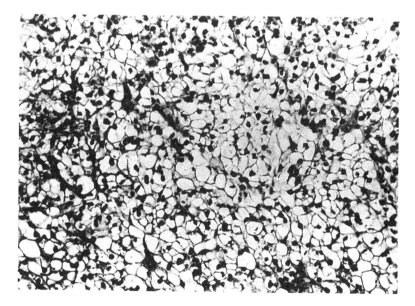

305.

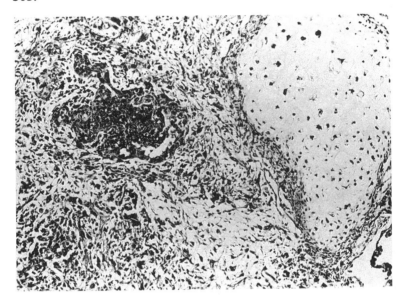

306.

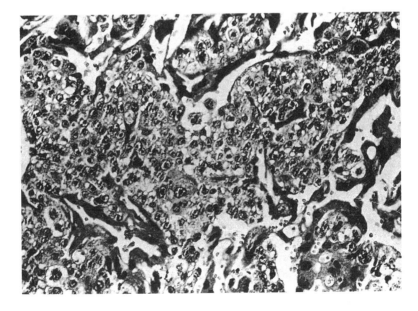

307.

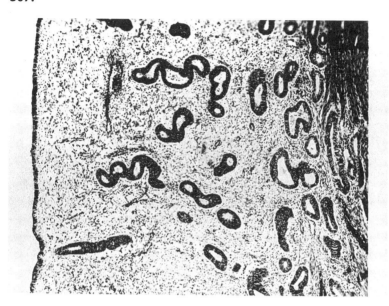

308.

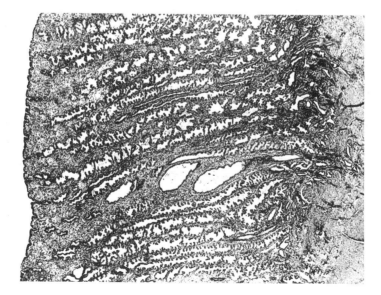

309. A patient is diagnosed with carcinoma of the breast. Which of the following is the most important prognostic factor in the treatment of this disease?

a. Age at diagnosis
b. Size of tumor
c. Axillary node metastases
d. Estrogen receptors on the tumor cells
e. Progesterone receptors on the tumor cells

310. A 25-year-old woman presents to you for routine well-woman examination. She has had two normal vaginal deliveries and is healthy. She smokes one pack of cigarettes per day. She has no gynecologic complaints. Her last menstrual period was 3 weeks ago. During the pelvic examination, you notice that her left ovary is enlarged to 5 cm in diameter. Which of the following is the best recommendation to this patient?

a. Order CA-125 testing
b. Schedule outpatient diagnostic laparoscopy
c. Return to the office in 1 to 2 months to recheck the ovaries
d. Schedule a CT scan of the pelvis
e. Admit to the hospital for exploratory laparotomy

311. A 23-year-old woman presents to your office complaining of a growth around her vaginal opening. Recently, the growth has been itching and bleeding. On physical examination, she has a broad-based lesion measuring 2 cm in diameter on the posterior fourchette. Although there is no active bleeding, the lesion has some crusted blood along the right lateral margin. Which of the following is the best way to treat this patient?

a. Weekly application of podophyllin in the office
b. Injection of 5-fluorouracil into the lesions
c. Self-application of imiquimod to the lesions by the patient
d. Weekly application of trichloroacetic acid in the office
e. Local excision of the lesion

312. At the time of annual examination, a patient expresses concern regarding possible exposure to sexually transmitted diseases. During your pelvic examination, a single, indurated, nontender ulcer is noted on the vulva. Venereal Disease Research Laboratory (VDRL) and fluorescent treponemal antibody (FTA) tests are positive. Without treatment, the next stage of this disease is clinically characterized by which of the following?

a. Optic nerve atrophy and generalized paresis
b. Tabes dorsalis
c. Gummas
d. Macular rash over the hands and feet
e. Aortic aneurysm

313. A 24-year-old patient recently emigrated from the tropics. Four weeks ago she noted a small vulvar ulceration that spontaneously healed. Now there is painful inguinal adenopathy associated with malaise and fever. You are considering the diagnosis of lymphogranuloma venereum (LGV). The diagnosis can be established by which of the following?

a. Staining for Donovan bodies
b. The presence of serum antibodies to *Chlamydia trachomatis*
c. Positive Frei skin test
d. Culturing *Haemophilus ducreyi*
e. Culturing *Calymmatobacterium granulomatis*

314. One day after a casual sexual encounter with a bisexual man recently diagnosed as antibody-positive for human immunodeficiency virus (HIV), a patient is concerned about whether she may have become infected. An HIV antibody titer is obtained and is negative. To test for seroconversion, when is the earliest you should reschedule repeat antibody testing after the sexual encounter?

a. 1 to 2 weeks
b. 3 to 4 weeks
c. 4 to 10 weeks
d. 12 to 15 weeks
e. 26 to 52 weeks

315. A 32-year-old G3P0030 obese woman comes to your office for a routine gynecologic examination. She is single, but is currently sexually active. She has a history of five sexual partners in the past, and became sexually active at the age of 15 years. She has had three first-trimester pregnancy terminations. She uses Depo-Provera for birth control, and reports occasionally using condoms. She has a history of genital warts, but has never had an abnormal Pap smear. The patient says she does not use illicit drugs, but admits to smoking about one pack of cigarettes a day. Her physical examination is normal. Three weeks later, you receive the results of her Pap smear, which was reported as a HSIL. Which of the following factors in this patient's history does not increase her risk for cervical dysplasia?

a. Young age at initiation of sexual activity
b. Multiple sexual partners
c. History of genital warts
d. Use of Depo-Provera
e. Smoking

Questions 316 to 320

Select the management option from the following list that is most appropriate as the next step in the treatment of the patient described. Each lettered option may be used once, more than once, or not at all.

a. Perform a cone biopsy of the cervix
b. Repeat the Pap smear to obtain endocervical cells
c. Order reflex HPV typing on the initial Pap smear
d. Perform a hysterectomy
e. Perform a colposcopy and directed cervical biopsies
f. Repeat the Pap smear in 1 year
g. Perform a colposcopy, endometrial biopsy, and endocervical curettage

316. A 23-year-old woman presents for a routine annual examination. Her Pap smear returns as HSIL.

317. A 21-year-old woman presents for her first Pap smear. The following week, the results return as low grade squamous intraepithelial lesion (LSIL).

318. A 55-year-old postmenopausal woman has a Pap smear that returns as atypical glandular cells of undetermined significance (AGUS).

319. A 35-year-old with an LSIL Pap smear undergoes colposcopy. Directed biopsies return showing severe dysplasia (CIN III).

320. A 43-year-old has negative cytology results but absent endocervical cells are reported.

Questions 321 and 322

321. A 24-year-old G0 presents to your office complaining of vulvar discomfort, with intense burning and pain during intercourse. The discomfort occurs at the vaginal introitus, primarily with penile insertion into the vagina. The patient also experiences the same pain with tampon insertion and when the speculum is inserted during a gynecologic examination. The problem has become so severe that she can no longer have intercourse, which is causing problems in her marriage. She is otherwise healthy. She has regular menses without dysmenorrhea. On physical examination, the region of the vulva around the vaginal vestibule has several punctate, erythematous areas of epithelium measuring 3 to 8 mm in diameter. Most of the lesions are located on the skin between the two Bartholin glands. Each inflamed lesion is tender to touch with a cotton swab. Which of the following is the most likely diagnosis?

a. Vulvodynia
b. Atrophic vaginitis
c. Contact dermatitis
d. Lichen sclerosus
e. Vulvar intraepithelial neoplasia (VIN)

322. You recommended that she wear loose clothing and cotton underwear and stop using tampons. After 1 month she returns, reporting that her symptoms of intense burning and pain with intercourse have not improved. Which of the following treatment options is the best next step in treating this patient's problem?

a. Podophyllin
b. Surgical excision of the vestibular glands
c. Topical lidocaine
d. Topical trichloroacetic acid
e. Valtrex therapy

Questions 323 and 324

323. A 29-year-old G0 comes to your office complaining of a vaginal discharge for the past 2 weeks. The patient describes the discharge as thin in consistency and of a grayish white color. She has also noticed a slight fishy vaginal odor that seems to have started with the appearance of the discharge. She reports no vaginal or vulvar pruritus or burning. She admits to being sexually active in the past, but has not had intercourse during the past year. She has no history of sexually transmitted diseases. The only medication she takes are oral contraceptives. Last month, she took a course of amoxicillin for the treatment of sinusitis. On physical examination, the vulva appears normal. There is a discharge present at the introitus. A copious, thin, whitish discharge is in the vaginal vault. The vaginal pH is 5.5. The cervix is not inflamed and there is no cervical discharge. Wet smear of the discharge indicates the presence of clue cells. Which of the following is the most likely diagnosis?

a. Candidiasis
b. Bacterial vaginosis
c. Trichomoniasis
d. Physiologic discharge
e. Chlamydia

324. In the patient described earlier, which of the following is the best treatment?

a. Reassurance
b. Oral diflucan
c. Doxycycline 100 mg PO twice daily for 1 week
d. Ampicillin 500 mg PO twice daily for 1 week
e. Metronidazole 500 mg PO twice daily for 1 week

Questions 325 and 326

325. A 20-year-old G2P0020 with an LMP 5 days ago presents to the emergency department with a chief complaint of a 24-hour history of increasing pelvic pain. This morning she experienced chills and fever, although she did not take her temperature. She reports no changes in her bladder or bowel habits. She has had nausea or vomiting, and has not been able to tolerate liquids. She reports no medical problems, and her only surgery was a laparoscopy performed last year for an ectopic pregnancy. She reports regular menses without dysmenorrhea. She is currently sexually active with a new sexual partner, and had intercourse with him just prior to her last menstrual period. She reports no history of abnormal Pap smears or sexually transmitted diseases. Urine pregnancy test is negative. Urinalysis is normal. WBC is 18,000. Temperature is 38.8°C (102°F). On physical examination, her abdomen is diffusely tender in the lower quadrants with rebound and voluntary guarding. Bowel sounds are present but diminished. Which of the following is the most likely diagnosis?

a. Ovarian torsion
b. Endometriosis
c. Pelvic inflammatory disease (PID)
d. Kidney stone
e. Ruptured ovarian cyst

326. Which of the following is the most appropriate initial antibiotic treatment regimen for this patient?

a. Doxycycline 100 mg PO twice daily for 14 days
b. Clindamycin 450 mg IV every 8 hours plus gentamicin 1 mg/kg load followed by 1 mg/kg every 12 hours
c. Cefoxitin 2 g IV every 6 hours with doxycycline 100 mg IV twice daily
d. Ceftriaxone 250 mg IM plus doxycycline 100 mg PO twice daily for 14 days
e. Ofloxacin 400 mg PO twice daily for 14 days plus Flagyl 500 mg PO twice daily for 14 days

327. A 43-year-old G2P2 comes to your office reporting intermittent right nipple discharge that is bloody. She says the discharge is spontaneous and not associated with any nipple pruritus, burning, or discomfort. On physical examination, you do not detect any dominant breast masses, skin changes, or axillary lymphadenopathy. Which of the following conditions is the most likely cause of this patient's problem?

a. Breast cancer
b. Duct ectasia
c. Intraductal papilloma
d. Fibrocystic breast disease
e. Pituitary adenoma

328. A 20-year-old G0, LMP 1 week ago, presents to your clinic reporting a mass in her left breast that she discovered during routine breast self-examination in the shower. When you perform a breast examination on her, you palpate a 2-cm firm, nontender mass in the upper inner quadrant of the left breast that is smooth, well-circumscribed, and mobile. You do not detect any skin changes, nipple discharge, or axillary lymphadenopathy. Which of the following is the most likely diagnosis?

a. Fibrocystic breast change
b. Fibroadenoma
c. Breast carcinoma
d. Fat necrosis
e. Cystosarcoma phyllodes

329. A 55-year-old G3P3 with a history of fibroids presents to you complaining of irregular vaginal bleeding. Until last month, she had not had a period in over 9 months. She thought she was in menopause, but because she started bleeding again last month she is not sure. Over the past month she has had irregular, spotty vaginal bleeding. The last time she bled was 1 week ago. She also complains of frequent hot flushes and emotional lability. She does not have any medical problems and is not taking any medications. She is a nonsmoker and does not consume alcohol or drugs. Her gynecologic history is significant for cryotherapy of the cervix 10 years ago for mild dysplasia. She has had three cesarean deliveries and a tubal ligation. On physical examination, her uterus is 12 weeks in size, mobile, nontender, and irregularly shaped. Her ovaries are not palpable. A urine pregnancy test is negative. Which of the following is the most reasonable next step in the evaluation of this patient?

a. Schedule her for a hysterectomy
b. Insert a progesterone-containing intrauterine device (IUD)
c. Arrange for outpatient endometrial ablation
d. Perform an office endometrial biopsy
e. Arrange for outpatient conization of the cervix

330. A 57-year-old menopausal patient presents to your office for evaluation of postmenopausal bleeding. She is morbidly obese and has chronic hypertension and adult onset diabetes. An office endometrial biopsy shows complex endometrial hyperplasia with atypia, and a pelvic ultrasound demonstrates multiple, large uterine fibroids. Which of the following is the best next step in management for this patient?

a. Myomectomy
b. Total abdominal hysterectomy
c. Hysteroscopy with dilation and curettage
d. Uterine artery embolization
e. Oral progesterone

Benign and Malignant Disorders of the Breast and Pelvis

Answers

271. The answer is c. Benign cystic teratomas (dermoids) are the most common germ cell tumors, and account for about 20% to 25% of all ovarian neoplasms. They occur primarily during the reproductive years, but may also occur in postmenopausal women and in children. Dermoids are usually unilateral, but 10% are bilateral. Usually the tumors are asymptomatic, but they can cause severe pain if there is torsion or if the sebaceous material perforates, spills, and creates a reactive peritonitis.

272. The answer is e. The survival of women who have ovarian carcinoma varies inversely with the amount of residual tumor left after the initial surgery. At the time of laparotomy, a maximum effort should be made to determine the sites of tumor spread and to excise all resectable tumor. Although the uterus and ovaries may appear grossly normal, there is a relatively high incidence of occult metastases to these organs; for this reason, they should be removed during the initial surgery. Ovarian cancer metastasizes outside the peritoneum via the pelvic or para-aortic lymphatics, and from there into the thorax and the remainder of the body. Therefore, a complete staging procedure also includes pelvic washings, pelvic and abdominal exploration for metastatic disease, appendectomy, and lymph node sampling.

273. The answer is c. Although rare, adenocarcinoma of the Bartholin gland must be excluded in women older than 40 years of age who present with a cystic or solid mass in this area. The incidence peaks in women in their sixties. The appropriate treatment in these cases is surgical excision of the Bartholin gland to allow for a careful pathologic examination. In cases of abscess formation, both marsupialization of the sac and incision with drainage as well as appropriate antibiotics are accepted modes of therapy. In the case of the asymptomatic Bartholin cyst, no treatment is necessary.

274. The answer is a. Cervical cancer is still staged clinically, not surgically. Physical examination, routine x-rays, barium enema, colposcopy, cystoscopy, proctosigmoidoscopy, and IVP are used to stage the disease. CT scan results, while clinically useful, are not used to stage the disease. The stage does not include information about lymph node involvement. Stage I disease is limited to the cervix. Stage Ia disease is preclinical (ie, microscopic), while stage Ib denotes macroscopic disease that is clinical visible. Stage II invades beyond the uterus but not to the pelvic side wall or lower third of the vagina. It may involve the upper vagina and/or the parametrium. Stage IIa denotes tumor without parametrial invasion or involvement of the lower third of the vagina, while stage IIb denotes parametrial extension. Stage III involves the lower one-third of the vagina or extends to the pelvic side wall; there is no cancer-free area between the tumor and the pelvic wall. Stage IIIa lesions have not extended to the pelvic wall, but involve the lower one-third of the vagina. Stage IIIb tumors have extension to the pelvic wall and/or are associated with hydronephrosis or a nonfunctioning kidney caused by tumor. Stage IV is outside the reproductive tract, such as invasion of the mucosa of the bladder or rectum.

275. The answer is c. An adequate colposcopy requires that the entire squamocolumnar junction and all lesions be visualized, and that the biopsies of the lesion explain the abnormal cytology. Since her colposcopy was not adequate, an excisional procedure is required.

276. The answer is c. Stage Ia1, or microinvasive carcinoma of the cervix, includes lesions stromal invasion 3 mm or less in depth and 7 mm or less in horizontal spread, with no confluent tongues or lymphatic or vascular invasion. Stage Ia2 is stromal invasion more than 3 mm but less than 5 mm, and horizontal spread less than 7 mm.

277. The answer is d. The main routes of spread of cervical cancer include vaginal mucosa, myometrium, paracervical lymphatics, and direct extension into the parametrium. The prevalence of lymph node disease correlates with the stage of malignancy. Primary node groups involved in the spread of cervical cancer include the paracervical, parametrial, obturator, hypogastric, external iliac, and sacral nodes, essentially in that order. Less commonly, there is involvement in the common iliac, inguinal, and para-aortic nodes. The presence of lymph node involvement confers a worse prognosis and impacts how the patient is managed. In stage I, the pelvic nodes are positive in approximately 15% of cases and the para-aortic nodes in 6%. In stage II, pelvic nodes are positive in 28% of cases and para-aortic nodes in 16%. In stage III, pelvic nodes are positive in 47% of cases and para-aortic nodes in 28%.

278. The answer is c. The treatment of choice for microinvasive disease in a woman who has completed childbearing is extrafascial (or simple) hysterectomy. If the patient desired fertility sparing treatment, then stage Ia1 disease may be treated with cone biopsy.

279. The answer is e. Women who have invasive vulvar carcinoma usually are treated surgically. Tumors larger than 2 cm are staged as IB. If the lesion is unilateral, is not associated with fixed or ulcerated inguinal lymph nodes, and does not involve the urethra, vagina, anus, or rectum, then treatment usually consists of radical excision and unilateral inguinal lymphadenectomy. The risk of inguinal node metastasis is around 8%. Inguinal lymphadenectomy involves removal of the superficial inguinal and deep femoral lymph nodes. Unilateral rather than bilateral lymphadenectomy decreases postoperative morbidity. The lymph nodes should be sent intraoperatively for frozen section, and if positive, a bilateral lymphadenectomy should be performed. Radiation therapy, though not a routine part of the management of women who have early vulvar carcinoma, is employed in the treatment of women who have local, advanced carcinoma.

280. The answer is b. Patients with multiple comorbidities who are not considered surgical candidates should be treated with radiation therapy. In some institutions, chemoradiation is preferred, but there is not good data to recommend that routinely.

281. The answer is c. Breast cancer is the most common type of malignancy detected during pregnancy, affecting approximately 1 in 3,000 pregnant women. This is thought to be at least partially due to the fact that more women are choosing to have children later in life, and the risk of breast cancer increases with age.

282. The answer is b. Cervical cancer is one of the more common malignancies found during pregnancy. Management of cervical intraepithelial lesions is complicated in pregnancy because of increased vascularity of the cervix and because of the concern that manipulation of and trauma to the cervix can compromise continuation of the pregnancy. A traditional cone biopsy is indicated in the presence of apparent microinvasive disease on a colposcopically directed cervical biopsy. Otherwise, more limited procedures such as shallow cervical biopsies are more appropriate. If invasive cancer is diagnosed, the decision to treat immediately or wait until fetal viability depends in part on the gestational age at which the diagnosis is made, and the severity of the disorder. Survival is decreased for malignancies discovered later in pregnancy. Radiation therapy almost always results in spontaneous abortion, in part because the fetus is particularly radiosensitive. Chemotherapy is associated with higher than expected rates of fetal malformations consistent with the antimetabolite effects of agents used. Specific malformations depend on the agent used and the time in pregnancy at which the exposure occurs.

283. The answer is c. Most ovarian malignancies are not found until significant spread has occurred; therefore it is not unreasonable to further evaluate patients as soon as there is a suspicion of an ovarian neoplasm. Pelvic ultrasonography, tumor markers, and even surgical exploration may be part of the evaluation of a patient with an ovarian mass. Pelvic ultrasound findings of internal ovarian papillary vegetations, ovarian size greater than 10 cm, the presence of ascites, possible ovarian torsion, or solid ovarian lesions are indications for exploratory laparotomy in the postmenopausal patient. In a younger woman, a cyst can be followed past one menstrual cycle to determine if it is a follicular cyst, since a follicular cyst should regress after onset of the next menstrual period. If regression does not occur, then surgery is appropriate. Doppler ultrasound imaging allows visualization of arterial and venous flow patterns superimposed on the image of the structure being examined; arterial and venous flow are expected in a normal ovary.

284. The answer is b. An important feature of the lymphatic drainage of the vulva is the existence of drainage across the midline. The vulva drains first into the superficial inguinal lymph nodes, then into the deep femoral nodes, and finally into the external iliac lymph nodes. The clinical significance of this sequence for patients with carcinoma of the vulva is that the iliac nodes are probably free of the disease if the deep femoral nodes are not involved. Unlike the lymphatic drainage from the rest of the vulva, the drainage from the clitoral region bypasses the superficial inguinal nodes and passes directly to the deep femoral nodes. Thus, while the superficial nodes usually also have metastases when the deep femoral nodes are implicated, it is possible for only the deep nodes to be involved if the carcinoma is in the midline near the clitoris.

285. The answer is a. One half to two-thirds of ovarian neoplasms in young women in their teens and early twenties are of germ cell origin. Epithelial tumors of the ovary are quite rare in prepubertal girls. Papillary serous cystadenocarcinoma is an example of a malignant epithelial tumor and would be very uncommon in a girl of this age. Stromal tumors (such as fibrosarcoma) and Brenner tumors are not usually seen in this age group. Sarcoma botryoides, a tumor seen in children, is a malignancy associated with Müllerian structures such as the vagina and uterus, including the uterine cervix.

286. The answer is c. Serous carcinoma is the most common epithelial tumor of the ovary. Bilateral involvement characterizes about one-third of all serous carcinomas.

287. The answer is e. The prevalence of lichen sclerosus is unknown, because some women with this condition may be asymptomatic. The exact etiology is unknown, but there may be an autoimmune or genetic component. Patients with lichen sclerosus of the vulva tend to be older, and they typically present with pruritus, irritation, burning, dyspareunia, and tearing. On examination, the lesions are usually white papules and plaques, often with areas of ecchymosis or purpura. The skin often appears thinned, whitened, and crinkling. There may also be fusion of the labia minora, phimosis of the clitoral hood, and fissures, all of which can lead to narrowing of the introitus and dyspareunia. The histologic appearance of lichen sclerosus includes loss of the rete pegs within the dermis, chronic inflammatory infiltrate below the dermis, the development of a homogenous subepithelial layer in the dermis, a decrease in the number of cellular layers, and a decrease in the number of melanocytes. Lichen sclerosus is not a premalignant lesion; however, women with it have an increased risk of vulvar malignancy, and it must be distinguished from vulvar squamous cancer. Therefore, biopsy is necessary to confirm the diagnosis. First line therapy is ultrapotent corticosteroids such as clobetasol, halobetasol, or diflorasone. Topical estrogen may also be indicated if labial adhesions are present. Experience with intralesional corticosteroids is limited and is not recommended for first-line therapy. Surgical intervention is reserved for cases associated with malignancy or disease unresponsive to medical therapy.

288 and 289.   The answers are 288-c and 289-a. The HPVs are a group of double-stranded DNA viruses that infect epithelial cells. They do not cause systemic infection. There are numerous viruses within the group, and they are named by number according to the order of their discovery. HPVs can be sexually transmitted. HPV 16 has the highest carcinogenic potential and accounts for approximately 55% to 60% of cases of cervical cancer. HPV 18 is the next most carcinogenic type, and accounts for 10% to 15% of cases of cervical cancer. Approximately 10 other genotypes of HPV are associated with the remaining cases of cervical cancer. HPV types 6 and 11 are considered "low risk" subtypes, and are associated with benign condyloma and low grade cervical lesions. Women with condyloma are at an increased risk for anogenital cancers.

290 to 295.   The answers are 290-b, 291-a, 292-e, 293-d, 294-c, 295-e. Sertoli-Leydig cell tumors, which represent less than 1% of ovarian tumors, may produce symptoms of virilization. Histologically, they resemble fetal testes; clinically, they must be distinguished from other functioning ovarian neoplasms as well as tumors of the adrenal glands, since both adrenal tumors and Sertoli-Leydig tumors produce androgens. The androgen production can result in seborrhea, acne, menstrual irregularity, hirsutism, breast atrophy, alopecia, deepening of the voice, and clitoromegaly. Granulosa and theca cell tumors are often associated with excessive estrogen production, which may cause pseudoprecocious puberty, postmenopausal bleeding, or menorrhagia. These tumors are associated with endometrial carcinoma in 15% of patients. Because these tumors are quite friable, affected women may present with symptoms caused by tumor rupture and intraperitoneal bleeding. Gonadoblastomas frequently contain calcifications that can be detected by plain radiography of the pelvis. Women who have gonadoblastomas often have ambiguous genitalia. The tumors are usually small, and are bilateral in one-third of affected women. The malignant potential of immature teratomas correlates with the degree of immature or embryonic tissue present. The presence of choriocarcinoma can be determined histologically as well as by human chorionic gonadotropin (hCG) assays. The presence of choriocarcinoma in an immature teratoma worsens the prognosis. Krukenberg tumors are typically bilateral, solid masses of the ovary that nearly always represent metastases from another organ, usually the stomach or large intestine. They contain large numbers of signet ring adenocarcinoma cells within a cellular hyper-plastic but nonneoplastic ovarian stroma.

296 to 301. The answers are 296-a, 297-b, 298-j, 299-e, 300-h, 301-i. Cyclophosphamide is an alkylating agent that cross-links DNA and also inhibits DNA synthesis. Hemorrhagic cystitis and alopecia are common side effects. Cisplatin causes renal damage and neural toxicity, therefore patients must be well hydrated. Its mode of action does not fit a specific category. Paclitaxel can produce allergic reactions and bone marrow depression. Bleomycin and doxorubicin are antibiotics whose side effects are pulmonary fibrosis and cardiac toxicity, respectively. Vincristine arrests cells in metaphase by binding microtubular proteins and preventing the formation of mitotic spindles. Peripheral neuropathy is a common side effect.

302 to 308. The answers are 302-f, 303-a, 304-g, 305-e, 306-c, 307-b, 308-d. The tumor in question 302 is an opened mature cystic teratoma (dermoid tumor), in which hair is visible.

The microscopic section in question 303 is a classical example of well-differentiated adenocarcinoma of the endometrium, showing cellular pleomorphism, nuclear atypia with mitoses, and back-to-back crowding of glands with obliteration of intervening stroma; the glandular architecture of the tissue is maintained. Endometrial cancer is categorized by both stage and grade. The differentiation of a carcinoma is expressed as its grade. Grade I lesions are well-differentiated; grade II lesions are moderately well-differentiated; grade III lesions are poorly differentiated. An increasing grade (ie, a decreasing degree of differentiation) implies worsening prognosis. Tumors may be of a mixed cell type—for example, squamous and adenocarcinoma—or may be mucinous, serous, or clear.

Question 304 shows clear cell adenocarcinoma with large, pale staining cells. Clear cell carcinoma of the endometrium is similar to that arising in the cervix, vagina, and ovary, and the histologic appearance is similar in each of these organs. Diethylstilbestrol exposure has been associated with an increased incidence of vaginal and cervical clear cell carcinomas. The tumor's origins are suggested to be mesonephric duct remnants. The microscopic appearance of clear cell carcinoma is related to deposits of periodic acid–Schiff (PAS) stain–positive glycogen. These tumors characteristically occur in older women and are very aggressive.

The section in question 305 shows uterine carcinosarcoma, which used to be called mixed Müllerian tumors. These tumors have a combination of heterologous elements—that is, tissue of different sources (cartilage in this picture).

Question 306 is an example of choriocarcinoma, showing sheets of malignant trophoblasts. Malignant choriocarcinoma is a transformation of molar tissue or a de novo lesion arising from the placenta. There are significant degrees of cellular pleomorphism and anaplasia. Choriocarcinoma can be differentiated from invasive mole by the fact that the latter has chorionic villi and the former does not.

Questions 307 and 308 show early to midproliferative endometrium and late secretory endometrium, respectively. Proliferative and late secretory endometrium can be differentiated by the development of glandular tissue and secretory patterns. In question 307, the glands are just beginning to proliferate, and the section cuts through several coils as they course toward the surface epithelium on the left. In question 309, the glands are dilated and filled with amorphous (glycogen) material.

309. The answer is c. Recognition of the high risk associated with axillary node metastases for early death and poor 5-year survival has led to the use of postsurgical adjuvant chemotherapy in these patients. Patients who have estrogen- or progesterone-receptive tumors (ie, receptor present or receptor-positive) are particular candidates for this adjuvant therapy, as 60% of estrogen-positive tumors will respond to hormonal therapy. Age and size of the tumor are certainly factors of importance, but they are secondary to the presence or absence of axillary metastases.

310. The answer is c. In young, menstruating women the most common reason for an enlargement of one ovary is the presence of a functional ovarian cyst. Functional cysts are physiologic, forming during the normal functioning of the ovaries. Follicular cysts are usually asymptomatic, unilateral, thin-walled, and filled with a watery, straw-colored fluid. Corpus luteum cysts are less common than follicular cysts. They are usually unilateral, but often appear complex, as they may be hemorrhagic. Patients with a corpus luteum cyst may complain of dull pain on the side of the affected ovary. Theca lutein cysts are the least common of the three types of functional ovarian cysts. They are almost always bilateral and are associated with pregnancy. Since the most common cause of a unilateral, asymptomatic ovarian cyst in a young, menstruating woman is a functional cyst, it is most reasonable to follow the patient conservatively and have her return after 1 to 2 months to recheck her ovary. More aggressive primary management with surgery is not indicated in a young, asymptomatic patient. CT scanning or pelvic ultrasonography may be indicated if the cyst is persistent. CA-125 is a cancer antigen expressed by approximately 80% of ovarian epithelial carcinomas. CA-125 testing is not very specific in women of childbearing age and is not useful for primary evaluation of an ovarian cyst in a young, asymptomatic patient. CA-125 testing is valuable in evaluating postmenopausal women with pelvic masses and in assessing treatment response in women undergoing treatment for CA-125 producing ovarian cancers.

311. The answer is e. The lesions are most likely condyloma acuminata, also known as venereal warts. Condyloma acuminata are squamous lesions caused by a HPV, most commonly HPV 6 and 11. Treatment options include chemical or physical destruction, immune therapy, and surgical therapy. Self treatment with imiquimod, an immune modulator, is considered first line treatment for most simple condyloma. Other options for chemical destruction include in-office application of podophyllin or trichloroacetic acid. Surgical therapy could include laser therapy or excision. Podophyllum is not recommended for extensive disease because of toxicity (peripheral neuropathy). As this patient has large, bleeding lesions, local excision is the best treatment option.

312. The answer is d. Syphilis is a chronic disease produced by the spirochete *Treponema pallidum*. Because of the spirochete's extreme thinness, it is difficult to detect by light microscopy; therefore, spirochetes in the lesion exudate or tissue are diagnosed by use of a specially adapted technique known as dark-field microscopy. Clinically, syphilis is divided into primary, secondary, and tertiary (or late) stages. In primary syphilis a chancre develops. This is a painless ulcer with raised edges and an indurated base that is usually found on the vulva, vagina, or cervix. Secondary syphilis is the result of hematogenous dissemination of the spirochetes and thus is a systemic disease. There are a number of systemic symptoms depending on the major organs involved. The classic rash of secondary syphilis is red macules and papules over the palms of the hands and the soles of the feet. Secondary syphilis may also be manifest by mucocutaneous lesions or lymphadenopathy. The manifestations of tertiary, or late, syphilis include optic atrophy, tabes dorsalis, generalized paresis, aortic aneurysm, and gummas of the skin and bones.

313. The answer is b. LGV is a chronic infection produced by *C trachomatis*. It is most commonly found in the tropics. The primary infection begins as a painless ulcer on the labia or vaginal vestibule; the patient usually consults the physician several weeks after the development of painful adenopathy in the inguinal and perirectal areas. Diagnosis can be established by culture or by demonstrating the presence of serum antibodies to *C trachomatis*. The differential diagnosis includes syphilis, chancroid, granuloma inguinale, carcinoma, and herpes. Chancroid is a sexually transmitted disease caused by *H ducreyi* that produces a painful, tender ulceration of the vulva. Donovan bodies are present in patients with granuloma inguinale, which is caused by *C granulomatis*. Therapy for both granuloma inguinale and LGV is administration of doxycycline. Chancroid is successfully treated with either azithromycin or ceftriaxone.

314. The answer is c. Persons at high risk for infection by HIV include homosexuals, bisexual males, women having sex with a bisexual or homosexual male partner, intravenous drug users, and hemophiliacs. African Americans are the racial/ethnic group most affected by HIV in the United States. Gay, bisexual, and other men who have sex with men account for the majority of new infections despite making up only 2% of the population. The virus can be transmitted through sexual contact, use of contaminated needles or blood products, and perinatal transmission from mother to child. The antibody titer usually becomes positive 2 to 8 weeks after exposure, and the presence of the antibody provides no protection against AIDS. Because of occasional delayed appearance of the antibody after initial exposure, if the initial test is negative, a repeat HIV screening test should be repeated at least 3 months after the likely exposure.

315. The answer is d. The occurrence of cervical squamous dysplasia/carcinoma is caused by infection with the HPV, which is sexually transmitted. HPV causes genital warts as well. Women who begin sexual activity at a young age, have multiple sexual partners, do not use condoms, and have a history of sexually transmitted diseases are at an increased risk for cervical neoplasia. Alterations in immune function (such as in patients with HIV or on immunosuppressive therapy) place a patient at an increased risk of cervical neoplasia. Women who smoke tobacco have an increased risk of developing cervical dysplasia. There is no known increased risk of cervical dysplasia caused by the use of Depo-Provera.

316 to 320. The answers are 316-e, 317-f, 318-g, 319-a, 320-c. Knowledge of the natural history, epidemiology, and basic science of HPV and precancerous lesions of the cervix is rapidly evolving; in fact, the guidelines have been revised many times over the last 10 years to incorporate this new evidence. Women younger than 21 years should not be screened. The guidelines have changed significantly for the management of abnormal Pap smears in women between the ages of 21 and 24 years. For women aged 21 to 24 years with LSIL cytology results, follow up Pap smear is recommended in 1 year because the risk of malignancy is low and the rate of viral clearance is high. However, for women in this age range with HSIL cytology results, colposcopy is recommended. Approximately 0.5% of Pap smears come back with glandular cell abnormalities such as atypical glandular cells (AGC). These abnormalities can be associated with squamous lesions, adenocarcinoma in situ, or invasive adenocarcinoma. Therefore, any patient with AGS should undergo colposcopy and endocervical curettage. In addition, women older than 35 years, or women younger than 35 with clinical risk of endometrial neoplasia (ie, unexplained vaginal bleeding, chronic anovulation), should undergo endometrial sampling. Women with biopsy proven CIN III should undergo excisional procedure such as a cone biopsy. The indications for a cone biopsy would be as follows: (1) unsatisfactory colposcopic examination (ie, the entire transformation zone cannot be seen), (2) a colposcopically directed cervical biopsy that indicates severe dysplasia or the possibility of invasive disease, (3) neoplasm in the endocervix, or (4) cells seen on cervical biopsy that do not adequately explain the cells seen on cytologic examination (ie, the Pap). A woman with normal cytology but a report of absent endocervical cells suggests that there is adequate cellularity for interpretation but lack of adequate cells from the transformation zone. These women may be at an increased risk for missed disease, but there is not a higher risk for CIN II or higher over time. Therefore, the next step is to perform an HPV test, and if negative, return to routine screening.

321 and 322. The answers are 321-a, 322-c. Vulvodynia is a syndrome of unknown etiology that is defined as vulvar discomfort in the absence of reliable visible findings or a specific neurologic disorder. It may be provoked (ie, with intercourse), unprovoked, or mixed. To treat vulvodynia, the first step is to avoid tight clothing, tampons, hot tubs, and soaps, which can all act as vulvar irritants. If this fails, topical treatments include lidocaine, estrogen, and steroids. Tricyclic antidepressants and intralesional interferon injections have also been used. For women refractory to medical therapy, surgical excision of the vestibular mucosa may be helpful. Valtrex (valacyclovir) is an antiviral medication used in the treatment of genital herpes and is not indicated for vulvodynia. Contact dermatitis is an inflammation and irritation of the vulvar skin caused by a chemical irritant. The vulvar skin is usually red, swollen, and inflamed, and may become weeping and eczemoid. Women with a contact dermatitis usually experience chronic vulvar tenderness, burning, and itching that can occur even when they are not engaging in intercourse. Atrophic vaginitis is a thinning and ulceration of the vaginal mucosa that occurs as a result of hypoestrogenism; thus this condition is usually seen in postmenopausal women not on hormone replacement therapy. Lichen sclerosus is another atrophic condition of the vulva. It is characterized by diffuse, thin, whitish epithelial areas on the labia majora, minora, clitoris, and perineum. In severe cases, it may be difficult to identify normal anatomic landmarks. The most common symptom of lichen sclerosus is chronic vulvar pruritus. VIN are precancerous lesions of the vulva that are usually HPV related and can progress to cancer. Women with VIN complain of vulvar pruritus, chronic irritation, and raised lesions. These lesions are most commonly located along the posterior vulva and in the perineal body and have a whitish cast and rough texture.

323 and 324. The answers are 323-b, 324-e. Bacterial vaginosis (BV) is a condition in which there is an overgrowth of anaerobic bacteria in the vagina, displacing the normal lactobacillus. Women with this type of vaginitis complain of an unpleasant vaginal odor that is described as musky or fishy, and a thin, gray-white vaginal discharge. Vulvar irritation and pruritus are rarely present. To confirm the diagnosis of bacterial vaginosis, a wet prep is performed by mixing with the vaginal discharge, spreading it on a glass slide, and identifying clue cells on microscopy. Clue cells are vaginal epithelial cells with clusters of bacteria adherent to their surfaces. In addition, a whiff test can be performed by mixing potassium hydroxide with the vaginal discharge. In cases of bacterial vaginosis, an amine-like (ie, fishlike) odor will be detected. The treatment of choice for BV is metronidazole (Flagyl) 500 mg given twice daily for 7 days. Pregnant women with symptomatic BV should be treated the same way as nonpregnant women with BV. In cases of a normal or physiologic discharge, vaginal secretions are white and odorless. In addition, normal vaginal secretions do not adhere to the vaginal side walls. In cases of candidiasis, patients commonly complain of vulvar burning, pain, pruritus, and erythema. The vaginal discharge tends to be white, clumpy, and adherent to the vaginal walls. A wet prep with potassium hydroxide can confirm the diagnosis by the identification of hyphae. Treatment of candidiasis can be achieved with the administration of topical imidazoles or triazoles, or the oral medication Diflucan (fluconazole). *Trichomonas vaginitis* is the most common nonviral, nonchlamydial sexually transmitted disease in women. It is caused by the anaerobic, flagellated protozoan *T vaginalis.* Women with *T vaginitis* commonly complain of a copious vaginal discharge that may be white, yellow, green, or gray, and that has an unpleasant odor. Some women complain of vulvar pruritus, which is primarily confined to the vestibule and labia minora. On physical examination, the vulva and vagina frequently appear red and swollen. Only a small percentage of women possess the classically described "strawberry cervix." The diagnosis of trichomoniasis is confirmed with a wet saline smear. Under the microscope, the Trichomonas organisms can be visualized; these organisms are unicellular protozoans that are spherical in shape with three to five flagella extending from one end. The recommended treatment for trichomoniasis is a one-time dose of metronidazole 2 g orally. *C trachomatis* is an intracellular parasite that can cause an infection that may be manifested as cervicitis, urethritis, or salpingitis. Patients with chlamydial infections may be asymptomatic. On physical examination, women with chlamydial infections may demonstrate a mucopurulent cervicitis. The diagnosis of chlamydia is suspected on clinical examination and confirmed with cervical cultures. Treatment for a chlamydial cervicitis is with oral azithromycin 1 g or doxycycline 100 mg twice daily for 7 days.

325 and 326. The answers are 325-c, 326-c. The patient is most likely to have PID. Ovarian torsion, appendicitis, and acute salpingitis are all commonly associated with fever, abdominal pain, and elevated white blood cell count. Ruptured ovarian cysts present with acute abdominal pain without fever. Ovarian torsion usually presents as waxing and waning pain that is associated with an adnexal mass. Pain from ruptured ovarian cysts may occur at any time throughout the menstrual cycle but often present around the time of ovulation. Although appendicitis is in the differential diagnosis in any woman presenting with abdominal pain and fever, this patients specific pain history, examination, and associated symptoms are less consistent with appendicitis. In cases of kidney stone, urinalysis usually indicates the presence of blood and there is often flank pain. PID should be managed as an inpatient with intravenous antibiotics in cases where the patient cannot tolerate oral therapy, has not been compliant with oral therapy, has failed oral therapy, or has severe illness with high fever and pain. Outpatient oral therapy may be appropriate for patients with PID who have more mild to moderate symptoms. The decision for inpatient versus outpatient treatment of a patient with PID depends on several factors such as patient compliance, tolerance of oral medications, and certainty of diagnosis. Given this patient's symptoms, the best treatment for this patient is inpatient intravenous antibiotics. A TOA may form in a patient with untreated PID. A patient with a TOA should also be initially hospitalized and treated with intravenous antibiotics. Patients with TOAs, who do not improve on broad-spectrum antibiotics, may require drainage of the abscesses by laparotomy, laparoscopy, or percutaneously under CT guidance.

The recommendation of Centers for Disease Control for inpatient management of PID includes the following:

1. Cefoxitin 2 g IV every 6 hours OR cefotetan 2 g IV every 12 hours PLUS doxycycline 100 mg PO or IV twice daily

OR

2. Clindamycin 900 mg IV every 8 hours PLUS gentamicin loading dose IV or IM (2 mg/kg) followed by maintenance dose (1.5 mg/kg) every 8 hours. Single daily dosing (3-5mg/kg) may be substituted.

The recommendation of Centers for Disease Control for the outpatient management of PID includes the following:

1. Cefoxitin 2 g IM plus probenecid 1 g PO in a single dose concurrently OR ceftriaxone 250 mg IM PLUS doxycycline 100 mg PO twice daily for 14 days WITH OR WITHOUT metronidazole 500 mg PO twice daily for 14 days.

327. The answer is c. Nipple discharge can occur in women with either benign or malignant breast conditions. Approximately 10% to 15% of women with benign breast disease complain of nipple discharge. Nipple discharge is present in only about 3% of women with breast malignancies. The most worrisome nipple discharges tend to be spontaneous, unilateral, and persistent. The color of nipple discharge does not differentiate benign from malignant breast conditions. The most common breast disorder associated with a bloody nipple discharge is an intraductal papilloma. However, breast carcinoma must always be ruled out in any patient complaining of a bloody nipple discharge. Sanguineous or serosanguineous nipple discharges can also be seen in women with duct ectasia and fibrocystic breast disease. Women with hyperprolactinemia caused by a pituitary adenoma experience bilateral milky white nipple discharges.

328. The answer is b. This patient's breast mass is characteristic of a fibroadenoma. Fibroadenomas are the second most common benign breast disorder, after fibrocystic changes. Fibroadenomas are characterized by the presence of a firm, solid, well-circumscribed, nontender, freely mobile mass, and have an average diameter of 2.5 cm. These lesions most commonly occur in adolescents and women in their twenties. Fibrocystic changes occur in about one-third to one-half of reproductive-age women and represent an exaggerated response of the breast tissue to hormones. Patients with fibrocystic changes complain of bilateral mastalgia and breast engorgement preceding menses. On physical examination, diffuse bilateral nodularity is typically encountered. Cystosarcoma phyllodes are rare fibroepithelial tumors that constitute 1% of breast malignancies. These rapidly growing tumors are the most frequent breast sarcoma and occur most frequently in women in the fifth decade of life. Trauma to the breast can result in fat necrosis. Women with fat necrosis commonly present to the physician with a firm, tender mass that is surrounded by ecchymosis. Occasional skin retraction can occur, making this lesion difficult to differentiate from cancer. It is unlikely that this patient who presents in her twenties has breast cancer. Fine-needle aspiration or excisional biopsy may be performed to rule out the rare chance of malignancy, but breast cancer is not the most likely diagnosis based on the patient's age and lack of any other breast changes consistent with carcinoma (such as a fixed mass, skin retraction, or lymphadenopathy).

329. The answer is d. Given this patient's age and symptoms, she is probably undergoing menopausal transition or "perimenopause." Menopause is defined as the absence of menses for 12 months. Women with perimenopausal or postmenopausal bleeding should be evaluated with an endometrial biopsy to rule out hyperplasia or malignancy. A pelvic ultrasound may also be helpful to provide information regarding the size and location of any uterine fibroids. In addition, the endometrial stripe thickness could be evaluated (it should be less than 5 mm in a postmenopausal patient). Endometrial polyps as a cause for her irregular bleeding may be diagnosed with an office hysteroscopy or a saline infusion sonohysterogram. Conization of the cervix is performed for evaluation and treatment of severe cervical dysplasia, and is not indicated in this patient. Progesterone-containing IUDs may be used for contraception or for the treatment of menorrhagia. Endometrial ablation is used to treat heavy menstrual bleeding in premenopausal patients. There is no indication for hysterectomy.

330. The answer is c. Postmenopausal patients with atypical complex hyperplasia of the endometrium have a 25% to 30% risk of having an associated endometrial carcinoma in the uterus. Given the high risk of malignancy, the next best step in management is hysteroscopy with dilation and curettage. This allows the entire uterus to be evaluated for malignancy. If there is no malignancy on the D&C pathology, the next best step in a patient who has completed childbearing or who is menopausal is simple hysterectomy. If a malignancy is identified on the D&C specimen, the patient would be referred to a gynecologic oncologist for a staging surgery, which includes hysterectomy. If hysterectomy is not medically advisable, progesterone treatment can be used. Myomectomy, or surgical removal of fibroid, is a treatment option for premenopausal women with symptomatic uterine fibroids. There is no role for the use of oral contraceptives in the treatment of postmenopausal bleeding.

Suggested Readings

American College of Obstetricians and Gynecologists. *Diagnosis and Management of Vulvar Skin Disorders.* Practice Bulletin Number 93, May 2008, reaffirmed 2013.

American College of Obstetricians and Gynecologists. *Management of Abnormal Cervical Cancer Screening Test Results and Cervical Cancer Precursors.* Practice Bulletin Number 140, December 2013.

American College of Obstetricians and Gynecologists. *Management of Adnexal Masses.* Practice Bulletin Number 83, July 2007, reaffirmed 2013.

2015 Sexually Transmitted Disease Treatment Guidelines. Centers for Disease Control. www.cdc.gov

DiSaia PJ, Creasman WT. Chapter 3: Invasive cervical cancer; Chapter 8: Invasive cancer of the vulva; Chapter 11: Epithelial ovarian cancer; Chapter 15: Cancer in pregnancy; Chapter 16: Complication of disease and therapy; Chapter 17: Basic principles of chemotherapy. *Clinical Gynecologic Oncology.* Philadelphia, PA: Elsevier Saunders, 2012.

Infertility, Endocrinology, and Menstrual Dysfunction

Questions

331. A mother brings her 14-year-old daughter to the office for consultation. The mother is concerned that her daughter is shorter than her friends, and should have started her period by now. On physical examination, the girl is 4 ft 10 in tall. She shows evidence of breast development at Tanner stage 2. She has no axillary or pubic hair. You reassure the mother that her daughter seems to be developing normally. Educating the mother and daughter, your best advice is to tell them which of the following?

a. The daughter will start her period when her breasts reach Tanner stage 5.
b. The daughter will start her period, then have her growth spurt.
c. The daughter's period should start within 1 to 2 years since she has just started developing breast buds.
d. The daughter will have her growth spurt, then pubic hair will develop, heralding the onset of menstruation.
e. The daughter's period should start by the age of 18 years, but if she has not had her period by then, she should come back for further evaluation.

332. A mother brings her 12-year-old daughter to your office for consultation. She is concerned because most of the other girls in her daughter's class have already started their period. She thinks her daughter hasn't shown any evidence of going into puberty yet. Knowing the usual first sign of the onset of puberty, you should ask the mother which of the following questions?

a. Has your daughter had any acne?
b. Has your daughter started to develop breasts?
c. Does your daughter have any axillary or pubic hair?
d. Has your daughter started her growth spurt?
e. Has your daughter had any vaginal spotting?

333. A 9-year-old girl presents for evaluation of regular vaginal bleeding. History reveals thelarche at the age of 7 and adrenarche at the age of 8. Which of the following is the most common cause of this condition in girls?

a. Idiopathic
b. Gonadal tumors
c. McCune-Albright syndrome
d. Hypothyroidism
e. Tumors of the central nervous system (CNS)

Questions 334 to 336

A 68-year-old Caucasian woman comes to your office for advice regarding her risk factors for developing osteoporosis. She is 5 ft 1 in tall and weighs 105 lb. She stopped having periods at the age of 42 years. She is healthy and walks on a treadmill daily. She does not take any medications. She has never taken hormone replacement therapy (HRT). Her mother died at the age of 71 after she suffered a spontaneous hip fracture.

334. Which of the following will have the least effect on this patient's risk for developing osteoporosis?

a. Her family history
b. Her race
c. Her level of physical activity
d. Her early menopause status
e. Her weight

335. The patient asks how and if she should be tested for osteoporosis. What is the best method to screen her for osteoporosis?

a. Peripheral measurement of her heel with photon absorptiometry
b. Standard x-ray of her spine
c. Dual-energy x-ray absorptiometry (DEXA)
d. Measure biochemical markers of bone remodeling
e. CT scan to measure the bone density

336. The patient has a DEXA study that demonstrates a T-score of –2.0. What is the best next step in management?

a. Begin a bisphosphonate
b. Encourage her to engage in weight bearing exercise and take a calcium supplement
c. Repeat the study in 1 year
d. Begin raloxifene therapy
e. Recommend she begin combined HRT

Questions 337 and 338

For each of the following patient, select the most ideal treatment for dysmenorrhea. Each lettered option may be used once, more than once, or not at all.

a. Acupuncture
b. Prostaglandin inhibitors
c. Gonadotropin-releasing hormone (GnRH) analogues
d. Oral contraceptives
e. Narcotic analgesics

337. A 17-year-old consults you for evaluation of disabling pain with her menstrual periods. The pain has been present since menarche, and is accompanied by nausea and headache. Her medical history is otherwise unremarkable, and pelvic examination is normal. She is not currently sexually active, and she has not tried any therapy for her dysmenorrhea.

338. A 19-year-old college student is seen for severe primary dysmenorrhea. She has no medical problems and a normal pelvic examination. A heating pad has not helped her pain. She has recently become sexually active and does not currently desire pregnancy.

339. An 18-year-old patient presents to you for evaluation because she has not yet started her period. On physical examination, she is 5 ft 7 in tall. She has minimal breast development and no axillary or pubic hair. On pelvic examination, she has a normally developed vagina. A cervix is visible. The uterus is palpable, as are normal ovaries. Which of the following is the best next step in the evaluation of this patient?

a. Draw her blood for a karyotype.
b. Test her sense of smell.
c. Draw her blood for TSH, FSH, and LH levels.
d. Order an MRI of the brain to evaluate the pituitary gland.
e. Prescribe a progesterone challenge to see if she will have a withdrawal bleed.

Questions 340 and 341

A 7-year-old girl is brought in to see you by her mother because the girl has developed breasts and a few pubic hairs. Evaluation demonstrates a pubertal response to a GnRH-stimulation test and a prominent increase in luteinizing hormone (LH) pulses during sleep.

340. These findings are characteristic of patients with which of the following?
a. Theca cell tumors
b. Iatrogenic sexual precocity
c. Premature thelarche
d. Granulosa cell tumors
e. Central precocious puberty

341. Which of the following is the best treatment for the girl's condition?
a. Exogenous gonadotropins
b. Ethinyl estradiol
c. GnRH agonists
d. Clomiphene citrate
e. No treatment; reassure the mother that pubertal symptoms at the age of 7 years are normal

342. A mother brings her daughter to see you for consultation. The daughter is 17 years old and has not started her period. She is 4 ft 10 in tall. On physical examination, she has no breast buds or pubic hair. Her pelvic examination demonstrates a uterus and cervix, but the ovaries are not palpable. As part of the workup, serum FSH and LH levels are drawn and both are high. Which of the following is the most likely reason for delayed puberty in this patient?
a. Testicular feminization
b. McCune-Albright syndrome
c. Kallmann syndrome
d. Gonadal dysgenesis
e. Müllerian agenesis

343. While evaluating a 30-year-old woman for infertility, you diagnose a bicornuate uterus. You explain that additional testing is necessary because of the woman's increased risk of congenital anomalies in which organ system?
a. Skeletal
b. Hematopoietic

c. Urinary
d. Central nervous
e. Tracheoesophageal

344. A 47-year-old G3P3 complains of severe menstrual cramps and heavy menstrual bleeding. Her dysmenorrhea has worsened since the birth of her last child. Pelvic examination demonstrates a tender, diffusely enlarged uterus with no adnexal tenderness. Results of endometrial biopsy are normal. Which of the following is the most likely diagnosis?

a. Endometriosis
b. Endometritis
c. Adenomyosis
d. Uterine sarcoma
e. Leiomyoma

345. A 28-year-old G3P0 has a history of severe menstrual cramps, prolonged, heavy periods, chronic pelvic pain, and painful intercourse. All of her pregnancies were spontaneous abortions in the first trimester. A hysterosalpingogram (HSG) she just had as part of the evaluation for recurrent abortion showed a large uterine septum. You have recommended surgical repair of the uterus. Of the patient's symptoms, which is most likely to be corrected by resection of the uterine septum?

a. Habitual abortion
b. Dysmenorrhea
c. Menometrorrhagia
d. Dyspareunia
e. Chronic pelvic pain

346. In the evaluation of a 26-year-old patient with 4 months of secondary amenorrhea, you order serum prolactin and β-hCG assays. The β-hCG test is positive, and the prolactin level is 100 ng/mL (normal is < 25 ng/mL in nonpregnant women in this assay). This patient requires which of the following?

a. Routine obstetric care
b. Computed tomography (CT) scan of her brain to rule out pituitary adenoma
c. Repeat measurements of serum prolactin to ensure that values do not increase more than 300 ng/mL
d. Bromocriptine to suppress prolactin
e. Evaluation for possible hypothyroidism

347. You have just performed diagnostic laparoscopy on a 28-year-old patient with chronic pelvic pain and dyspareunia. At the time of the laparoscopy, there were multiple implants of endometriosis on the uterosacral ligaments and ovaries. At the time of the procedure, you ablated all of the visible lesions on the peritoneal surfaces with the CO_2 laser. Because of the extent of the patient's disease, you recommend postoperative medical treatment. Which of the following medications is the best option for the treatment of this patient's endometriosis?

a. Continuous oral estrogen
b. Non-steroidal anti-inflammatories (NSAIDs)
c. Danazol
d. A GnRH agonist
e. Combined oral contraceptive pills

348. A 28-year-old nulligravid patient complains of bleeding between her periods and increasingly heavy menses. Over the past 9 months, a trial of oral contraceptives and NSAIDs have failed to decrease the heavy bleeding. Which of the following options is most appropriate at this time?

a. Perform a hysterectomy.
b. Perform hysteroscopy.
c. Perform endometrial ablation.
d. Treat with a GnRH agonist.
e. Start the patient on a high-dose progestational agent.

349. A 26-year-old P0 presents to you for evaluation of infertility. She and her husband have been trying to get pregnant for 2 years. As part of the workup, her husband had a normal semen analysis. The patient has a history of endometriosis diagnosed by laparoscopy at the age of 17 due to severe pelvic pain and dysmenorrhea. After the surgery, the patient was told she had a few small implants of endometriosis on her ovaries and fallopian tubes and several others in the posterior cul-de-sac. She also had a left ovarian cyst, filmy adnexal adhesions, and several subcentimeter subserosal fibroids. You have recommended that she should have an HSG as part of her evaluation for infertility. Which of the patient's following conditions can be diagnosed with an HSG?

a. Endometriosis
b. Ovarian cyst
c. Subserosal fibroids
d. Minimal pelvic adhesions
e. Hydrosalpinx

350. During the evaluation of infertility in a 25-year-old woman, a HSG showed evidence of Asherman syndrome. Which one of the following symptoms would you expect this patient to have?

a. Amenorrhea
b. Menometrorrhagia
c. Menorrhagia
d. Metrorrhagia
e. Dysmenorrhea

351. During the evaluation of secondary amenorrhea in a 24-year-old woman, hyperprolactinemia is diagnosed. Which of the following conditions could cause increased circulating prolactin concentration and amenorrhea in this patient?

a. Stress
b. Primary hyperthyroidism
c. Anorexia nervosa
d. Congenital adrenal hyperplasia
e. Polycystic ovarian disease

352. A 36-year-old morbidly obese woman presents to your office for evaluation of irregular, heavy menses occurring every 3 to 6 months. An office endometrial biopsy shows complex hyperplasia of the endometrium without atypia. The hyperplasia is most likely related to the excess formation in the patient's adipose tissue of which of the following hormones?

a. Estriol
b. Estradiol
c. Estrone
d. Androstenedione
e. Dehydroepiandrosterone

353. A couple presents for evaluation of primary infertility. The evaluation of the woman is completely normal. The husband is found to have a left varicocele. If the husband's varicocele is the cause of the couple's infertility, what would you expect to see when evaluating the husband's semen analysis?

a. Decreased sperm count with an increase in the number of abnormal forms
b. Decreased sperm count with an increase in motility
c. Increased sperm count with an increase in the number of abnormal forms
d. Increased sperm count with absent motility
e. Azoospermia

354. Your patient delivers a 7-lb male infant at term. On physical examination, the baby has normal-appearing male external genitalia. However, the scrotum is empty, and no testes are palpable in the inguinal canals. At 6 months of age, the boy's testes still have not descended. A pelvic ultrasound shows the testes in the pelvis, and there appears to be a uterus present as well. The presence of a uterus in an otherwise phenotypically normal male is caused by which of the following?

a. Lack of Müllerian-inhibiting factor (MIF)
b. Lack of testosterone
c. Increased levels of estrogens
d. 46, XX karyotype
e. Presence of ovarian tissue early in embryonic development

Questions 355 and 356

A 45-year-old G2P2 presents for management of heavy menses. She reports her periods occur once a month, last 6 days, and are very heavy and painful. She has tried oral contraceptives, but she does not like having to take a pill every day. She had a levonorgestrel-containing intrauterine device (IUD) in the past, but did not like it due to symptoms of cramping. Her medical history is unremarkable, and her only surgery is a postpartum tubal ligation. Her evaluation has included a normal Pap smear, normal endometrial biopsy, and normal pelvic ultrasound.

355. What is the best next step in management of this patient's bleeding?

a. Recommend a hysterectomy
b. Try to talk her into another IUD
c. Recommend an endometrial ablation
d. Prescribe daily oral progesterone
e. Refer her for uterine artery embolization (UAE)

356. A 45-year-old woman who had two normal pregnancies 15 and 18 years ago presents with the complaint of amenorrhea for 7 months. She expresses the desire to become pregnant again. After exclusion of pregnancy, which of the following tests is next indicated in the evaluation of this patient's amenorrhea?

a. Hysterosalpingogram
b. Endometrial biopsy
c. Thyroid function studies
d. Testosterone and DHEA-S levels
e. FSH level

Questions 357 and 358

A 22-year-old woman consults you for treatment of hirsutism. Physical examination demonstrates facial acne, as well as dark, course hair on her upper lip, chin, and midsternum. She has a BMI of 35 kg/m². Serum LH level is 35 mIU/mL and FSH is 9 mIU/mL. Androstenedione and testosterone levels are mildly elevated, but serum DHEA-S is normal. The patient does not wish to conceive at this time.

357. Which of the following single agents is the most appropriate treatment of her condition?

a. Oral contraceptives
b. Corticosteroids
c. GnRH agonists
d. Metformin
e. Spironolactone

358. The patient returns 3 years later. She discontinued the oral contraceptives 1 year ago because she and her husband wanted to get pregnant. Since that time, her periods have been very unpredictable, usually every 3 to 6 months. She would like your advice about the best way to conceive. Which of the following is the most appropriate first line therapy to help her conceive?

a. Intrauterine insemination
b. In vitro fertilization
c. Metformin
d. Clomiphene citrate
e. Laparoscopic ovarian drilling

359. A 20-year-old woman with Müllerian agenesis is undergoing laparoscopic appendectomy by a general surgeon. You are consulted intraoperatively because the surgeon sees several lesions in the pelvis suspicious for endometriosis. You should tell the surgeon which of the following?

a. Endometriosis cannot occur in patients with Müllerian agenesis since they do not have a uterus.
b. Endometriosis is common in women with Müllerian agenesis since they have menstrual outflow obstruction.
c. Endometriosis probably occurs in patients with Müllerian agenesis as a result of retrograde menstruation.
d. Endometriosis may arise in patients with Müllerian agenesis as a result of coelomic metaplasia.
e. Endometriosis cannot occur in patients with Müllerian agenesis because they have a 46, XY karyotype.

360. A 19-year-old patient presents to your office with primary amenorrhea. She has normal breast and pubic hair development, but the uterus and vagina are absent. Diagnostic possibilities include which of the following?

a. XYY syndrome
b. Gonadal dysgenesis
c. Müllerian agenesis
d. Klinefelter syndrome
e. Turner syndrome

Questions 361 and 362

A 23-year-old woman presents for evaluation of a 7-month history of amenorrhea. She has no other major medical problems. Examination discloses bilateral galactorrhea and normal breast and pelvic examinations. Pregnancy test is negative. Serum prolactin is ordered and the result is elevated at 47ng/mL.

361. What is the next step in management?

a. Repeat the serum prolactin in 1 month
b. Order an MRI of the brain
c. Provide reassurance
d. Refer her to a breast surgeon
e. Check a hemoglobin (HbA1c)

362. Which of the following classes of medication is also a possible cause of galactorrhea?

a. Antiestrogens
b. Gonadotropins
c. Phenothiazines
d. Prostaglandins
e. GnRH analogues

363. Which of the following pubertal events in girls is not estrogen dependent?

a. Menses
b. Vaginal cornification
c. Hair growth
d. Reaching adult height
e. Production of cervical mucus

364. An infertile couple presents to you for evaluation. A semen analysis from the husband is ordered. The sample of 2.5 cc contains 25 million sperm per mL; 65% of the sperm show normal morphology; 20% of the sperm show progressive forward mobility. You should tell the couple which of the following?

a. The sample is normal, but of no clinical value because of the low sample volume.
b. The sample is normal and should not be a factor in the couple's infertility.
c. The sample is abnormal because the percentage of sperm with normal morphology is too low.
d. The sample is abnormal because of an inadequate number of sperm per milliliter.
e. The sample is abnormal owing to a low percentage of forwardly mobile sperm.

Questions 365 and 366

A 21-year-old woman presents to you for management of menstrual migraines. She has no other medical problems, does not smoke, and does not take any medications routinely. Her periods are regular and last 5 days. She says the flow is moderate and she does not have dysmenorrhea. She is sexually active with her partner of 1 year, and she uses condoms for contraception. She says she develops a debilitating migraine for the first 2 days of her period every month. She describes her headaches as unilateral, throbbing, and associated with nausea and photophobia. She has missed work due to these symptoms.

365. What is the best next step in management of her migraines?

a. Refer her to a neurologist
b. Recommend that she discontinue caffeine use
c. Prescribe her a combined oral contraceptive
d. Recommend that she take NSAIDs every 6 hours during the 5 days when she is menstruating
e. Prescribe her a narcotic to take during the 2 days she has the migraine every month

366. What change in her management would be indicated if she reported that 2 days before the onset of her migraine, she develops an aura consisting of bright spots in her vision?

a. No changes in her management are warranted.
b. Estrogen should be avoided.
c. Progesterone should be avoided.
d. She should be referred to an ophthalmologist.
e. She should not be offered any hormonal therapy.

367. A 16-year-old P0 presents to your office accompanied by her mother to discuss options for management of heavy menstrual bleeding. She has been on oral contraceptives for the last 9 months, but admits she often forgets to take her pills and develops breakthrough bleeding. They have both researched the options on the Internet, and are interested in depo provera (depot medroxyprogesterone acetate, or DMPA) because of the possibility of amenorrhea and the ease of use. How should you counsel this patient?

a. Depo provera is a reasonable option to manage heavy periods in the adolescent population.
b. Depo provera is contraindicated in the adolescent population due to adverse effects on bone density.
c. Depo provera does not cause amenorrhea.
d. She will need to return once a month for a depo provera injection.
e. DMPA is associated with an increased risk of fracture due to bone loss.

368. You ask a patient to call your office during her next menstrual cycle to schedule an HSG as part of her infertility evaluation. Which day of the menstrual cycle is best for performing an HSG?

a. Day 3
b. Day 8
c. Day 14
d. Day 21
e. Day 26

369. You have recommended that your infertility patient return to your office during her next menstrual cycle to have her serum progesterone level checked. Which is the best day of the menstrual cycle to check her progesterone level if you are trying to confirm ovulation?

a. Day 3
b. Day 8
c. Day 14
d. Day 21
e. Day 26

370. Your patient is 43 years old and is concerned that she may be too close to menopause to get pregnant. You recommend that her FSH level be tested. Which is the best day of the menstrual cycle to check an FSH in this situation?

a. Day 3
b. Day 8
c. Day 14
d. Day 21
e. Day 26

Questions 371 and 372

A 26-year-old G0P0 comes to your office with a chief complaint of being "too hairy." She reports that her menses started at the age of 13 years, and have always been very irregular, occurring every 2 to 6 months. She also complains of acne, but reports no other medical problems. Her only surgery was an appendectomy at the age of 8 years. Her height is 5 ft 5 in, her weight is 180 lb, and her blood pressure is 100/60 mm Hg. On physical examination, there are a few coarse, dark hairs around the nipples, chin, and upper lip. No galactorrhea, thyromegaly, or temporal balding is noted. Pelvic examination is normal and there is no evidence of clitoromegaly.

371. Which of the following is the most likely explanation for this patient's problem?

a. Idiopathic hirsutism
b. Polycystic ovarian syndrome (PCOS)
c. Late-onset congenital adrenal hyperplasia
d. Sertoli-Leydig cell tumor of the ovary
e. Adrenal tumor

372. Which of the following blood tests has no role in the evaluation of this patient?

a. Total testosterone
b. 17 α-hydroxyprogesterone
c. Dehydroepiandrostenedione (DHEA-S)
d. Estrone
e. Thyroid-stimulating hormone (TSH)

Questions 373 and 374

A patient in your practice calls you in a panic because her 14-year-old daughter has been bleeding heavily for the past 2 weeks. The daughter experienced menarche about 6 months ago, and since that time her periods have been irregular and very heavy. You instruct the mother to bring her daughter to the emergency department so that you can evaluate her. When they arrive, you note that she appears fatigued. Her blood pressure and pulse are 110/60 mm Hg and 70 beats per minute, respectively. When you stand her up, her blood pressure and pulse remain stable. While in the emergency room, you obtain a more detailed history. She reports no medical problems or prior surgeries, and is not taking any medications. She says that she has never been sexually active. On physical examination, her abdomen is soft and nontender. She will not let you perform a speculum examination, but the bimanual examination is normal. She is 5 ft 4 in tall and weighs 95 lb.

373. Which of the following blood tests is not indicated in the evaluation of this patient?

a. BHCG
b. Bleeding time
c. CBC
d. Blood type and screen
e. Estradiol level

374. What is the most appropriate next step in management?

a. Prescribe a combined oral contraceptive taper to be started as an outpatient, and followed by cyclic oral contraceptive therapy.
b. Perform a dilation and curettage.
c. Recommend a blood transfusion.
d. Admit her to the hospital for intravenous iron therapy.
e. Admit her to the hospital for intravenous estrogen therapy.

375. A 32-year-old P0 morbidly obese diabetic woman presents to your office with a chief complaint of prolonged vaginal bleeding. Her periods were regular, monthly, and light until 2 years ago. At that time, she started having periods every 3 to 6 months. Her last normal period was 5 months ago. She started having vaginal bleeding again 3 weeks ago. It started as light bleeding, but over the last week, she has been bleeding heavily and passing large clots. On pelvic examination, the external genitalia is normal. The vagina is filled with blood and large clots. A large clot is seen protruding through the cervix. On bimanual examination, the uterus is at the upper limit of normal size, and the ovaries feel normal. Her urine pregnancy test is negative. Which of the following is the most likely cause of her abnormal uterine bleeding (AUB)?

a. Uterine fibroids
b. Cervical polyp
c. Incomplete abortion
d. Chronic anovulation
e. Coagulation defect

376. A 26-year-old P0 with PCOS presents to the emergency department with a chief complaint of prolonged, heavy vaginal bleeding. She was taking oral contraceptives to regulate her periods until 4 months ago, when she stopped taking them because she and her spouse want to try to get pregnant. She thought she might be pregnant because she had not had a period since her last one on the birth control pills 4 months ago. She started having vaginal bleeding 8 days ago. Her bleeding has been very heavy, requiring her to double up on her sanitary napkins and change them five to six times daily since the bleeding began. In the emergency department, the patient has a supine blood pressure of 102/64 mm Hg with a pulse of 96 beats per minute. Upon standing, the patient feels light-headed. Her blood pressure while standing is 108/66 mm Hg with an increase in her pulse to 126 beats per minute. While you wait for laboratory work to come back, you order intravenous hydration. After 2 hours, she is no longer orthostatic. Her pregnancy test comes back negative, and her Hct is 31%. A transvaginal ultrasound showed an atrophic appearing endometrial stripe. Which of the following is the best next step in the management of this patient?

a. Perform a dilation and curettage.
b. Administer a blood transfusion to treat her severe anemia.
c. Send her home with a prescription for iron therapy.
d. Administer high-dose estrogen therapy.
e. Administer antiprostaglandins.

377. A 29-year-old P0 presents to your office with a chief complaint of symptoms of premenstrual syndrome (PMS). A detailed history reveals that she experiences emotional lability and depression for about 10 days prior to her menses. Once her period starts, she feels "back to normal." She also reports a long history of premenstrual fatigue, breast tenderness, and bloating. Her previous physician prescribed oral contraceptives to treat her PMS 6 months ago, and she reports that the pills have alleviated all her PMS symptoms except for the depression and emotional symptoms. Which of the following is the best next step in the treatment of this patient's problem?

a. Spironolactone
b. Evening primrose oil
c. Fluoxetine
d. Progesterone supplements
e. Vitamin B_6

Questions 378 to 381

A 51-year-old woman G3P3 presents to your office with a 6-month history of amenorrhea. She complains of debilitating hot flushes that awaken her at night; and she wakes up the next day feeling exhausted and irritable. She tells you she has tried herbal supplements for her hot flushes, but nothing has worked. She is interested in beginning HRT, but is hesitant to do so because of its possible risks and side effects. The patient is very healthy. She has no medical problems, and the only medication she takes are calcium supplements. She has a family history of osteoporosis. Her height is 5 ft 5 in and her weight is 115 lb.

378. In counseling this patient regarding the risks and benefits of HRT, you should tell her that HRT (estrogen and progesterone) has been associated with which of the following?

a. An increased risk of colon cancer
b. An increased risk of uterine cancer
c. An increased risk of thromboembolic events
d. An increased risk of developing Alzheimer disease
e. An increased risk of malignant melanoma

379. She tells you she is worried about how HRT might impact her lipid panel. You should counsel her to expect which of the following?

a. An increase in her LDL
b. An increase in her HDL
c. An increase in her total cholesterol
d. A decrease in her triglycerides
e. A decrease in her HDL

380. The patient asks you what she should expect in regard to her hot flushes if she does not take hormone replacement. How should you counsel her?

a. Hot flushes usually resolve spontaneously within 1 year of the last menstrual period.
b. Hot flushes are normal and rarely interfere with a woman's well-being.
c. Hot flushes usually resolve within 1 week after the initiation of HRT.
d. Hot flushes can begin several years before actual menopause.
e. Hot flushes are the final manifestation of ovarian failure and menopause.

381. What should you tell her regarding the psychologic symptoms of menopause?

a. They are not related to her changing levels of estrogen and progesterone.
b. They commonly include depression, irritability, poor concentration, and impaired memory.
c. They are related to a drop in gonadotropin levels.
d. They are not affected by environmental factors.
e. They are primarily a reaction to the cessation of menstrual flow.

Questions 382 to 387

For each following description, select the type of precocious puberty with which it is most likely to be associated. Each lettered option may be used once, more than once, or not at all.

a. Central (true) precocious puberty
b. Incomplete precocious puberty
c. Isosexual peripheral (or pseudo) precocious puberty
d. Contrasexual peripheral (or pseudo) precocious puberty
e. Precocious puberty caused by gonadotropin-producing tumors

382. Defined by the presence of virilizing signs in girls

383. Characterized by the presence of premature adrenarche, pubarche, or thelarche

384. Can arise from cranial tumors or hypothyroidism

385. Results from premature activation of the hypothalamic-pituitary system

386. Is frequently caused by ovarian tumors

Questions 387 to 391

Match each HSG with the correct description. Each lettered option may be used once, more than once, or not at all.

a. Bilateral hydrosalpinx
b. Unilateral hydrosalpinx with intrauterine adhesions
c. Unilateral hydrosalpinx with a normal uterine cavity
d. Bilateral proximal occlusion
e. Salpingitis isthmica nodosa
f. Bilateral normal spillage

387.

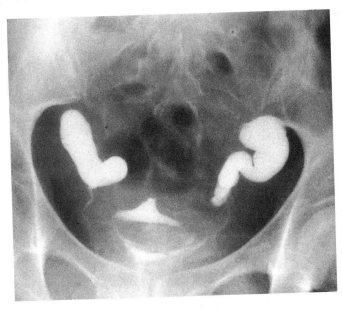

388.

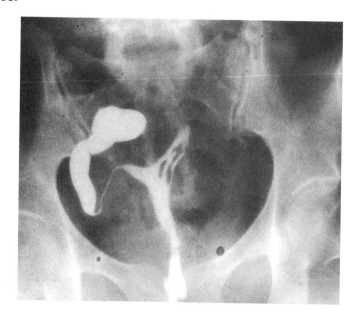

389.

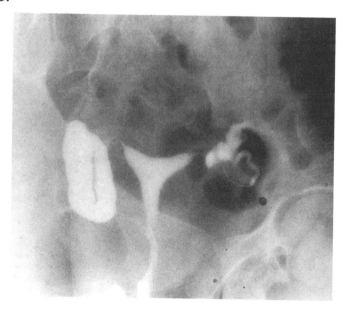

390.

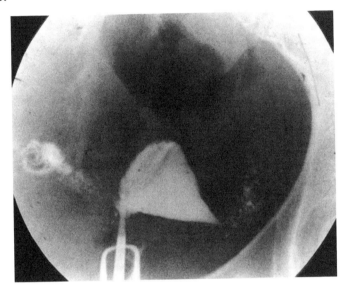

391.

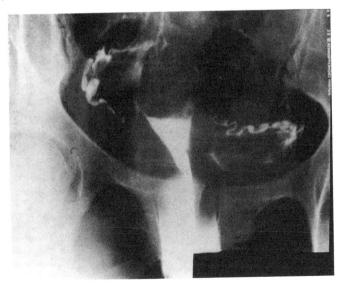

Infertility Endocrinology and Menstrual Dysfunction

Answers

331. The answer is c. Significant emotional concerns develop when puberty is delayed. By definition, if breast development has not begun by the age of 13 years, delayed puberty should be suspected. Menarche usually follows about 1 to 2 years after the beginning of breast development; if menarche is delayed beyond the age of 16 years, delayed puberty should be investigated. Appropriate laboratory tests include circulating pituitary and steroid hormone levels, karyotypic analysis, and CNS imaging when indicated. An FSH value greater than 40 mIU/mL defines hypergonadotropic hypogonadism as a cause of delayed pubertal maturation. Hypergonadotropic hypogonadism is seen in girls with gonadal dysgenesis, such as with Turner syndrome.

332. The answer is b. In the United States, the appearance of breast buds (thelarche) is usually the first sign of puberty, generally occurring between the ages of 9 and 11 years. This is subsequently followed by the appearance of pubic and axillary hair (adrenarche or pubarche), the adolescent growth spurt, and finally menarche. On average, the sequence of developmental changes requires a period of 4.5 years to complete, with a range of 1.5 to 6 years. The average ages of adrenarche/pubarche and menarche are 11.0 and 12.8 years, respectively; however, puberty onset is slightly earlier in African-American girls and in overweight girls. These events are considered to be delayed if thelarche has not occurred by the age of 13 years, adrenarche by the age of 14, or menarche by the age of 16. Girls with delayed sexual development should be fully evaluated for delayed puberty, including central, ovarian, systemic, or constitutional causes.

333. The answer is a. In North America, pubertal changes before the age of 8 years in girls and 9 years in boys are regarded as precocious. Although the most common type of precocious puberty in girls is idiopathic, it is essential to ensure close long-term follow-up of these patients to ascertain that there is no serious underlying pathology, such as tumors of the CNS or ovary. Only 1% to 2% of patients with precocious puberty have an estrogen-producing ovarian tumor as the causative factor. McCune-Albright syndrome (polyostotic fibrous dysplasia) is also relatively rare and consists of fibrous dysplasia and cystic degeneration of the long bones, sexual precocity, and café au lait spots on the skin. Hypothyroidism is a cause of precocious puberty in some children, making thyroid function tests mandatory in these cases. Tumors of the CNS as a cause of precocious puberty occur more commonly in boys than in girls; they are seen in about 11% of girls with precocious puberty.

334. The answer is e. Osteoporosis is defined as decreased bone mass and microarchitectural disruption which leads to an increased risk of fractures. Fractures may occur in the vertebra, distal forearm (Colles' fracture), or femur head. Although all races experience osteoporosis, white and Asian women lose bone earlier and at a more rapid rate than black women. Thin women and those who smoke are at increased risk for developing osteoporosis. Other risk factors include advanced age, history of prior fracture, long-term steroid therapy, or excessive alcohol use. Physical activity increases the mineral content of bone in postmenopausal women.

335. The answer is c. DEXA is the best method to measure bone density because it is precise, uses low doses of radiation, and has been well studied in terms of how the DEXA results correlate to risk of fracture. In addition, the World Health Organization (WHO) criteria for diagnosis for osteoporosis and osteopenia are based on DEXA results. CT scan may measure bone density, but requires much higher doses of radiation. Peripheral measurement may correlate to DEXA, but the results are difficult to interpret. X-ray is not used to assess bone density.

336. The answer is a. Osteopenia is defined as a T-score between −1 and −2.5 standard deviations from the mean (SD). Osteoporosis is defined as a T-score below −2.5 SD. A T-score is the standard deviation between the patient and the peak young adult bone mass. The more negative, the greater the risk of fracture. This patient has osteopenia based on her DEXA, and she also has risk factors for fracture (low body weight, family history, of fracture), making her a good candidate for pharmacologic therapy to reduce her risk of fracture. Bisphosphonates are considered first line therapy as they are well tolerated, relatively low cost, and have a favorable safety profile. Raloxifene, a selective estrogen receptor modulator (SERM), is effective at reducing the risk of vertebral fractures, but is associated with an increased risk of thromboembolism; therefore, it is usually used in situations where bisphosphonates are not well tolerated. HRT is not indicated for the management of osteoporosis or osteopenia.

337 and 338. The answers are 337-b and 338-d. Primary dysmenorrhea is painful menstruation associated with a normal pelvic examination and with ovulatory cycles. Dysmenorrhea is considered secondary if it is associated with pelvic disease such as endometriosis, uterine myomas, or pelvic inflammatory disease. The pain of dysmenorrhea may be accompanied by other symptoms (nausea, fatigue, diarrhea, and headache), which may be related to excess of prostaglandin $F_{2\alpha}$. In patients with dysmenorrhea, there is a significantly higher than normal concentration of prostaglandins in the endometrium and menstrual fluid. Conservative measures for treating dysmenorrhea include heating pads and exercise. The two major drug therapies effective in dysmenorrhea are oral contraceptives and antiprostaglandins. Nonsteroidal anti-inflammatory drugs (NSAIDs) function as prostaglandin synthase inhibitors, and are very effective for treatment of dysmenorrhea. These medications may include naproxen, ibuprofen, and mefenamic acid and are very effective in these patients. They are a reasonable first step to manage dysmenorrhea in a patient who does not require contraception. However, for patients who are sexually active, oral contraceptives will provide both protection from unwanted pregnancy and will alleviate the dysmenorrhea, and should be considered first-line therapy. GnRH analogues are sometimes used in several gynecologic pain conditions, but would not be first-line therapy for primary dysmenorrhea. Narcotics would generally be employed only in very severe cases when no other treatment provides adequate relief. There is inconsistent data about the usefulness of acupuncture to treat dysmenorrhea.

339. The answer is b. The evaluation and diagnosis of the patient with abnormal development of secondary sex characteristics is challenging as there are many potential causes. The evaluation of the patient should note the presence or absence of a uterus, breast buds, and pubic and axillary hair. Testicular feminization is a syndrome of androgen insensitivity in genetic males, characterized by a normal 46, X genotype, normal female phenotype during childhood, tall stature, and "normal" breast development with absence of axillary and pubic hair. Breast development (gynecomastia) occurs in these males because high levels of circulating testosterone (which cannot act at its receptor) are aromatized to estrogen, which then acts on the breast. The external genitalia develop as those of a female because testosterone cannot masculinize them, while the Müllerian structures are absent because of testicular secretion of MIF in utero. Gonadal dysgenesis (eg, 45, X Turner syndrome) is characterized by short stature and absence of pubertal development; in these girls the ovaries are either absent or streak gonads that are nonfunctional. In either case, estrogen production is possible, and therefore isosexual pubertal development does not occur. Kallmann syndrome (hypogonadotropic hypogonadism), the most likely diagnosis in this patient, should be suspected in an amenorrheic patient of normal stature with delayed or absent pubertal development, especially when associated with the classic finding of anosmia. Testing the sense of smell with coffee or perfume is a simple way to screen for this disorder. These individuals have a structural defect of the CNS involving the hypothalamus and the olfactory bulbs (located in close proximity to the hypothalamus) such that the hypothalamus does not secrete GnRH in normal pulsatile fashion, if at all. Other causes of minimal or absent pubertal development with normal stature include malnutrition; anorexia nervosa; severe systemic disease; and intensive athletic training, particularly ballet and running.

340 and 341. The answers are 340-e and 341-c. Precocious puberty is diagnosed if a young girl develops pubertal changes before the age of 8 years. This patient is most likely to have true central precocious puberty. The GnRH results and LH pulses described in the question are seen in normal puberty. Normal signs of puberty involve breast budding (thelarche), pubic hair (pubarche or adrenarche), and menarche. Besides an increase in androgens and a moderate rise in FSH and LH levels, one of the first indications of puberty is an increase in the amplitude and frequency of nocturnal LH pulses. In patients with idiopathic central precocious puberty, the pituitary response to GnRH is identical to that in girls undergoing normal puberty. Iatrogenic sexual precocity (ie, the accidental ingestion of estrogens), premature thelarche, and ovarian tumors are examples of sexual precocity independent of GnRH, FSH, and LH function. Precocious puberty can be treated by agents that reduce gonadotropin levels by exerting negative feedback in the hypothalamic—pituitary axis or that directly inhibit gonadotropin secretion from the pituitary gland. Currently, the most effective treatment for central precocious puberty is the use of a long-acting

GnRH agonist, such as leuprolide (Lupron) and others. These drugs act by downregulating pituitary gonadotropes, eventually decreasing the secretion of FSH and LH, which are inappropriately stimulating the ovaries of these patients. As a result of this induced hypogonadotropic state, ovarian steroids (estrogens, progestins, and androgens) are suppressed back to prepubertal levels and precocious pubertal development stops or regresses. During the first 1 or 2 weeks of therapy there is a flare-up effect of increased gonadotropins and sex steroids, a predicted side effect of these medications. At the time of expected puberty, the GnRH analogue is discontinued and the pubertal sequence resumes.

342. The answer is d. Delayed puberty is a rare condition, and is usually differentiated into hypergonadotropic (high FSH and LH levels) hypogonadism or hypogonadotropic (low FSH and LH) hypogonadism. The most common cause of hypergonadotropic hypogonadism is gonadal dysgenesis (ie, 45X Turner syndrome). Hypogonadotropic hypogonadism can be seen in patients with hypothalamic-pituitary or constitutional delays in development. Kallmann syndrome presents with amenorrhea, delayed sexual development, low gonadotropins, normal female karyotype, and anosmia (a defect in smell). In addition to these conditions, many other types of medical and nutritional problems can lead to this type of delayed development (eg, malabsorption, diabetes, regional ileitis, and other chronic illness). Congenital adrenal hyperplasia leads to early pubertal development, although in girls the development is not isosexual (not of the expected sex) and would therefore include hirsutism, clitoromegaly, and other signs of virilization. Complete Müllerian agenesis is a condition in which the Müllerian ducts either fail to develop or regress early in fetal life. These patients have a blind vaginal pouch and no upper vagina, cervix, or uterus, and they present with primary amenorrhea. However, because ovarian development is not affected, secondary sexual characteristics develop normally despite the absence of menarche, and gonadotropin levels are normal. The McCune-Albright syndrome involves the constellation of precocious puberty, café au lait spots, and polyostotic fibrous dysplasia.

343. The answer is c. A bicornuate uterus results from partial lack of fusion of the Müllerian ducts, which produces a single cervix with varying degrees of separation in the two uterine horns. This condition is associated with a higher risk of obstetric complications, such as an increase in the rate of second-trimester abortion, preterm labor, malpresentation, and labor abnormalities. An intravenous pyelogram or urinary tract ultrasound is mandatory in patients with Müllerian anomalies since approximately 30% of patients have coexisting congenital urinary tract anomalies.

344. The answer is c. Adenomyosis is a condition in which normal endometrial glands grow into the myometrium. Symptomatic disease primarily occurs in multiparous women over the age of 35 years, compared to endometriosis, in which onset is considerably younger. Patients with adenomyosis complain of dysmenorrhea and menorrhagia, and the classical examination findings include a tender, symmetrically enlarged uterus without adnexal tenderness. Although patients with endometriosis can have similar complaints, the physical examination of these patients more commonly reveals a fixed, retroverted uterus, adnexal tenderness and scarring, and tenderness along the uterosacral ligaments. Leiomyoma is the most common pelvic tumor, but most are asymptomatic, and the uterus is irregular in shape on examination. Patients with endometritis can present with abnormal bleeding, but endometrial biopsies show an inflammatory pattern. Uterine sarcoma is rare, and presents in older women with postmenopausal bleeding and nontender uterine enlargement.

345. The answer is a. Uterine anomalies such as a uterine septum may cause recurrent miscarriage; thus, women with recurrent miscarriages should have their uterine cavity evaluated. A septate uterus results from partial lack of resorption of the midline septum between the two Müllerian ducts, and may present with varying degrees of septation. Hysterosalpingography, hysteroscopy, ultrasound, CT, and magnetic resonance imaging (MRI) are all potentially useful imaging modalities in this investigation. Hysteroscopic resection of the septum is the method of choice to surgically repair this problem. Dysmenorrhea, dyspareunia, and menometrorrhagia are typically not caused by the presence of a uterine septum.

346. The answer is a. There is a marked increase in levels of serum prolactin during pregnancy to over 10 times those values found in nonpregnant women. This woman's pregnancy test is positive. If she were not pregnant, the prolactin value could easily explain the amenorrhea, and further evaluation of the cause of the hyperprolactinemia would be necessary. The physiologic significance of increasing prolactin in pregnancy appears to involve preparation of the breasts for lactation. As this patient is pregnant, there is no need for further evaluation of the elevated prolactin level and she should begin routine prenatal care.

347. The answer is e. Medical treatment of endometriosis may be recommended as suppressive therapy following ablative surgery. Combined oral contraceptives remain the mainstay of therapy; however, continuous oral progesterone is also a reasonable option. There is some data that a progesterone-containing IUD results in decreased rates of dysmenorrhea. If these therapies are not effective, aGnRH agonists may be used, although it is associated with more adverse side effects, because they produce a medically induced and reversible menopause state. Danazol has been shown to improve pain related to endometriosis, but is not used often due to significant androgenic side effects such as weight gain, hirsutism, and depression.

348. The answer is b. In patients with abnormal bleeding who are not responding to standard therapy, hysteroscopy should be performed. Hysteroscopy can rule out the presence endometrial polyps or small fibroids by direct visualization. If these lesions are present, they can be resected or removed. In patients with heavy abnormal bleeding who no longer desire fertility, an endometrial ablation may be performed. If a patient has completed childbearing and is having significant abnormal bleeding, a hysteroscopy and possible endometrial ablation, rather than a hysterectomy, would still be the procedure of choice to rule out easily treatable disease and manage the bleeding in a minimally invasive manner. Treatment with a GnRH agonist would induce a menopausal state and only temporarily relieve symptoms.

349. The answer is e. An HSG is a procedure in which 3 mL to 6 mL of either an oil or water-soluble contrast medium is injected through the cervix in a retrograde fashion to outline the uterine cavity and fallopian tubes. Spill of contrast medium into the peritoneal cavity proves patency of the fallopian tubes. By outlining the uterine cavity, abnormalities such as bicornuate or septate uterus, uterine polyps, or submucous myomas can be diagnosed, while tubal opacification allows identification of such conditions as salpingitis isthmica nodosum and hydrosalpinx. However, pelvic abnormalities outside the uterine cavity and fallopian tube (such as subserosal fibroids, ovarian tumors, endometriosis, or minimal pelvic adhesions) are not visible with this study. Some studies have shown a therapeutic effect resulting in an increased rate of pregnancy in the months immediately following the HSG.

350. The answer is a. Asherman syndrome refers to a condition where intrauterine adhesions are present. These adhesions can often cause symptoms such as amenorrhea or infertility. Because of the decreased amount of functional endometrium present in this setting, progressive hypomenorrhea (lighter menstrual flow) or amenorrhea is common. Oligomenorrhea is defined as infrequent, irregular uterine bleeding for more than 35 days apart, often attributed to anovulation. Ovulation is not affected in Asherman syndrome; therefore, ovulatory patients with Asherman syndrome may continue to have regular periods. The best diagnostic study to confirm intrauterine adhesions is an HSG under fluoroscopy. Hysteroscopy with lysis of adhesions is the treatment of choice. Prophylactic antibiotics may improve success rates.

351. The answer is a. Physical or psychological stress may result in an increase in prolactin. Prolactin is under the control of prolactin-inhibiting factor (PIF), which is produced in the hypothalamus. Many drugs (eg, the phenothiazines), stress, hypothalamic lesions, stalk lesions, and stalk compression decrease PIF. In anorexia nervosa, prolactin, TSH, and thyroxine levels are normal, FSH and LH levels are low, and cortisol levels are elevated. In hypothyroidism, elevated TRH acts as a prolactin-releasing hormone to cause release of prolactin from the pituitary; hyperthyroidism is not associated with hyperprolactinemia. There are many other conditions, such as acromegaly and pregnancy, that are associated with elevated prolactin levels. Hyperandrogenic conditions such as congenital adrenal hyperplasia or polycystic ovarian disease are not typically associated with hyperprolactinemia.

352. The answer is c. In premenopausal adult women, most of the estrogen in the body is derived from ovarian secretion of estradiol, but a significant portion also comes from the peripheral conversion of androstenedione to estrone in adipose tissue. When there is an increase in fat cells, as in obese persons, estrogen levels—particularly estrone—will be higher, provoking anovulation and endometrial hyperplasia.

353. The answer is a. A varicocele is an abnormal tortuosity and dilation of the veins of the pampiniform plexus within the spermatic cord. The incidence of varicoceles in the general population is about 15%, but 40% of males with infertility are found to have varicoceles. Varicoceles are more likely to occur on the left side due to the direct insertion of the spermatic vein into the renal vein. There is no correlation between the size of the varicocele and the prognosis for fertility. The characteristic semen analysis seen with varicoceles shows a decrease in the number of spermatozoa with decreased motility and increased abnormal forms. How the varicocele causes abnormal semen quality, and the relationship between varicocele, semen abnormalities, and male infertility (especially when semen quality appears normal) is unclear.

354. The answer is a. Bilateral nonpalpable testes in a phenotypically normal male newborn require prompt evaluation due to the possibility of a disorder of sexual development. Müllerian structures appear during embryonic development in both males and females. Female gonads do not secrete Müllerian-inhibiting substance (MIS), and therefore the Müllerian structures persist. Male testes secrete MIF, which causes regression of Müllerian structures. Anything that prevents MIF secretion in genetic males will result in persistence of Müllerian structures into the postnatal period. Persons who appear to be normal males but who possess a uterus and fallopian tubes have such a failure of MIF. Their karyotype is 46, XY, testes are present, and testosterone production is normal.

355. The answer is c. This patient has had a normal workup, and has failed conservative treatment. She had adverse symptoms with an IUD in the past, so this is not the best option. Daily oral progesterone is a very reasonable option to manage her bleeding, but she does not want to take a pill every day. UAE is a reasonable treatment option for women with fibroids, but this patient had a normal ultrasound. Hysterectomy will certainly manage her bleeding, but there is another option that is more conservative and minimally invasive. Endometrial ablation has a high success rate, with roughly a 50% amenorrhea rate at 1 year, and over a 90% patient satisfaction rate based on normalization of menstrual flow. It is an outpatient procedure that requires very little time for recovery.

356. The answer is e. This patient has secondary amenorrhea, which excludes etiologies associated with primary amenorrhea, such as chromosomal abnormalities and congenital Müllerian abnormalities. Pregnancy is the most common cause of amenorrhea in a woman of reproductive age, and this should be assessed first. Other possibilities include chronic endometritis or scarring of the endometrium (Asherman syndrome), hypothyroidism, and ovarian failure. The latter is the most likely diagnosis in a woman at this age. In addition, emotional stress, extreme weight loss, and adrenal cortisol insufficiency can cause secondary amenorrhea. An HSG is part of an infertility workup that may demonstrate Asherman syndrome as a cause of amenorrhea, but it is not indicated until ovarian failure has been excluded. Persistently elevated FSH levels (especially when accompanied by low serum estradiol levels) are diagnostic of ovarian failure.

357. The answer is a. This patient has PCOS, diagnosed by the clinical picture and laboratory values, including abnormally high LH-to-FSH ratio (which should normally be approximately 1:1), elevated androgens, and normal DHEA-S. DHEA-S is a marker of adrenal androgen production; when normal, it essentially excludes adrenal sources of hyperandrogenism. Several medications have been used to treat hirsutism associated with PCOS. Oral contraceptives are the most frequently used agents to treat hirsutism in a patient who does not desire pregnancy. They act by increasing sex hormone binding globulin and suppressing LH-driven ovarian androgen production, thereby reducing levels of free circulating androgen. GnRH agonists suppress ovarian steroid production, but they are expensive, cause bone demineralization, and result in menopausal symptoms by causing a medical menopause. Metformin may be used to treat women with PCOS who want to conceive, as it has been shown to improve ovulation rages in women with a high BMI; however, it has not been shown to improve hirsutism. Spironolactone is an anti-androgen that may be used to treat hirsutism; however, it is rarely selected as first line therapy due to the possibility of adverse effects on a developing male fetus in utero.

358. The answer is d. Clomiphene citrate is first line therapy for anovulatory women, including women with PCOS. Most women with PCOS will ovulate with clomiphene citrate, and approximately 50% will conceive. Intrauterine insemination is not an ideal treatment in a setting where ovulation is unpredictable. Metformin may improve ovulation, and is sometimes used in combination with clomiphene citrate. Clomid had been shown to be superior to metformin alone for ovulation induction. Laparoscopic ovarian drilling is not used as much anymore since there are so many other pharmacologic options to induce ovulation. In vitro fertilization would be considered in patients who failed medical therapy.

359. The answer is d. Retrograde menstruation is currently believed to be the major cause of endometriosis. Supporting this belief are the following findings: inversion of the uterine cervix into the peritoneal cavity can cause monkeys to develop endometriosis; endometrial tissue is viable outside the uterus; and blood can expel from the ends of the fallopian tubes of some women during menstruation. There is an increased incidence of endometriosis in girls who have genital tract obstructions that prevent the blood flow from exiting the uterus, and increase the incidence of retrograde flow out of the tubes. The fact that endometrial implants can occur in the lung implies that lymphatic or vascular routes of spread of the disease also are possible. Another theory of the etiology of endometriosis entails the conversion of coelomic epithelium into glands resembling those of the endometrium. Endometriosis in men, or in women without Müllerian structures, is an example of this causative mechanism.

360. The answer is c. Since this patient has other signs of pubertal development that are sex steroid–dependent, we can conclude that some ovarian function is present. This excludes such conditions as gonadal dysgenesis and hypothalamic-pituitary failure as possible causes of her primary amenorrhea. Müllerian defects are the only plausible cause, and the diagnostic evaluation in this patient would be directed toward both confirmation of this diagnosis and establishment of the exact nature of the Müllerian defect. Müllerian agenesis, also known as Mayer-Rokitansky-Küster-Hauser syndrome, presents as amenorrhea with absence of a vagina. The incidence is approximately 1 in 10,000 female births. The karyotype is 46,XX. There is normal development of breasts, sexual hair, ovaries, tubes, and external genitalia. There are associated skeletal (12%) and urinary tract (33%) anomalies. Treatment generally consists of progressive vaginal dilation or creation of an artificial vagina with split-thickness skin grafts (McIndoe procedure). Testicular feminization, or congenital androgen insensitivity syndrome, is an X-linked recessive disorder with a karyotype of 46,XY. These genetic males have a defective androgen receptor and/or downstream signal transduction mechanism (in the genome) such that the androgenic signal does not have its normal tissue-specific effects. This accounts for 10% of all cases of primary amenorrhea. The patient presents with an absent uterus and blind vaginal pouch. However, in these patients, the amount of sexual hair is significantly decreased. Although there is a 25% incidence of malignant tumors in these patients, gonadectomy should be deferred until after full development is obtained. In other patients with a Y chromosome, gonadectomy should be performed as early as possible to prevent masculinization. Patients with gonadal dysgenesis present with lack of secondary sexual characteristics. Patients with Klinefelter syndrome typically have a karyotype of 47, XXY and a male phenotype. Causes of primary amenorrhea, in descending order of frequency, are gonadal dysgenesis, Müllerian agenesis, and testicular feminization. XYY syndrome and Turner syndrome often present with menstrual abnormalities, but these patients have a uterus.

361. The answer is a. Modest increased in serum prolactin should be reevaluated at least once prior to ordering an imaging study, because prolactin can be transiently increased by many factors such as stress, breast stimulation, or eating. If it is persistently elevated, she should undergo MRI of the pituitary. It is also important to check a TSH to rule out thyroid disease and an FSH to rule out ovarian failure (as a cause of the amenorrhea). There is no indication to refer her to a breast surgeon or to check a HbA1c.

362. The answer is c. Amenorrhea and galactorrhea may be seen when something causes an increase in prolactin secretion or action. The differential diagnosis involves several possible causes. Excessive estrogens, such as with birth control pills, can reduce PIF, thus raising serum prolactin level. Similarly, intensive suckling during lactation can activate the reflex arc that results in hyperprolactinemia. Many antipsychotic medications, especially the phenothiazines, are also known to have mammotropic properties. Hypothyroidism appears to cause galactorrhea secondary to thyrotropin-releasing hormone (TRH) stimulation of prolactin release. When prolactin levels are persistently elevated without obvious cause (eg, in breastfeeding), evaluation for pituitary adenoma becomes necessary.

363. The answer is c. The presence of estrogen in a pubertal girl stimulates the formation of secondary sex characteristics, including development of breasts, production of cervical mucus, and vaginal cornification. As estrogen levels increase, menses begins and ovulation is maintained for several decades. Ovarian estrogen production late in puberty is at least in part responsible for termination of the pubertal growth spurt, thereby determining adult height. Decreasing levels of estrogen are associated with lower frequency of ovulation, eventually leading to menopause. Hair growth during puberty is caused by androgens from the adrenal gland and, later, the ovary.

364. The answer is e. Semen analysis is an important part of an infertility evaluation. This specimen should ideally be collected at a doctor's office by masturbation following at least 48 hours of abstinence. Because of the variability in semen specimens from the same person, at least two samples should be collected over 1 to 2 weeks during the course of an investigation for infertility. A normal semen analysis will demonstrate at least 20 million sperm per milliliter, over 60% of the sperm with a normal shape, a volume of between 2 mL and 6 mL, and at least 50% of the sperm with progressive forward motility.

365. The answer is c. Menstrual migraines occur in 8% to 14% of women. They occur exclusively during menses, and are absent during other times of the cycle. They are thought to be caused by hormonal fluctuations, specifically the premenstrual decline in estrogen. Use of combined oral contraceptives stabilizes these hormone fluctuations, and provides relief for many women. There is no indication for narcotics, and continuous NSAIDs may cause gastrointestinal side effects. Referral to a neurologist for consideration of abortive treatments such as triptans may be indicated if the patient fails other therapies.

366. The answer is b. A visual aura may present as an area of vision loss, bright spots in the vision, or flashing lights. There is some data that migraines with visual aura are associated with an increased risk of stroke, and therefore estrogen should be avoided.

367. The answer is a. DMPA inhibits secretion of pituitary gonadotropins, resulting in anovulation and decreased estrogen production. It is a highly effective contraceptive that affords privacy and a convenient dosing schedule (once every 12 weeks). In addition, the mechanism of action results in approximately 50% rate of amenorrhea, making it a reasonable option for management of heavy menses in the adolescent population. DMPA has been associated with bone loss, but not with an increase in fracture risk. The FDA issued a "black box" warning in 2004 regarding the prolonged use of DMPA causing significant bone loss. The stance of ACOG is that practitioners should notify patients about this potential side effect of long-term use of DMPA, but it should not prevent the use of this medication in the adolescent population.

368 to 370. The answers are 368-b, 369-d, 370-a. An infertility evaluation should be initiated in women younger than 35 years after 1 year of infertility (regular unprotected intercourse), and after 6 months in women older than 35 years. An HSG is performed in the mid-follicular phase, around day 8, in order to evaluate the patency of the fallopian tubes and the contour of the uterine cavity; it should not be done while the patient is menstruating or after ovulation has occurred. In women with normal menstrual cycles, ovulation may be confirmed with a day 21 serum progesterone level. Serum progesterone levels greater than 3ng/mL is consistent with ovulation. Ovarian reserve may be tested with a day 3 FSH. Women with adequate ovarian function will have sufficient production of ovarian hormones early in the menstrual cycle to keep the FSH at a low level, thus indicating an adequate pool of follicles and oocytes.

371 and 372. The answers are 371-b, 372-d. PCOS is the most common cause of androgen excess and hirsutism. Women with this syndrome often have irregular menstrual cycles due to anovulation. Given the history and physical examination in this patient, PCOS is the most likely diagnosis. Sertoli-Leydig cell tumors, also known as androblastomas, are testosterone-secreting ovarian neoplasms. These tumors usually occur in women between the ages of 20 and 40, tend to be unilateral, and can reach a size of 7 cm to 10 cm. Women with a Sertoli-Leydig cell tumor tend to have very high levels of testosterone (> 200 ng/dL) and rapidly develop virilizing characteristics such as temporal balding, clitoral hypertrophy, voice deepening, breast atrophy, and terminal hair between the breasts and on the back. A total testosterone level can help differentiate between PCOS (elevated testosterone, but not as high as with a Sertoli-Leydig cell tumor). Very high levels of total testosterone would indicate the presence of an androgen-secreting ovarian tumor. Elevated levels of DHEA-S would be consistent with PCOS. There is no role for ordering an isolated estrone level in the workup and evaluation of hirsutism. Women with idiopathic hirsutism have greater activity of 5α-reductase than do unaffected women. They have hirsutism with a diagnostic evaluation that gives no explanation for the excess hair. Women with late-onset congenital adrenal hyperplasia are hirsute due to an increase in adrenal androgen production caused by a deficiency in 21-hydroxylase. In order to rule out congenital adrenal hyperplasia caused by a deficiency in 21-hydroxylase, a 17α-hydroxyprogesterone level should be drawn. Thyroid dysfunction and hyperprolactinemia can both be associated with hirsutism, and therefore it is important to check levels of TSH and prolactin.

373 and 374. The answers are 373-e, 374-a. The case presented is a typical representation of a patient with AUB due to ovulatory dysfunction.

This is a very common etiology of AUB during adolescence. The onset of menarche in young women is typically followed by approximately 12 to 18 months of irregular cycles that result from anovulation secondary to immaturity of the hypothalamic-pituitary-gonadal axis. Obesity is becoming an increasingly important contributor to anovulatory cycles in adolescents. The differential diagnosis for AUB in the adolescent patient is similar to that of other age groups, except that the risk of endometrial hyperplasia or malignancy is very low. Pregnancy should always be considered as a possible cause in all women of reproductive age. Appropriate laboratory tests to order in the emergency department would be a BHCG (to rule out pregnancy), a bleeding time (20% of adolescents with dysfunctional uterine bleeding have a coagulation defect, most commonly Von Willebrand disease), and blood type and screen (since she is orthostatic she may require a blood transfusion). A CBC will show the degree of blood loss this patient has suffered. Measuring an estradiol level would serve no purpose in the workup of this patient. Adolescents with chronic anovulation will typically respond well to outpatient therapy, most commonly oral contraceptives. If the patient is hemodynamically unstable, cannot tolerate outpatient management, or is symptomatic from anemia, a brief hospitalization with high dose estrogen may be necessary. In this patient, since she is clinically stable, outpatient treatment with combined oral contraceptives is the most appropriate therapy. It is reasonable to prescribe an OCP taper to try to stop the acute bleeding. There are many ways to do this taper, but one option is to recommend one tablet three times a day for 3 days, one tablet twice a day for 3 days, and then on to one tablet per day. Admission for treatment is not necessary since she is clinically and hemodynamically stable.

375. The answer is d. This patient presents an example of chronic anovulation in an older woman. She gives a classic history of changing from regular, monthly periods to irregular, infrequent episodes of vaginal bleeding. Patients with chronic anovulation often have underlying medical problems such as diabetes, thyroid problems, or PCOS. A patient with uterine fibroids may have heavy periods, but the regularity of the periods is usually not affected unless the patient has underlying ovulatory dysfunction. A cervical polyp would typically be seen on physical examination and, like uterine fibroids, would not affect the timing of menstruation. Patients with cervical polyps often complain of bleeding in between periods, sometimes provoked by intercourse. Since the patient's pregnancy test is negative, she cannot have an incomplete abortion. Patients with coagulation defects typically have problems with heavy periods from the time of menarche.

376. The answer is d. This patient is having bleeding due to ovulatory dysfunction related to PCOS. The transvaginal ultrasound helps direct the next step in the care of this patient. Her endometrial stripe is thin, suggesting that she has shed her endometrium to its basalis layer. Women who have experienced acute heavy bleeding and have an atrophic endometrium should be treated with 25 mg of conjugated estrogen every 4 hours until the bleeding subsides. Estrogen will help stop the bleeding by rebuilding the endometrium and stimulating clotting at the capillary level. Since this patient's bleeding is due to an atrophic endometrium, estrogen therapy is the preferred treatment. Had the transvaginal ultrasound shown a thickened endometrial stripe, hysteroscopy and D&C would be an option to stop the bleeding more rapidly than medical treatment. In older women, a D&C might be helpful in obtaining tissue for pathology to rule out endometrial hyperplasia or cancer. In this young patient who is resuscitated and stabilized with intravenous fluids, there is no indication for a blood transfusion as long as the bleeding abates. Iron therapy alone would not be adequate for this patient; the bleeding must be stopped first. Antiprostaglandins have no role in curtailing hemorrhage in a woman bleeding due to anovulation. They have been used with some success in ovulatory women who have heavy cycles, or in women with menorrhagia caused by use of the IUD. It is thought that prostaglandin synthetase inhibitors reduce the amount of bleeding by promoting vasoconstriction and platelet aggregation.

377. The answer is c. PMS is a constellation of physical, emotional, and behavioral symptoms that occur in a cyclic pattern, always in the same phase of the menstrual cycle. These symptoms usually occur 7 to 10 days before the onset of menses, and are relieved at some point following the onset of menses. Examples of symptoms include edema, mood swings, depression, irritability, breast tenderness, increased appetite, and cravings for sweets. The etiology is unclear. Selective serotonin reuptake inhibitors (SSRIs) are safe, well tolerated, and are considered first line therapy for PMS. For those who don't respond or cannot tolerate SSRIs, other therapies include oral contraceptives, GnRH agonists (with add-back estrogen/progesterone therapy), alprazolam, and aerobic exercise. Progesterone, diet modification, and vitamins have not been proven to be beneficial. The only medications that have been shown in randomized, double-blind, placebo-controlled trials to be consistently effective in treating the emotional symptoms of PMS are the SSRIs such as fluoxetine. Some women can be effectively treated by limiting use of the medication to the luteal phase.

378 to 381. The answers are 378-c, 379-b, 380-d, 381-b. The Women's Health Initiative helped establish that the use of ERT/HRT increases the user's risk of a thromboembolic event two to threefold. The use of combined HRT does not increase the risk of uterine cancer, colon cancer, melanoma, or Alzheimer disease. There is much literature that indicates that HRT reduces the risk of both colon cancer and Alzheimer disease. Estrogen use has a proven beneficial effect on serum lipid concentration. It decreases total cholesterol and LDL and increases HDL and triglycerides.

The hot flush is the first physical symptom of declining ovarian function. More than 95% of perimenopausal/menopausal women experience these vasomotor symptoms. Hot flushes may begin several years before the cessation of menstruation. When a woman experiences a hot flush, she typically feels a sudden sensation of heat over the chest and face that lasts between 1 and 2 minutes, followed by a sensation of cooling or a cold sweat. The entire hot flush lasts about 3 minutes total. Estrogen therapy will usually cause resolution of the hot flush within 3 to 6 weeks. Without estrogen therapy, hot flushes on average resolve spontaneously within 2 to 3 years after cessation of menstruation. Although hot flushes are normal, they may interfere with a woman's sleep, causing significant interference with her sense of well-being. Psychological symptoms during the climacteric occur at a time when much is changing in a woman's life. Steroid hormone levels are dropping, and the menses is stopping. However, studies show these two factors to be unrelated to emotional symptoms in most women. Many factors, such as hormonal, environmental, and psychiatric elements, combine to cause the symptoms of the climacteric such as insomnia; vasomotor instability (hot flushes, hot flashes); emotional lability; and genital tract atrophy with vulvar, vaginal, and urinary symptoms.

382 to 386. The answers are 382-d, 383-b, 384-a, 385-a, 386-c. Gonadotropin dependent precocious puberty is also known as central or true precocious puberty. It is characterized by normal gonadotropin levels (as opposed to expected low prepubertal gonadotropin levels) and a normal ovulatory pattern. It represents premature activation of a normally operating hypothalamic-pituitary axis. In these patients, the sexual characteristics are isosexual, or appropriate for the child's gender. Although it is usually idiopathic, true precocious puberty can arise from cerebral causes such as tumors, radiation, trauma, or inflammatory diseases. Gonadotropin independent precocious puberty is also called peripheral or pseudo precocious puberty. This may be caused by excess secretion of sex hormones (estrogens or androgens) from either intrinsic or exogenous sources. Gonadotropins are suppressed in the prepubertal range. This type of puberty may be isosexual (appropriate for the child's gender), or contrasexual (virilization of girls). Ovarian tumors are the most common cause of isosexual precocious pseudopuberty; some ovarian tumors, including dysgerminomas and choriocarcinomas, can produce so much gonadotropin that pregnancy tests are positive. Incomplete precocious puberty is usually idiopathic, and is characterized by only partial sexual maturity, such as premature thelarche or premature adrenarche (pubarche). Incomplete precocious puberty can be accompanied by abnormal function of the CNS. Gonadotropin levels are frequently normal in these patients. In gonadotropin-producing tumors, high levels of gonadotropins such as FSH are produced with subsequent production of estrogen.

387 to 391. The answers are 387-a, 388-b, 389-c, 390-e, 391-f. Hysterosalpingography is an important tool in the evaluation of infertility. It provides information regarding the shape of the uterine cavity and the patency of the tubes. Tubal factors, which may result from sexually transmitted diseases, are an important cause of infertility. The figure in question 387 displays bilateral hydrosalpinx and clubbing of the tubes, with no evidence of spillage into the peritoneal cavity. The uterine cavity appears normal. The figure in question 388 shows unilateral hydrosalpinx and evidence of adhesions within the uterine cavity consistent with Asherman syndrome. These adhesions appear as filling defects. There is no filling of the other tube, consistent with proximal occlusion. In the figure in question 389, one tube fills and has unilateral hydrosalpinx; the other shows loculation and minimal fluid accumulation. The uterine cavity here is normal. The figure in question 390 shows salpingitis isthmica nodosa, in which there is a characteristic "salt-and-pepper" pattern of tubal filling and evidence of a diverticulum of the tube on one side. The figure in question 391 shows normal filling and spillage of contrast media. This is a normal HSG. None of the figures show bilateral proximal occlusion.

Suggested Readings

American College of Obstetricians and Gynecologists. *Diagnosis of Abnormal Uterine Bleeding in Reproductive-Aged Women.* Practice Bulletin Number 128, July 2012, reaffirmed 2014.

American College of Obstetricians and Gynecologists. *Management of Abnormal Uterine Bleeding Associated with Ovulatory Dysfunction.* Practice Bulletin Number 136, July 2013.

American College of Obstetricians and Gynecologists. *Endometrial Ablation.* Practice Bulletin Number 81, May 2007, reaffirmed 2013.

American College of Obstetricians and Gynecologists. *Noncontraceptive Uses of Hormonal Contraception.* Practice Bulletin Number 110, January 2010, reaffirmed 2014.

American College of Obstetricians and Gynecologists. *Polycystic Ovary Syndrome.* Practice Bulletin Number 108, October 2009, reaffirmed 2013.

Cosman F, de Beur SJ, LeBoff MS, et al. Clinician's guide to prevention and treatment of osteoporosis. *Osteoporos Int.* 2014 Oct;25(10):2359-2381. Epub 2014 Aug 15.

Cushman M, Kuller LH, Prentice R, et al. Estrogen plus progestin and risk of venous thromboembolism. *JAMA.* 2004;292(13):1573.

Speroff L, Fritz M. Chapter 4: The uterus; Chapter 5: Neuroendocrinology; Chapter 9: Sexual development; Chapter 10: Puberty, Chapter 14: Menstrual disorders; Chapter 15: Dysfunctional uterine bleeding; Chapter 17: The perimenopausal transition; Chapter 30: Male infertility. *Clinical Gynecologic Endocrinology and Infertility.* 8th ed. Baltimore, MD: Lippincott, Williams & Wilkins; 2010.

Pelvic Relaxation and Urogynecology

Questions

Questions 392 and 393

A 46-year-old P3003 presents to your office with a chief complaint of leakage of urine. She reports that she leaks when she coughs or sneezes. She is otherwise healthy, does not smoke, and takes no medications. Her history is significant for three vaginal deliveries.

392. Which of the following is the most common cause of urinary incontinence in women of this age?

a. Functional incontinence
b. Urge incontinence
c. Stress urinary incontinence (SUI)
d. Urethral diverticulum
e. Overflow incontinence

393. If this woman were 78-year-old, what would be the most likely cause of urinary incontinence?

a. Anatomic stress urinary incontinence
b. Urethral diverticulum
c. Overflow incontinence
d. Urge incontinence
e. Fistula

394. A healthy 59-year-old woman with no history of urinary incontinence undergoes vaginal hysterectomy with anterior and posterior (A&P) repair for uterine prolapse, a large cystocele, and a rectocele. Two weeks postoperatively, she presents to your office with a new complaint of intermittent leakage of urine. What is the most likely cause of this complaint following her surgery?

a. Urethral diverticulum
b. Overflow incontinence
c. Rectovaginal fistula
d. Stress urinary incontinence
e. Vesicovaginal fistula

395. A 53-year-old postmenopausal woman, G3P3, presents for evaluation of new onset urinary leakage for the past 6 weeks. Which of the following is the most appropriate first step in this patient's evaluation?

a. Urinalysis and culture test
b. Urethral pressure profiles
c. Intravenous pyelogram
d. Cystourethrogram
e. Urethrocystoscopy

396. A 38-year-old woman G4P4 is undergoing evaluation for fecal incontinence. She has no known medical problems. Which of the following is the most likely cause of this patient's condition?

a. Rectal prolapse
b. Diabetes
c. Obstetric trauma
d. Early onset dementia
e. Excessive caffeine intake

397. You are discussing surgical options with the family of an elderly patient with symptomatic pelvic organ prolapse. Le Fort colpocleisis may be more appropriate than vaginal hysterectomy and A&P repair for patients in which of the following circumstances?

a. The patient is debilitated and in a nursing home
b. The patient has had postmenopausal bleeding
c. The patient has had endometrial hyperplasia
d. The patient has had cervical dysplasia that requires colposcopic evaluation
e. The patient has a history of urinary incontinence

398. A 65-year-old woman presents to your office for evaluation of pelvic organ prolapse (POP). Her past medical history is significant for chronic hypertension, which is well controlled with a calcium channel blocker. She also has chronic constipation which requires use of a laxative to have a bowel movement. She has smoked for over 30 years, and has a chronic cough. She entered menopause at the age of 52 years, but has never taken hormone replacement therapy. Her obstetric history includes three term vaginal deliveries. Her last baby weighed 9 lb, and required a forceps delivery. The delivery was complicated by a large tear that involved the vagina and rectum. Which of the following factors is least important in the subsequent development of POP in this patient?

a. Chronic cough
b. Chronic constipation
c. Chronic hypertension
d. Childbirth trauma
e. Menopause

399. A 43-year-old G2P2 woman is being evaluated for hysterectomy for abnormal uterine bleeding that has not responded to conservative management. She mentions during her evaluation that she has a 2-year history of leaking urine when she coughs, sneezes, or laughs. She does not appreciate a sense of urgency. She has to wear a pad when she leaves the house because of the leaking. She has tried Kegel exercises, but has not had any improvement. A urine culture and post void residual (PVR) are normal. A cough stress test in the office demonstrates leaking urine. What is the most appropriate surgical procedure to manage this problem?

a. Marshall-Marchetti-Krantz (MMK) procedure
b. Mid-urethral sling
c. Anterior colporrhaphy with Kelly plication
d. Burch retropubic colposuspension
e. Stamey transvaginal needle suspension

400. A 30-year-old G3P3 is being evaluated for urinary urgency, frequency, and dysuria. She also reports post-void dribbling of urine and insertional dyspareunia. Her history is significant for recurrent urinary tract infections (UTIs) as a teenager, but no other medical problems. She has had three term spontaneous vaginal deliveries, and her last baby weighed over 9 lb. She recalls having a vaginal laceration requiring multiple sutures after delivery of that child. On pelvic examination, she has a 1-cm tender suburethral mass. Palpation of the mass results in expression of a small amount of blood-tinged purulent discharge. Which of the following is the most likely cause of this patient's problem?

a. Urethral polyp
b. Urethral fistula
c. Urethral stricture
d. Urethral eversion
e. Urethral diverticulum

Questions 401 and 402

You evaluate a 39-year-old G2P2 on postoperative day 2 following a difficult abdominal hysterectomy for endometriosis. Her surgery was complicated by hemorrhage from the left uterine artery pedicle that required multiple sutures to control bleeding. Her estimated blood loss was 500 mL. Her only other medical problem is obesity, and her prior surgeries are two cesarean deliveries. The patient now has fever, left back pain, left costovertebral angle tenderness, and hematuria. Her vital signs are height 5 ft 2 in, weight 250 lb, temperature 38.2°C (100.8°F), blood pressure 110/80 mm Hg, respiratory rate 18 breaths per minute, and pulse 102 beats per minute. Her postoperative hemoglobin dropped from 11.2 g/dl to 9.8 g/dl, her white blood cell count is 9.5 L, and her creatinine rose from 0.6 mg/dL to 1.8 mg/dL.

401. What is next best step in the management of this patient?

a. Order chest x-ray
b. Order intravenous pyelogram
c. Order renal ultrasound
d. Start intravenous antibiotics
e. Transfuse two units of packed red blood cells

402. Which of the following aspects of the patient's history is the least likely to have contributed to this postoperative complication?

a. Her history of endometriosis
b. Her age
c. Her weight
d. Her prior cesarean deliveries
e. The hemorrhage at the time of her hysterectomy

Questions 403 and 404

A 59-year-old G4P4 presents to your office with a chief complaint of losing urine when she coughs, sneezes, or engages in certain types of strenuous physical activity. The problem has gotten increasingly worse over the past few years, to the point where she finds her activities of daily living compromised secondary to fear of embarrassment. Her review of symptoms is negative for urgency, frequency, hematuria, or problems with her bowel movements. Her past medical history is significant for type 2 diabetes, which is well controlled on oral Metformin. She does not take any other medications. Her prior surgeries include a tonsillectomy and appendectomy. Her obstetric history is significant for four vaginal deliveries, weighing between 8 lb and 9 lb. Her last delivery was forceps assisted, and was complicated by a third-degree laceration. She has been menopausal for 4 years, and has never taken hormone replacement therapy. Her height is 5 ft 6 in, and she weighs 190 lb. Her blood pressure is 130/80 mm Hg.

403. Based on the patient's history, which of the following is the most likely diagnosis?

a. Overflow incontinence
b. Stress urinary incontinence (SUI)
c. Urinary tract infection
d. Detrusor instability
e. Vesicovaginal fistula

404. Which of the following is the best next step in the initial management of this patient?

a. Recommend an incontinence pessary
b. Schedule her for a mid-urethral sling procedure
c. Refer the patient for formal urodynamic studies
d. Recommend lifestyle modification and Kegel exercises
e. Prescribe pharmacologic therapy

405. A 46-year-old woman presents to your office with a chief complaint of "something bulging" from her vagina. She first noticed it 1 year ago, and it has been getting progressively worse. She has also started to notice that she leaks urine when she laughs or sneezes. She has regular periods every 26 days, and her husband had a vasectomy for contraception. After appropriate evaluation and examination, you diagnose a grade 2 anterior vaginal wall defect (cystocele). She has no uterine prolapse or posterior vaginal wall defect (rectocele). Which of the following is the best treatment plan to offer this patient?

a. Anticholinergic medications
b. Antibiotic therapy with Bactrim
c. Le Fort colpocleisis
d. Anterior colporrhaphy and mid-urethral sling
e. Use of vaginal estrogen cream

406. An obese 46-year-old G6P1051 with type 1 diabetes since the age of 12 years presents to your office with a chief complaint of urinary incontinence. She has been menopausal since the age of 44 years. Her diabetes has been poorly controlled for many years. She often cannot tell when her bladder is full, and she will urinate on herself without warning. Which of the following factors in this patient's history has likely contributed the most to the development of her urinary incontinence?

a. Menopause
b. Obesity
c. Obstetric history
d. Age
e. Suboptimal diabetic control

Questions 407 and 408

A 42-year-old G3P3 presents to your office 2 weeks after undergoing a vaginal hysterectomy, anterior colporrhaphy, and mid-urethral sling for POP and stress incontinence. She is concerned because she has noticed that she constantly leaks urine throughout the day. She reports no urgency or dysuria.

407. Which of the following is the most likely explanation for this complaint?

a. Failure of the procedure
b. Urinary tract infection
c. Vesicovaginal fistula
d. Detrusor instability
e. Diabetic neuropathy

408. What is the next step to try to confirm you suspected diagnosis?

a. Order an intravenous pyelogram
b. Perform a cystoscopy
c. Refer her to urology for further evaluation
d. Perform a physical examination and an in-office dye study
e. Order a CT of the pelvis with contrast

Questions 409 to 410

A 90-year-old G5P5 with multiple medical problems is brought into your office accompanied by her granddaughter. Her medical history is significant for hypertension, chronic anemia, coronary artery disease, and osteoporosis. She is alert and oriented, and lives in an assisted living facility. She takes numerous medications, but is very functional at the current time. She is a widow and is not sexually active. Her chief complaint is a sensation of heaviness and pressure in the vagina. It is uncomfortable when she sits. She reports no significant urinary or bowel problems. On physical examination, you note that the cervix to the level just inside the introitus.

409. Based on the physical examination, which of the following is the most likely diagnosis?

a. Normal examination
b. First-degree uterine prolapse
c. Second-degree uterine prolapse
d. Third-degree uterine prolapse
e. Complete procidentia

410. What is the best next step in the management of this patient?

a. Reassurance
b. Placement of a pessary
c. Le Fort colpocleisis
d. Vaginal hysterectomy with apical repair
e. Anterior colporrhaphy

411. If instead of the scenario described earlier, this patient told you that she was asymptomatic from this pelvic organ prolapse, what would be the best next step in management?

a. Reassurance
b. Placement of a pessary
c. Vaginal hysterectomy
d. Le Fort colpocleisis
e. Anterior colporrhaphy

412. A 78-year-old woman with chronic obstructive pulmonary disease, chronic hypertension, and history of myocardial infarction requiring angioplasty presents to your office for evaluation of "something hanging out of her vagina." She had a hysterectomy for benign indications at the age of 48 years. For the past few months, she has been experiencing pelvic pressure and a bulge at the vaginal opening. She reports that 2 weeks ago, something fell out of her vagina. Pelvic examination demonstrates total eversion of the vagina. There is an arc of superficial ulceration at the vaginal apex measuring 2 to 3 cm in diameter. Which of the following is the best next step in the management of this patient?

a. Biopsy of the vaginal ulceration
b. Schedule abdominal sacral colpopexy
c. Place a pessary
d. Prescribe oral estrogen
e. Prescribe topical vaginal estrogen cream

Questions 413 to 415

A 40-year-old G3P3 presents for a routine annual examination. She tells you that she gets up several times during the night to void. She also reports that during the day she sometimes gets the urge to void, but cannot quite make it to the bathroom in time. She does not leak urine when she coughs or sneezes. Upon further questioning, she admits to drinking several large glasses of iced tea and water on a daily basis, because her mother always told her to drink lots of liquids to decrease her risk of developing a UTI. She attributes this to getting older and is not extremely concerned, although she often wears a pad when she goes out because she is afraid she will leak urine. The patient is otherwise healthy, and does not take any medication. She has had three vaginal deliveries of infants weighing between 7 lb and 8 lb. An office dipstick of her urine does not indicate any blood, bacteria, WBCs, or protein. Her urine culture is negative.

413. Based on her office presentation and history, which of the following is the most likely diagnosis?

a. Stress urinary incontinence (SUI)
b. Urinary tract infection
c. Urge incontinence
d. Vesicovaginal fistula
e. Mixed incontinence

414. Which of the following treatments should you recommend to the patient as the next step in the management of her problem?

a. Instruct her to start performing Kegel exercises.
b. Tell her to hold her urine for 6 hours at a time to enlarge her bladder capacity.
c. Instruct her to eliminate excess water and caffeine from her daily fluid intake.
d. Prescribe an anticholinergic.
e. Schedule a cystoscopy.

415. This patient returns to your office 3 months later, and continues to be symptomatic after following your advice for conservative self-treatment. Which of the following is the best next step in management?

a. Prescribe Ditropan (oxybutynin chloride)
b. Prescribe estrogen therapy
c. Schedule a mid-urethral sling
d. Refer her to an urologist for urethral dilation
e. Schedule a voiding cystourethrogram

416. An 18-year-old G0 comes to see you with a chief complaint of a 3-day history of urinary frequency, urgency, and dysuria. She panicked this morning when she noticed bright red blood in her urine. She also reports some midline lower abdominal discomfort. She had intercourse for the first time 5 days ago and reports that she used condoms. On physical examination, there are no lacerations of the external genitalia, there is no discharge from the cervix or in the vagina, and the cervix appears normal. Bimanual examination is normal except for mild suprapubic tenderness. There is no flank tenderness, and the patient's temperature is normal. Which of the following is the most likely diagnosis?

a. Chlamydia cervicitis
b. Pyelonephritis
c. Acute cystitis
d. Acute appendicitis
e. Monilial vaginitis

417. A 28-year-old woman presents to your office with symptoms of a UTI. This is her second infection in 2 months. You treated the last infection with Bactrim DS for 3 days. Her symptoms never really improved. Now she has worsening lower abdominal discomfort, dysuria, and frequency. She reports no fever or flank pain. Physical examination shows only mild suprapubic tenderness. Which of the following is the best next step in the evaluation of this patient?

a. Urine culture
b. Intravenous pyelogram
c. Cystoscopy
d. Wet smear
e. Treat her with a different antibiotic

418. You have diagnosed a healthy, sexually active 24-year-old female patient with an uncomplicated acute UTI. Which of the following is the most likely organism responsible for this patient's infection?

a. *Chlamydia*
b. *Pseudomonas*
c. *Klebsiella*
d. *Escherichia coli*
e. *Candida albicans*

419. A 32-year-old woman presents to your office with dysuria, urinary frequency, and urinary urgency for 24 hours. She is healthy but is allergic to sulfa drugs. Urinalysis shows large blood, leukocytes, and nitrites in her urine. Which of the following medications is the best to treat this patient's condition?

a. Dicloxacillin
b. Bactrim
c. Nitrofurantoin
d. Azithromycin
e. Flagyl

420. You are seeing a patient in the emergency department who presents with fever, chills, flank pain, and blood in her urine. She has had severe nausea and started vomiting after the fever developed. She was diagnosed with a UTI 3 days ago by her primary care physician, but she never took the antibiotics that were prescribed, because her symptoms improved after she started drinking cranberry juice. The patient has a temperature of 38.8°C (102°F). On physical examination, she has right-sided CVA tenderness and suprapubic tenderness. Her clean-catch urinalysis shows a large amount of ketones, RBCs, WBCs, bacteria, and squamous cells. Which of the following is the most appropriate next step in the management of this patient?

a. Tell her to take the oral antibiotics that she was prescribed and give her a prescription for Phenergan rectal suppositories.
b. Admit the patient for IV fluids and IV antibiotics.
c. Admit the patient for diagnostic laparoscopy.
d. Admit the patient for an intravenous pyelogram and consultation with an urologist.
e. Arrange for a home health agency to go to the patient's home to administer IV fluids and oral antibiotics.

421. A 22-year-old woman has been seeing you for treatment of recurrent UTIs over the past 6 months. She married 6 months ago and became sexually active at that time. She seems to become symptomatic shortly after having intercourse. Which of the following is the most appropriate treatment?

a. Refer her to an urologist
b. Schedule an IVP
c. Prescribe prophylactic urinary antispasmodic
d. Prescribe antibiotic suppression
e. Recommend that she use condoms to prevent recurrent UTIs

Pelvic Relaxation
and Urogynecology

Answers

392 and 393. The answers are 392-c, 393-d. SUI is the involuntary loss of urine when intravesical pressure exceeds the maximum urethral pressure in the absence of detrusor activity. It is often brought on by laughing, coughing, or sneezing. This incidence is highest in women between the ages of 45 and 50. SUI may be caused by urethral hypermobility or intrinsic sphincter deficiency (ISD). The other major cause of incontinence is urge incontinence. With urge incontinence, the bladder leaks urine due to involuntary, uninhibited detrusor contractions. The incidence of urge incontinence increases with age. Other causes of urinary incontinence are less common and include overflow incontinence secondary to urinary retention, congenital abnormalities, infections, fistulas, and urethral diverticula. Urethral diverticula classically present with dribbling incontinence after voiding. Functional incontinence occurs when a patient cannot reach the toilet in time due to physical, cognitive, or psychological limitations.

In the elderly population there are also many transient causes of incontinence that the physician should consider. These include dementia, medications (especially α-adrenergic blockers), decreased patient mobility, endocrine abnormalities (hypercalcemia, hypothyroidism), stool impaction, and UTIs.

394. The answer is d. Many patients who have uterine prolapse or a large protuberant cystocele will be continent because of urethral obstruction caused by the cystocele or prolapse. In fact, at times these patients may need to reduce the prolapse in order to void. Following surgical repair, if the urethrovesical junction is not properly elevated, SUI may result. This incontinence may present within the first few days to weeks following surgery. Typically, patients undergoing hysterectomy for prolapse will be evaluated with urodynamic or other studies to help determine if they are likely to leak once normal anatomy is restored following surgery. If they are shown to leak when the cystocele is reduced, the physician may recommend a concomitant procedure to support the mid urethra, such as a mid-urethral sling, to avoid the development of SUI postoperatively. Rectovaginal fistula would present with passage of stool from vagina. Vesicovaginal fistula would present with continuous leakage of urine from the vagina. Detrusor instability would have been present prior to her surgery.

395. The answer is a. When patients present with urinary incontinence, a urinalysis and culture tests should be performed to evaluate for acute cystitis. In patients diagnosed with a UTI, treatment should be initiated, and then the patient should be reevaluated. It is not uncommon for symptoms of urinary leakage to resolve after appropriate therapy. After obtaining the history and physical examination and evaluating a urinalysis and urine culture, only a few clinical tests are necessary in the initial evaluation of the incontinent patient. Most women with incontinence can begin conservative treatment based on history and examination alone. However, further conservative evaluation may include a PVR urine volume, cough stress test, and urinary diary. A PVR is determined by bladder catheterization after the patient has voided; when a large amount of urine remains after voiding, infection and incontinence may result. A cough stress test is performed by filling the bladder with fluid, asking the patient to cough or Valsalva, and directly visualizing the urethra to see if there is leakage.

396. The answer is c. The most common cause of fecal incontinence is obstetric trauma that causes direct damage to the anal sphincter or to the pudendal nerve. The rectal sphincter can be completely lacerated, but as long as the patient retains a functional puborectalis sling, a high degree of continence will be maintained. Anal sphincter weakness may also be caused by other nontraumatic etiologies, such as spinal cord injury. Other causes of fecal incontinence include conditions that decrease rectal sensation, such as dementia, central nervous system (CNS) disease, diabetes, or multiple sclerosis. Therapy for fecal incontinence includes bulk-forming and antispasmodic agents, especially in those patients presenting with diarrhea. All caffeinated beverages should be stopped. Biofeedback and electrical stimulation of the rectal sphincter are other possible conservative treatments. Surgical repair of a defect is indicated when conservative measures fail, when the defect is large, or when symptoms warrant a more aggressive treatment approach.

397. The answer is a. Partial colpocleisis by the Le Fort procedure is reasonable for elderly patients who are not good candidates for surgery as treatment for uterine prolapse. The technique is appropriate for women who have a uterus in situ, and involves partial denudation of opposing surfaces of the vaginal mucosa followed by surgical apposition, thereby resulting in partial obliteration of the vagina. Small strips of vaginal epithelium are left laterally, to allow an outlet for drainage or bleeding. Patients who are candidates for this procedure must have no evidence of cervical dysplasia or endometrial hyperplasia, and must have an atrophic endometrium. This type of obliterative procedure is ideal for women who cannot tolerate a more extensive surgery and who no longer plan to have vaginal intercourse. A similar obliterative procedure may be performed in women who have already undergone hysterectomy, as treatment for vaginal prolapse. Urinary incontinence can be a side effect of these procedures, so many surgeons perform a concomitant incontinence procedure at the same time. An A&P repair essentially involves excision of redundant mucosa along the A&P walls of the vagina, at the same time strengthening the vaginal walls by suturing the lateral paravaginal fascia together in the midline.

398. The answer is c. POP involves herniation of the pelvic organs to or beyond the vaginal walls. Chronic cough, constipation, obstetric trauma, and menopause are all risk factors for this condition. Undoubtedly, the most important factor is the actual quality of the tissue itself. There is a much lower incidence of POP in black women compared to white women. Any factors that increase intra-abdominal pressure can aggravate or further deteriorate the prolapse. Vaginal delivery is a risk factor for POP, and operative vaginal delivery may further increase the risk. High birth weight also contributes to development of POP. Chronic hypertension is not a risk factor for POP.

399. The answer is b. A mid-urethral sling is the procedure of choice in women undergoing primary surgery for uncomplicated SUI. For many years, the Burch retropubic colposuspension was considered the gold standard; however, mid-urethral slings have been shown to have comparable success rates, and are less invasive with a shorter operative time and faster recovery. The MMK is a type of bladder neck suspension, and the Stamey is a needle urethropexy; both procedures are no longer used. Anterior repair with Kelly plication is not an effective surgery for treatment of SUI.

400. The answer is e. Urethral diverticula occur in 3% to 4% of all women. Classic symptoms include urinary frequency, urgency, dysuria, hematuria, and dyspareunia. Patients often report a history of frequent UTIs, dribbling, or incontinence. A urethral diverticulum is often palpable as a tender mass on the anterior vaginal wall under the urethra. Although urethral polyps, eversion, fistula, and stricture may present with similar symptoms, there is no suburethral mass present on examination.

401. The answer is c. The patient most likely has a ureteral injury near the location of the left uterine artery. A noninvasive renal ultrasound is fast, inexpensive, and accurate way to make the diagnosis by evaluating for hydronephrosis and/or a retroperitoneal fluid collection. Cystoscopy with retrograde intravenous pyelogram has largely been replaced by computed tomography (CT). A CT scan with contrast gives excellent information about the integrity and function of the renal collecting system; however, when the serum creatinine is elevated, intravenous contrast can cause significant renal damage and is contraindicated in those circumstances. A chest x-ray would not be helpful in making the diagnosis. Intravenous antibiotics are not indicated at this time since there is not clear evidence of an infection (normal white blood cell count). The patient has a normal drop in hemoglobin for the surgical blood loss, and does not have signs of hemodynamic instability to warrant a blood transfusion at this time.

402. The answer is b. Postoperative ureteral injury is a potential complication following gynecologic surgery. Risk factors for ureteral injury include endometriosis, surgery for malignant conditions, prior pelvic radiation, obesity, prior pelvic surgery, and conditions that impair visualization or tissue planes (such as hemorrhage). Her age is not a risk factor for ureteral injury.

403 and 404. The answers are 403-b, 404-d. This patient's history is most consistent with a diagnosis of SUI. Stress incontinence is a condition of immediate involuntary loss of urine when intravesical pressure exceeds the maximum urethral pressure in the absence of detrusor activity. SUI is typically caused by urethral hypermobility, intrinsic sphincter deficiency, or a combination of both. Patients with this condition often complain of urine loss with anything that increases intra-abdominal pressure, such as vigorous physical activity, coughing, laughing, or sneezing. Overflow incontinence typically presents with continuous loss of a small amount of urine, often with associated symptoms of fullness and pressure. Overflow incontinence is usually caused by obstruction or loss of neurologic control. Women with detrusor instability/overactivity have a loss of bladder inhibition, and report symptoms of urgency, frequency, and nocturia. Vesicovaginal fistulas usually occur as a complication of benign gynecologic procedures. Women with this complication usually present with a painless and continuous loss of urine from the vagina. Sometimes the uncontrolled loss of urine is not continuous, but related to a change in position or posture. Women with UTIs usually present with symptoms of frequency, urgency, nocturia, dysuria, and hematuria. Initial treatment for uncomplicated SUI involves lifestyle modification and Kegel exercise. Behavioral modification may include weight loss, scheduled voiding, caffeine reduction and fluid management, smoking cessation, and relief of constipation. Kegel exercises may be taught to strengthen the voluntary urethral sphincter and levator ani muscles. This conservative approach to treatment should be attempted for several weeks before moving on to other forms of treatment such as an incontinence pessary or surgical treatment with a mid-urethral sling. Urodynamic studies do not have a role in the early management of uncomplicated SUI. Pharmacologic therapy, such as anticholinergic medications, is more often used to treat urge incontinence, not stress incontinence.

405. The answer is d. Surgical therapy for SUI and cystocele may be accomplished with anterior colporrhaphy and mid-urethral sling. Placement of a pessary is an option to relieve a cystocele, but is not ideal in this patient, who is sexually active, and feels her quality of life is being impacted. Antibiotics such as Bactrim would be used to treat a UTI, but would not treat a cystocele or SUI. A Le Fort colpocleisis is performed in patients with POP who are poor surgical candidates and not sexually active. The procedure involves obliterating the vaginal canal to provide support to the pelvic structures. Anticholinergic drugs such as Ditropan (oxybutynin chloride) are used to relax the bladder in the treatment of detrusor overactivity. The use of vaginal estrogen cream may relieve vaginal atrophy and improve patient comfort in postmenopausal patients, but it will not correct the cystocele or treat incontinence.

406. The answer is e. Poorly controlled diabetes can result in neuropathies to various organs, including the bladder. This can result in loss of bladder sensation and subsequent overflow urinary incontinence. Diabetes does not cause pelvic relaxation. Natural aging of the tissue, intrinsic weaknesses caused by genetics, birth trauma, hypoestrogenism, and chronic elevation of intra-abdominal pressure because of obesity, cough, or heavy lifting are all factors that contribute to pelvic relaxation.

407 and 408. The answer are 407-c, 408-d. Both vesicovaginal and ureterovaginal fistulas are complications that occur rarely after benign gynecologic procedures. Classically, urinary tract fistulas present with painless and continuous loss of urine 8 to 12 days after surgery. UTIs and detrusor overactivity present with dysuria, urgency, and frequency. Since this patient has no symptoms of stress incontinence, failure of the procedure would not be the correct answer. The first step in evaluation for a vesicovaginal fistula is a careful physical examination. It may be possible to identify a fistula as a defect in the mucosa, or as a erythematous area of granulation tissue. In many cases, the actual fistula cannot be seen. An in-office dye study may be performed by retrograde filling the bladder with a mixture of saline and indigo carmine dye. Speculum examination may then be performed to evaluate for a fistula directly, and the patient may be asked to Valsalva to encourage leakage. Alternatively, a tampon may be placed in the vagina, and evaluated to see if it stains blue, indicating a fistula.

409 to 411. The answers are 409-c, 410-b, 411-a. The degree or severity of pelvic relaxation is rated on a scale of 1 to 3, based on the descent of the organ or structure involved. First-degree prolapse involves descent limited to the upper two-thirds of the vagina. Second-degree prolapse is present when the structure is at the vaginal introitus. In cases of third-degree prolapse, the structure is outside the vagina. Total procidentia of the uterus is the same as a third-degree prolapse, which means that the uterus would be located outside the body.

Uterine prolapse that does not bother the patient or cause her any great discomfort does not require treatment. This especially applies to patients who are elderly or poor surgical candidates. Placement of a pessary provides mechanical support to pelvic tissue, while hysterectomy and the Le Fort procedure are surgical treatments for prolapse. An anterior colporrhaphy is a surgical method to reduce a cystocele. Pessaries provide mechanical support for the pelvic organs. These devices come in a variety of sizes and shapes and are placed in the vagina to provide support. Pessaries are ideal for patients who are not good surgical candidates. Potential complications from pessaries include vaginal trauma, necrosis, discharge from inflammation, and urinary stress incontinence.

412. The answer is c. Vaginal vault prolapse occurs in up to 18% of patients who have undergone hysterectomy. Symptoms include pelvic pressure, backache, and a mass protruding from the vagina. Depending on the duration and degree of the prolapse, the patient may also have vaginal ulcerations from the prolapsed vagina rubbing against the undergarments. This patient is a poor surgical candidate given her multiple medical problems; therefore abdominal sacral colpopexy is not the ideal treatment. Her age and medical history also preclude oral estrogen treatment. The preferred treatment is to place a pessary to prevent the vagina from rubbing against clothing and to relieve her sense of pelvic pressure and vaginal bulge. The patient could also apply a topical estrogen cream to the lesion and the prolapsed vagina to help with healing of the ulcer. If the ulcer does not resolve, biopsy is indicated.

413 to 415. The answers are 413-c, 414-c, 415-a. This patient's presentation is most consistent with urge incontinence. Urge incontinence is the involuntary loss of urine associated with a strong desire to void. Most urge incontinence is caused by detrusor overactivity, in which there is an involuntary contraction of the bladder during distension with urine. The initial management includes lifestyle modification such as weight loss, smoking cessation, relief of constipation, minimizing caffeine, and normalizing fluid intake. Other conservative treatments may include bladder training or biofeedback. If conservative measures fail, treatment with anticholinergic medications such as oxybutynin chloride may be successful. These medications inhibit the contractile activity of the bladder. Kegel exercises may strengthen the pelvic musculature and improve bladder control in women with SUI.

416 to 421. The answers are 416-c, 417-a, 418-d, 419-c, 420-b, 421-d. Approximately 11% of women report at least one documented UTI per year, and up to 60% of women will have UTI during the course of their lifetime. Acute cystitis usually presents with the symptoms of dysuria, frequency, and urgency. In contrast, patients with pyelonephritis may have the same symptoms accompanied by fever, chills, and/or flank pain. A UTI may be diagnosed by evaluating a clean, mid-stream urine sample and finding at least 100,000 single isolate bacteria per mL. A urine dipstick is a fast and inexpensive way to diagnose a simple UTI, and has a sensitivity of 75%. Women with a normal urine dipstick who are symptomatic should have a urine culture, because false negative results are common. The most common causative organism is *E coli*, which is responsible for 80% to 95% of infections. Other organisms include *Proteus, Pseudomonas, Klebsiella, Enterobacter,* and *Staphylococcus Saprophyticus.* Uncomplicated UTIs may be treated with a 3-day course of an antibiotic regimen with trimethoprim-sulfamethoxazole or nitrofurantoin, which have good coverage against *E coli* and are relatively inexpensive. Patients treated for a UTI who have persistent symptoms after treatment should have a urine culture performed to evaluate for the presence of resistant organisms. Patients with acute pyelonephritis may be treated on an outpatient basis unless they cannot tolerate oral antibiotic therapy or show evidence of sepsis. Women who experience recurrent UTIs with intercourse benefit from voiding immediately after intercourse. If this treatment method fails, then postcoital prophylactic treatment with an antibiotic effective against *E coli* may help prevent recurrent UTIs. Urinary antispasmodics do not prevent infection.

Suggested Readings

American College of Obstetricians and Gynecologists. *Episiotomy.* Practice Bulletin Number 71. April 2006, reaffirmed 2013.

American College of Obstetricians and Gynecologists. *Pelvic Organ Prolapse.* Practice Bulletin Number 85. September 2007, reaffirmed 2013.

American College of Obstetricians and Gynecologists. *Treatment of Urinary Tract Infections in Nonpregnant Women.* Practice Bulletin Number 91. March 2008, reaffirmed 2014.

American College of Obstetricians and Gynecologists. *Urinary Incontinence in Women.* Practice Bulletin Number 63. June 2005, reaffirmed 2015.

Human Sexuality and Contraception

Questions

423. A 20-year-old G0 and her partner, a 20-year-old man, present for counseling for sexual dysfunction. Prior to their relationship, neither had been sexually active. Both report no medical problems. In medical experience, which type of male or female sexual dysfunction has the lowest cure rate?

a. Premature ejaculation
b. Vaginismus
c. Primary impotence
d. Secondary impotence
e. Female orgasmic dysfunction

424. A 28-year-old G3P3 presents to your office for contraceptive counseling. She has no history of medical problems or sexually transmitted diseases. You counsel her on the risks and benefits of all contraceptive methods. Which of the following is the most common form of contraception used by reproductive-age women in the United States?

a. Pills
b. Condom
c. Diaphragm
d. Intrauterine device (IUD)
e. Sterilization

425. A 21-year-old woman presents to your office for her well-woman examination. She has recently become sexually active and desires an effective contraceptive method. She has no medical problems, but family history is significant for breast cancer in a maternal aunt at the age of 42 years. She is worried about getting cancer from taking birth control pills. You discuss with her the risks and benefits of contraceptive pills. You tell her that which of the following neoplasms has been associated with the use of oral contraceptives?

a. Breast cancer
b. Ovarian cancer
c. Endometrial cancer
d. Hepatic cancer
e. Hepatic adenoma

Questions 426 to 428

426. A 35-year-old G2P2 presents for a contraceptive counseling visit. She and her husband desire a long-term contraceptive method, and are uncertain if they want more children. She has been happily married for 10 years. Her only medical problem is mild hypertension, for which she takes a diuretic, and she has never had a sexually transmitted disease. She is considering the copper IUD and wants to know how it works. Which of the following mechanisms does not potentially contribute to the mechanism of the action of the copper IUD?

a. Decreased tubal motility inhibits ovum transport.
b. An inflammatory response within the endometrium damages the fertilized ovum.
c. Premature endometrial sloughing associated with menorrhagia causes early abortion.
d. An inflammatory response within the endometrium kills sperm.
e. Thickened cervical mucus blocks sperm transport.

427. The patient asks if she is a good candidate for an IUD. In which of the following situations would use of an IUD be contraindicated?

a. Uterine abnormalities that distort the uterine cavity
b. A history of chorioamnionitis in her last pregnancy
c. A history of *Chlamydia* infection treated 4 months ago
d. History of a loop electro-excision procedure (LEEP)
e. History of recurrent vulvar candidiasis

428. The patient decided to have the copper IUD placed. It is inserted without difficulty, and she returned 1 month later, at which time it was confirmed that her IUD string was in place. One year later, she returned because she had a positive pregnancy test. On examination, the IUD string is seen protruding from the cervical os. Ultrasound demonstrates a 10-week intrauterine pregnancy. The patient and her husband express a strong desire for the pregnancy to be continued. What is the best next step in management?

a. Leave the IUD in place without any other treatment.
b. Leave the IUD in place and continue prophylactic antibiotics throughout pregnancy.
c. Remove the IUD immediately.
d. Terminate the pregnancy because of the high risk of infection.
e. Perform a laparoscopy to rule out a heterotopic ectopic pregnancy.

429. A 21-year-old G0 presents to your office because her menses is 2 weeks late. She states that she is taking her birth control pills correctly; she may have missed a day at the beginning of the pack, but took it as soon as she remembered. She has no medical problems, but 3 weeks ago she had a "viral stomach flu," and missed 2 days of work due to nausea, vomiting, and diarrhea. Her cycles are usually regular, even without oral contraceptive pills. She has been on the pill for 5 years, and recently developed some midcycle bleeding, which usually lasts about 2 days. She has been sexually active with the same partner for the past 3 months, and has a history of chlamydia 3 years ago. She has had a total of 10 sexual partners. A urine pregnancy test is positive. Which of the following is the major cause of unplanned pregnancies in women using oral contraceptives?

a. Breakthrough ovulation at midcycle
b. High frequency of intercourse
c. Incorrect use of oral contraceptives
d. Gastrointestinal malabsorption
e. Development of antibodies

430. A 34-year-old G1P1 with a history of pulmonary embolism presents to your office to discuss contraception. Her cycles are regular. She has a history of pelvic inflammatory disease (PID) last year, for which she was hospitalized. She has currently been sexually active with the same partner for 1 year. She wants to use condoms and a spermicide. You counsel her on the risks and benefits. Which of the following statements correctly describes spermicides found in vaginal foams, creams, and suppositories?

a. The active agent in spermicides is nonoxynol-9.
b. Spermicides are protective against sexually transmitted infections.
c. Effectiveness is higher in younger users.
d. Effectiveness is higher than that of the diaphragm.
e. These agents are associated with an increased incidence of congenital malformations.

431. A 32-year-old woman presents for her annual examination. She is worried because she has not been able to achieve orgasm with her new partner, with whom she has had a relationship for the past 3 months. She had three prior sexual partners, and was able to achieve orgasm with each of them. Her medications include a combined oral contraceptive (COC) pill for birth control, clonidine for chronic hypertension, and fluoxetine for depression. She smokes one pack per day and drinks one drink per week. She had a cervical cone biopsy for severe cervical dysplasia 6 months ago. Which of the following is the most likely cause of her sexual dysfunction?

a. Alcohol
b. Birth control pills
c. Clonidine
d. Disruption of cervical nerve pathways
e. Fluoxetine

432. A 22-year-old woman presents to your office for a well-woman examination. She has been sexually active with one male partner for the past year. She is concerned because she has not achieved orgasm with her partner. On further questioning, she reveals that she has never achieved orgasm with any other partners, or with masturbation or the use of a vibrator. Which of the following statements correctly describes her condition?

a. It is unrelated to partner behavior.
b. The influence of religious beliefs is a major etiology.
c. It is unrelated to partner's sexual performance.
d. It is not associated with a history of rape.
e. It always has an underlying physical etiology.

433. A 23-year-old woman presents to your office with the complaint of a red splotchy rash on her chest that occurs during intercourse. It is nonpuritic and painless. She states that it usually resolves within a few minutes to a few hours after intercourse. Which of the following is the most likely cause of the rash?

a. Allergic reaction to her partner's pheromones
b. Decreased systolic blood pressure during the plateau phase
c. Increased estrogen during the excitement phase
d. Vasocongestion during the excitement phase
e. Vasoconstriction during the orgasmic phase

434. A 19-year-old woman presents for elective termination of pregnancy at 8 weeks' gestation. She previously had regular menses every 28 days. Pregnancy is confirmed by β-human chorionic gonadotropin (β-hCG), and ultrasound confirms expected gestational age. Which of the following techniques for termination of pregnancy would be safe and effective in this patient at this time?

a. Dilation and evacuation (D&E)
b. Hypertonic saline infusion
c. Suction dilation and curettage (D&C)
d. Misoprostol
e. Hysterotomy

435. A 48-year-old woman presents to your office with the complaint of vaginal dryness during intercourse. She reports no medical problems or prior surgeries, and she does not take any medications. She has regular menstrual cycles every 28 days, and has never had asexually transmitted disease. She describes her sexual relationship with her husband as satisfying. Her physical examination is normal. Components of the natural lubrication produced by the female during sexual arousal and intercourse include which of the following?

a. Fluid from Skene glands
b. Mucus produced by endocervical glands
c. Viscous fluid from Bartholin glands
d. Transudate-like material from the vaginal walls
e. Uterotubal fluid

436. A 62-year-old woman presents for annual examination. Her last menstrual period was 9 years ago, and she never used postmenopausal hormone replacement because of a strong family history of breast cancer. She now complains of diminished interest in sexual activity. Which of the following is the most likely cause of her complaint?

a. Decreased vaginal length
b. Decreased ovarian function
c. Alienation from her partner
d. Untreatable sexual dysfunction
e. Physiologic anorgasmia

437. A 22-year-old nulliparous woman has recently become sexually active. She consults you because of painful intercourse. She says her pain occurs with insertion, and is accompanied by cramping of her pelvic muscles. She says it is so painful that she does not want to have intercourse with her boyfriend, which is causing problems in their relationship. Other than confirmation of these findings, the pelvic examination is normal. Which of the following is the most common cause of this condition?

a. Endometriosis
b. Psychogenic causes
c. Bartholin gland abscess
d. Vulvar atrophy
e. Ovarian cyst

438. A 23-year-old woman presents for her postpartum visit and contraception management. She delivered by spontaneous vaginal delivery 6 weeks ago and is breastfeeding. After reviewing her history and performing physical examination, you discuss the various methods of contraception with the patient. She opts for depot medroxyprogesterone acetate (Depo-Provera). Which of the following is a disadvantage of Depo-Provera?

a. Impairment of lactation
b. Increased risk of hepatic cancer
c. Iron deficiency anemia
d. Irreversible bone loss
e. Prolonged anovulation

439. A 36-year-old woman presents to your office to discuss contraception. She has had three vaginal deliveries without complications. Her medical history is significant for hypertension, well controlled with a diuretic, and a seizure disorder. Her last seizure was 12 years ago. Currently she does not take any antiepileptic medications. She also reports stress-related headaches that are relieved with an over-the-counter pain medication. She has never had any surgery. She is divorced, smokes one pack of cigarettes per day, and has three to four alcoholic drinks per week. On examination, her vital signs include weight 90 kg, blood pressure 126/80 mm Hg, pulse 68 beats per minute, respiratory rate 16 breaths per minute, and temperature 36.4°C (97.6°F). Her examination is normal except for some lower extremity nontender varicosities. She has taken birth control pills in the past and wants to restart them because they help with her cramps. Which of the following would contradict the use of combination oral contraceptive pills in this patient?

a. Varicose veins
b. Tension headache
c. Seizure disorders
d. Smoking in a woman older than 35 years
e. Mild essential hypertension

440. A 32-year-old woman presents to your office to discuss contraception. She has recently stopped breastfeeding her 8-month-old son, and wants to stop her progestin-only pill (mini pill) because her cycles are irregular on it. You recommend a combination pill to help regulate her cycle. You also mention that with estrogen added, the contraceptive efficacy is also higher. In combination oral contraceptives, which of the following is the primary contraceptive effect of the estrogenic component?

a. Conversion of ethinyl estradiol to mestranol
b. Atrophy of the endometrium
c. Suppression of cervical mucus secretion
d. Suppression of luteinizing hormone (LH) secretion
e. Suppression of follicle-stimulating hormone (FSH) secretion

441. A 22-year-old woman presents to your office for her well-woman examination and contraception. She has no medical problems or prior surgeries. She does not smoke or drink. Her vital signs and physical examination are normal. You explain the risks and benefits of combination oral contraceptive pills to the patient. She wants to know how they will keep her from getting pregnant. Which of the following mechanisms best explains the contraceptive effect of birth control pills that contain both synthetic estrogen and progestin?

a. Direct inhibition of oocyte maturation
b. Inhibition of ovulation
c. Production of uterine secretions that are toxic to developing embryos
d. Impairment of implantation hyperplastic changes of the endometrium
e. Impairment of sperm transport caused by uterotubal obstruction

442. A 34-year-old G3P3 presents to discuss options for permanent sterilization. She has read about hysteroscopic sterilization, and is interested in having this procedure. Which of the following is a contraindication to this procedure?

a. Nickel allergy
b. Grand multiparity
c. History of postpartum endometritis
d. History of pelvic inflammatory disease (PID)
e. History of deep vein thrombosis (DVT)

443. A 30-year-old woman presents to your office for her well-woman examination and contraception. She has two prior vaginal deliveries without any complications. Her medical history is significant for DVT in her right leg after her last delivery. Her family history is significant for coronary artery disease in her father, and breast cancer in her mother diagnosed at the age of 62 years. After a discussion of her choices for contraception, she opts for a mini-pill. Which of the following is true regarding the use of mini pills?

a. Contraindicated in women with migraine headaches
b. Decrease risk of ovarian cysts
c. Inhibition of ovulation is the main mechanism of action
d. May worsen acne
e. More effective than injectable progestins

444. A 19-year-old patient calls in your office requesting emergency contraception because a condom she and her boyfriend were using broke during intercourse last night. You counsel the patient appropriately and provide a suitable method of contraception. Which of the following statements correctly describes emergency contraception?

a. If an established pregnancy is present use of Plan B will cause an abortion.
b. Mifepristone is less effective than the Yuptze method.
c. Out of 100 women using emergency contraception 10 will become pregnant.
d. The emergency contraceptive, Plan B, requires a prescription.
e. The major mechanism of action of emergency hormone contraceptives is inhibition or delay of ovulation.

445. A couple presents to your office to discuss sterilization. They are very happy with their four children and do not want any more. You discuss with them the pros and cons of both female and male sterilization. The 34-year-old man undergoes a vasectomy. Which of the following is the most frequent immediate complication of this procedure?

a. Infection
b. Impotence
c. Hematoma
d. Spontaneous reanastomosis
e. Sperm granulomas

Questions 446 to 450

For each female patient seeking contraception, select the method that is medically contraindicated for that patient. Each lettered option may be used once, more than once, or not at all.

a. Progestin-only contraceptive pills
b. Intrauterine device (IUD)
c. Condoms
d. Laparoscopic tubal ligation
e. Diaphragm

446. A woman with Wilson disease

447. A woman with a history of breast cancer

448. A woman with moderate cystocele

449. A woman with severely reduced functional capacity as a result of chronic obstructive pulmonary disease

450. A woman with a known latex allergy

Questions 451 to 457

For the following clinical scenarios, select the most appropriate sexual dysfunction disorder. Each lettered option may be used once, more than once, or not at all.

a. Dyspareunia
b. Female orgasmic disorder
c. Female sexual arousal disorder
d. Hypoactive sexual desire disorder
e. Sexual aversion disorder
f. Vaginismus

451. A 35-year-old G2P2 states she just doesn't want to have sex with her current partner. It is causing difficulties in the relationship. Upon further questioning, she reports an absence of sexual fantasies or dreams. She has no medical problems and takes no medications. Her physical examination is normal.

452. A 22-year-old G0 presents for sexual counseling. She has been dating the same 23-year-old man for 3 months. She really likes him and enjoys being with him; however, when sexual opportunity arises, she has intense anxiety and cannot continue the sexual encounter.

453. A 40-year-old G3P3 reports she is having difficulty with adequate lubrication and stimulation during sexual activity with her current partner of 10 years. She wants to have sex and reports having sexual dreams. She has no medical problems, takes no medications, and her physical examination is normal.

454. A 52-year-old G3P3 reports an inability to climax during intercourse with her husband over the last 6 months. She denies any changes in their relationship or psychosocial stressors. She states that she has some vaginal dryness, but satisfactorily uses a lubricant. She states she gets aroused, has a strong desire for sex, and feels that stimulation is adequate. She is otherwise healthy and only takes a multivitamin.

455. A 25-year-old G1P1 woman presents with pain and difficulty having intercourse for the last 3 months. She gave birth via an uncomplicated vaginal delivery 5 months ago and recently stopped breast feeding. She states the pain occurs with penetration, and at times she cannot complete the sexual act because the pain is so intense. Her relationship with her husband is being affected.

456. A 33-year-old woman presents with complaints of painful inter-course. She has a new sexual partner for the last month. She states that the pain usually occurs with deep penetration and in certain positions. She reports normal feelings of arousal, climax, and normal lubrication. She denies any vaginal discharge and reports using condoms for contraception. She has no medical problems or prior surgeries and doesn't take any medications.

457. A 42-year-old G1P1 has recently started dating again after her divorce 3 years ago. She has been seeing the same man for the last 3 months. They have had several sexual encounters, but she reports a lack of interest in having sex. She reports a normal sexual desire when she was younger and wonders if hormonal changes are causing her lack of interest. She has a history of hypertension which is well controlled with metoprolol. She says she is not depressed, but she has been taking fluoxetine since her divorce to help her cope with the stresses of her life change.

Questions 458 to 462

For each situation involving oral contraceptives, select the most appropriate response. Each lettered option may be used once, more than once, or not at all.

a. Stop pills and resume after 7 days.
b. Continue pills as usual.
c. Continue pills and use an additional form of contraception.
d. Take an additional pill.
e. Stop pills and seek a medical examination.

458. Nausea during first cycle of pills

459. No menses during 7 days following 21-day cycle of correct use

460. Pill forgotten for 1 day

461. Pill forgotten for 3 continuous days

462. Light bleeding at midcycle during first month on pill

Human Sexuality and Contraception

Answers

423. The answer is c. In a 5-year follow-up study of couples treated by Masters and Johnson, the cure rates for vaginismus and premature ejaculation approached 100%. Orgasmic dysfunction was corrected in 80% of women, and secondary impotence (impotence despite a history of previous coital success) resolved in 70% of men. Primary impotence (chronic and complete inability to maintain an erection sufficient for intercourse) had the worst prognosis, with cure reported in only approximately 50% of cases. Other therapists report very similar statistics.

424. The answer is a. The most recent report from the CDC in 2010 demonstrated that the pills remain the most commonly used form of contraception among reproductive-age women in the United States with 28% of women choosing this method. Female sterilization (27%) and condoms (16%) were the next most commonly used methods of contraception used by women in the United States.

425. The answer is e. COC pills have been extensively studied to determine if there is an increased risk of neoplasms or cancer with use of these medications. Epidemiologic studies demonstrate that use of COCs actually decreases the risk of ovarian and endometrial cancers. There have been no studies that clearly demonstrate an association between the use of COCs and breast cancer. A slightly higher risk of cervical cancer has been observed in some studies of users of oral contraceptives. The risk of developing benign liver adenomas (which can cause life-threatening hemorrhage if they rupture) is increased somewhat in users of oral contraceptives, but the risk of hepatic carcinoma is not increased.

426 to 428. The answers are 426-c, 427-a, 428-a. Several mechanisms of action have been proposed for a copper IUD. These include inhibition of sperm migration and viability, change in transport speed of the ovum, and damage to or destruction of the ovum. The data demonstrates that these prefertilization mechanisms constitute the primary mechanism of action for prevention of pregnancy with the copper IUD; however, postfertilization effects, including damage or destruction of the fertilized ovum, may also occur. All of these effects occur before implantation. IUDs have few contraindications, and almost all women are eligible. Paragard should not be used in the following situations: pregnancy or suspected pregnancy, uterine abnormalities resulting in distortion of the uterine cavity, acute pelvic inflammatory disease, postpartum endometritis in the last 3 months, genital bleeding of unknown etiology, known or suspected uterine or cervical malignancy, mucopurulent cervicitis, or Wilson disease. The reported failure rate of a copper IUD at 1 year is very low, at 0.8 per 100 women. Although there is an increased risk of spontaneous abortion, and a small risk of infection, an intrauterine pregnancy can occur and continue successfully to term with an IUD in place. However, if the patient wishes to keep the pregnancy and if the string is visible, the IUD should be removed in an attempt to reduce the risk of infection, abortion, or both. Although the incidence of ectopic pregnancies with an IUD was at one time thought to be increased, it is now recognized that in fact the overall incidence is unchanged. The apparent increase is the result of the dramatic decrease in intrauterine implantation without affecting ectopic implantation. Thus, while the overall probability of pregnancy is dramatically decreased, when a pregnancy does occur with an IUD in place, there is a higher probability that it will be ectopic. With this in mind, in the absence of signs and symptoms suggestive of an ectopic pregnancy, especially after ultrasound documentation of an intrauterine pregnancy, laparoscopy is not indicated. The incidence of heterotopic pregnancy, in which intrauterine and extrauterine implantation occur simultaneously, is not increased.

429. The answer is c. The pregnancy rate with birth control pills, based on theoretical effectiveness, is 0.1%. However, the pregnancy rate in actual use is 0.7%. This increase is typically due to incorrect use of the pills. Breakthrough ovulation on combination birth control pills, when the pills are taken correctly, is thought to be a very rare occurrence. Unintended pregnancy in women correctly using oral contraceptive pills is not related to sexual frequency, gastrointestinal disturbances, or the development of antibodies.

430. The answer is a. Spermicides available in the United States contain nonoxynol-9, which immobilizes or kills sperm on contact. They do not provide protection against sexually transmitted infections. Spermicides provide a mechanical barrier (ie, gel, cream, foam, film) and need to be placed high in the vagina in contact with the cervix before each act of intercourse. They are available without a prescription. They are not highly effective when used alone, and effectiveness increases with concomitant use of barrier methods such as condoms. High pregnancy rates typically associated with spermicides are mostly due to inconsistent use rather than method failure. Their effectiveness increases with increasing age of the women who use them, probably because of increased motivation. The effectiveness of spermicides is similar to that of the diaphragm. Although it has been reported that contraceptive failures with spermicides may be associated with an increased incidence of congenital malformations, this finding has not been confirmed in several large studies and is not believed to be valid.

431. The answer is c. Clonidine, an antihypertensive agent, can cause inhibition of orgasm in women. Studies have shown that it decreases vaginal blood volume and inhibits sexual arousal. Selective serotonin reuptake inhibitors usually decrease libido. In women sensitive to hormonal changes, combination contraceptive pills can decrease free testosterone and decrease libido. Masters and Johnson identified the clitoris as the center of sexual satisfaction in women. Orgasm and sexual gratification has been associated with nerve endings in the clitoris, mons pubis, labia, and pressure receptors in the pelvis. Even though the cervix has a rich nerve supply, there is no scientific evidence that it plays a role in the sexual response.

432. The answer is b. Many factors can contribute to the development of primary orgasmic dysfunction in women. By definition, these women will not have been able to achieve orgasm through any means at any time in their lives; reasons for their dysfunction can include the influence of orthodox religious or rigid familial beliefs, dissatisfaction with their partner's behavioral or social traits, or past trauma such as rape. Sexual dysfunction, particularly premature ejaculation in a male partner, can reinforce a woman's orgasmic dysfunction.

433. The answer is d. The response of women to sexual stimulation is generalized and affects many different organ systems. During the excitement or seduction phase, vasocongestion leads to breast engorgement and possibly the development of a rash on the breasts, chest, and epigastric area, which is called the "sex flush." Heart rate and blood pressure also increase during this phase. Vasocongestion also occurs in the clitoris, labia, and vagina, and a transudative lubricant develops in the vagina. The plateau phase is marked by greater vasocongestion throughout the body and retraction of the clitoris. During the orgasmic phase, the sexual tension is released via muscular contractions throughout the body, but notably in the vagina, anus, and uterus. Changes in hormones such as estrogen are not part of the sexual response.

434. The answer is c. Surgical abortion is a safe and effective method for pregnancy termination, with a serious complication rate in the first trimester of less than 1%. It is the most common form of termination for pregnancies less than 14 weeks. Outpatient medical abortion is a safe and acceptable alternative to surgical abortion in select women with pregnancies less than 10 weeks' gestation. Three medications have been used. These are: mifepristone (antiprogestin), methotrexate (antimetabolite), and misoprostol (prostaglandin). Various regimens have been found to be effective. Usually mifepristone or methotrexate is initially administered followed by misoprostol. Intra-amniotic injection of hypertonic saline is no longer used regularly, because it has a much higher incidence of serious complications, including death, hyperosmolar crisis, cardiac failure, peritonitis, hemorrhage, and coagulation abnormalities. D&E is a surgical procedure similar in concept to a D&C. However, instead of curettage (scraping) to remove the products of conception, various forceps are placed into the uterine cavity to remove the products of conception. D&E is performed for termination of later pregnancies, generally those in the second trimester. Hysterotomy is a surgical procedure in which the uterus is opened transabdominally and the contents evacuated. It is a procedure done for termination of more advanced pregnancies when all other methods of termination are unsuccessful or contraindicated.

435. The answer is d. Masters and Johnson initially observed a transudate-like fluid emanating from the vaginal walls during sexual response. This mucoid material, which is sufficient for complete vaginal lubrication, is produced by transudation from the venous plexus surrounding the vagina and appears seconds after the initiation of sexual excitement. No activity by Skene glands was noted, and production of cervical mucus during sexual stimulation was observed in only a few subjects. Fluid from Bartholin glands appears long after vaginal lubrication is well established;

in addition, it appears to make only a minor contribution to lubrication in the late plateau phase. Uterine and tubal secretions do not contribute to this lubrication.

436. The answer is b. Sexuality continues despite aging. However, there are physiologic changes that must be recognized. Lack of estrogen from diminished ovarian function leads to decreased genital blood flow, decreased vaginal lubrication, and atrophy of vaginal tissues. These can lead to discomfort with intercourse. Vaginal lubricants and topical estrogen therapy may help. Topical estrogen has been shown to improve lubrication, blood flow, and vaginal compliance. Sexual dysfunction can be physiologic (ie, from decreased libido). Because aging does not alter the capacity for orgasm or produce vaginismus, further evaluation should be initiated if these symptoms persist after treatment is initiated.

437. The answer is b. Vaginismus is both an emotional and pain disorder. It involves involuntary painful spasm of the pelvic muscles and vaginal outlet that precludes intercourse, and causes stress or interpersonal difficulty. The patient is averse to vaginal penetration due to anticipated or actual pain. It usually has a large psychogenic component. It is different from dyspareunia, which is defined as genital pain associated with sexual activity that is not caused by a problem with lubrication or vaginismus. Treatment of vaginismus is primarily a combination of cognitive and behavioral therapy.

438. The answer is e. DMPA, or Depo-Provera is a highly effective form of contraception. It is injectable, private, convenient, and reversible. The failure rate is less than 1%. Its mechanisms of action include ovulation suppression, cervical mucus thickening, and decidualization of endometrium, making it unfavorable for implantation. It has no impairment of lactation, and iron deficiency anemia is less likely due to amenorrhea which develops in 80% of users. Its principal disadvantages are irregular bleeding and prolonged anovulation, which results in delayed return of fertility after discontinuation of the medication. Weight gain is often attributed to depot medroxyprogesterone, but conclusive evidence is lacking. Cervical and hepatic cancers do not appear to be increased, and ovarian and endometrial cancers are decreased. Loss of bone mineral density is one concern, but this loss is reversible after discontinuation of the medication, and has not been associated with an increased risk of pathologic fracture.

439. The answer is d. Women with absolute contraindications should not take COCs pills. Relative contraindications to the use of COCs require clinical judgment and informed consent.

Absolute contraindications	Relative contraindications
(1) Thromboembolic disorders DVT cerebrovascular accident (CVA) myocardial infarction (MI) vascular complications of lupus or diabetes	(1) Migraine headaches
	(2) Depression
	(3) Gall bladder disease
	(4) Seizure disorder
(2) Markedly impaired liver function	(5) Sickle cell disease
(3) Known or suspected carcinoma of the breast or other estrogen-dependent malignancies	(6) Pituitary adenoma
	(7) Surgery or prolonged immobilization
(4) Undiagnosed abnormal genital bleeding	
(5) Elevated triglycerides	
(6) Known or suspected pregnancy	
(7) Smokers older than 35 years	
(8) Uncontrolled hypertension	
(9) Congestive heart failure	

440. The answer is e. Ethinyl estradiol is the estrogen used in almost all currently available COCs. The estrogenic component of oral contraceptive pills was originally added to control irregular endometrial desquamation, resulting in undesirable vaginal bleeding. However, these estrogens imposed possible risks that would not be inherent in the progestational component alone. For example, thrombosis, the most serious side effect of the pill, is directly related to the dose of estrogen. The higher the estrogen dose, the more likely there will be thrombotic complications. The combination pill prevents ovulation by inhibiting gonadotropin secretion and exerting its principal effect on pituitary and hypothalamic centers. Progesterone primarily suppresses LH secretion, while estrogen primarily suppresses FSH secretion. Progestins are responsible for endometrial changes that result in an environment not conducive to implantation, and production of cervical mucus that inhibits sperm migration.

441. The answer is b. The marked effectiveness of the COC pill, which contains a synthetic estrogen and a progestin, is related to its multiple antifertility actions. The primary effect is to suppress gonadotropins at the time of the midcycle LH surge, thus inhibiting ovulation. The prolonged progestational effect also causes thickening of the cervical mucus and atrophic (not hyperplastic) changes of the endometrium, thus impairing sperm penetrability and ovum implantation, respectively. Progestational agents in oral contraceptives work by a negative feedback mechanism to inhibit the secretion of LH and, as a result, prevent ovulation. They also cause decidualization and atrophy of the endometrium, thereby inhibiting implantation. Some evidence indicates that progestational agents may change ovum and sperm migration patterns within the reproductive system. Progestins do not prevent irregular bleeding. Estrogen in birth control pills enhances the negative feedback of the progestins and stabilizes the endometrium to prevent irregular menses. Oral contraceptives have no direct effect on oocyte maturation and do not cause uterotubal obstruction.

442. The answer is a. Hysteroscopic sterilization is highly effective and low risk. It may be done in the office setting, without the need for general anesthesia. It should not be used if acute infection is suspected, but a history of PID or endometritis is not a contraindication. It is nonhormonal, so it is not contraindicated in women with a history of DVT. The most widely available method in the United States is the Essure, which was FDA approved in 2002. Essure involves the hysteroscopic placement of stainless steel and nickel coils into the fallopian tubes. Therefore, a nickel allergy would be a contraindication to its use. Tubal occlusion occurs by an inflammatory response, and is confirmed 12 weeks later with a hysterosalpingogram. Backup contraception must be used until tubal occlusion is documented.

443. The answer is d. Mini-pills are ideal for women with contraindications to estrogen and increased risk of cardiovascular complications, such as women with a history of thrombosis, hypertension, migraine headaches, or smokers older than 35 years. They are also a good choice for lactating women. Mini-pills do not reliably inhibit ovulation and their effectiveness relies more heavily on cervical mucus alterations and endometrial effects. Irregular bleeding is a common side effect, as is the risk of contraceptive failure. They have a higher pregnancy rate than combination pills or other methods such as injectable progestins or intrauterine devices. With failures, there is an increased risk of ectopic pregnancy. Another disadvantage is that it needs to be taken at the same time every day. If a mini-pill is taken even 4 hours late, an additional contraceptive must be used for the next 2 days. The mini-pill does not improve acne and may actually worsen it, with reports of a "acne flare." Functional ovarian cysts develop with a greater frequency in women using mini pills, but intervention is rarely needed.

444. The answer is e. Emergency contraception is warranted for prevention of unwanted pregnancy following unprotected sexual intercourse. Two hormonal methods are available. These are: the Yuptze method (estrogen and progestin pills) and plan B (progestin only). A number of combined (estrogen-progestin) contraceptives are FDA-approved for use as emergency contraception. The tablets are taken within 72 hours of intercourse, in two doses 12 hours apart. This method is highly effective and decreases pregnancy by 94%. Typically if 100 women had unprotected intercourse during the second or third week of their menstrual cycle, 8 would become pregnant. If they used this emergency contraception regimen, only two would conceive. Nausea and vomiting are common due to the high doses of estrogen; therefore, it is common to prescribe an anti-emetic to take before each dose. Plan B is a progestin-only emergency contraceptive method which contains 0.75 mg of levonorgestrel. The first dose is taken within 72 hours, and a second dose is repeated in 12 hours. Since it does not contain estrogen, nausea and emesis are not common, and it is better tolerated than the Yuptze method. It also has a slightly higher efficacy (1.1 pregnancies). Plan B is FDA-approved to be sold over the counter to women 18 years of age and older without a prescription. The major mechanism of action of both of these methods is inhibition or delay of ovulation. Other mechanisms suggested are endometrial effects that prevent implantation, sperm penetration, or tubal motility. Established pregnancies are not harmed by either method. Another method of emergency contraception is to insert a copper-containing IUD up to 5 days after unprotected intercourse. The failure rate is about 1%. Mifepristone (RU-486) is a potent anti-progesterone that can be used as emergency contraception. It interferes with implantation and a single dose is more effective and has fewer side effects than the Yuptze regimen.

445. The answer is c. Vasectomy is performed by isolating the vas deferens, cutting it, and closing the ends by either fulguration or ligation. It may be performed in the office setting under local anesthesia. Complications that may arise include hematoma (5%), sperm granulomas (inflammatory responses to sperm leakage), spontaneous reanastomosis, and, rarely, infections. Sexual function following healing is rarely affected. Vasectomy should not be considered effective until an examination of the ejaculate is sperm-free on two successive occasions. The failure rate is 1%. It has a lower complication rate and cost than outpatient laparoscopic sterilizations in females.

446 to 450. The answers are **446-b, 447-a, 448-e, 449-d, 450-c.** Mini pills are contraindicated in women with unexplained uterine bleeding or breast cancer. Both condoms and the diaphragm, used in conjunction with spermicides, are effective contraceptives. The diaphragm should carefully fit in the vagina and is therefore not applicable to women with anatomic distortion of the vagina. Latex condoms should not be used in women with a known latex allergy. Manufacturer's contraindications to IUD use include history of acute PID, unexplained genital bleeding, suspected pregnancy, uterine cavity distortion, or recent postpartum endometritis. Wilson disease or a copper allergy are contraindications to the use of a copper-containing IUD. Although tubal ligation may be considered in the patient with chronic obstructive lung disease, the risk of general anesthesia and surgical intervention in this patient is probably high enough to indicate a more conservative approach, such as the use of an IUD.

451 to 457. The answers are **451-d, 452-e, 453-c, 454-b, 455-f, 456-a, 458-d.** Female sexual dysfunction disorders are characterized by painful intercourse or disturbances in desire, arousal, orgasm or resolution that causes marked distress or interpersonal difficulty. Sexual dysfunction is not better accounted for by another psychiatric disorder, and is not due exclusively to a substance or medical condition. Hypoactive sexual desire disorder is the persistent or recurrent absence of sexual fantasies or desire for sexual activity. Alcohol and drugs may interfere with sexual desire. Medications such as antihypertensives, anticholinergics, antidepressants, narcotics, sedatives, and others may decrease arousal and inhibit sexual interest. Sexual aversion disorder is a persistent or recurrent extreme aversion to or avoidance of sexual genital contact. Sexual prompts or advances by a partner are dismissed. It may be acquired following sexual or physical abuse or trauma, and may be life-long. When presented with a sexual opportunity, the individual may experience panic attacks or extreme anxiety. Sexual arousal disorder is the persistent inability to attain or maintain until completion of sexual activity an adequate lubrication-swelling response of sexual excitement. The inability to become aroused also may be related to anxiety or inadequate stimulation. Vaginismus is the recurrent involuntary spasm of the musculature of the lower third of the vagina that interferes with sexual intercourse and penetration. Usually at the root of vaginismus is a combination of physical or nonphysical triggers that cause the body to anticipate pain. Reacting to the anticipation of pain, the body automatically tightens the vaginal muscles, and sex becomes painful. Penile entry may be more difficult or impossible depending on the severity muscle contraction. Dyspareunia is recurrent or persistent genital/pelvic pain associated with sexual intercourse (not caused by vaginismus or lack of lubrication).

458 to 462. The answers are **458-b, 459-b, 460-d, 461-c, 462-b.** Common side effects of birth control pills include nausea, breakthrough bleeding, bloating, and leg cramps. If these side effects are experienced in the first two or three cycles of pills—when they are most common—the pills may be safely continued, as these effects usually remit spontaneously. On occasion, following correct use of a full cycle of pills, withdrawal bleeding may fail to occur (silent menses). Pregnancy is a very unlikely explanation for this event; therefore, pills should be resumed as usual (after 7 days) just as if bleeding had occurred. However, if a second consecutive period has been missed, pregnancy should be more seriously considered and ruled out by a pregnancy test, medical examination, or both. Women occasionally forget to take pills; however, when only a single pill has been omitted, it can be taken immediately in addition to the usual pill at the usual time. This single-pill omission is associated with little if any loss in effectiveness. If two or more pills are omitted, the pill should be resumed as usual, but an additional contraceptive method (eg, condoms) should be used through one full cycle. Although most side effects caused by birth control pills can be considered minor, serious side effects do sometimes occur. A painful, swollen calf may signal a deep vein thrombosis.

Suggested Readings

American College of Obstetricians and Gynecologists. *Benefits and Risks of Sterilization.* Practice Bulletin Number 133, February 2013, reaffirmed 2015.

American College of Obstetricians and Gynecologists. *Female Sexual Dysfunction.* Practice Bulletin Number 119, April 2001, reaffirmed 2015.

American College of Obstetricians and Gynecologists. *Long Acting Reversible Contraception: Implants and Intrauterine Devices.* Practice Bulletin Number 121, July 2011, reaffirmed 2013.

Mosher WD, Jones J. *Use of Contraception in the United States: 1982-2008.* Centers for Disease Control Vital and Health Statistics 23, No. 29 (2010).

Sexual Abuse and Intimate Partner Violence

Questions

463. A 20-year-old woman presents to your office with a chief complaint of abdominal pain. Upon further questioning, the woman reveals that she was sexually assaulted at a party 3 weeks ago by a male friend whom she recently started dating. She tells you that she has not revealed this to anyone else, and has not informed the police because she was drinking. Her abdominal and pelvic examinations are normal. Which of the following is the best management to offer this patient?

a. Counsel patient to sue the male friend.
b. Provide an antidepressant.
c. Provide emergency contraception.
d. Test for and treat sexually transmitted infections.
e. Order CT of the abdomen and pelvis.

Questions 464 and 465

464. An 18-year-old undergraduate student presents to the emergency department at 5 AM on a Saturday morning reporting that she was the victim of sexual assault while attending a fraternity party the evening before. When you first encounter this patient to take a detailed history, she remains very calm, but has trouble remembering the details of the experience. She reports that she has not used any alcohol or illicit drugs. The victim's inability to think clearly and remember things is best explained by which of the following?

a. Alcohol use
b. Head injury
c. Illicit drug use
d. Rape trauma syndrome
e. Secondary gain

465. Which of the following is most likely a component of the acute phase of the rape trauma syndrome?

a. No physical complaints.
b. Duration for up to 6 months after the event.
c. Always in control of emotions.
d. The reaction of the victim may be influenced by victim's relationship to the attacker.
e. The victim's coping mechanisms usually remain intact.

466. You are called to the emergency department to evaluate an 18-year-old woman for a vulvar laceration. She is accompanied by her mother and father. The father explains that the injury was caused by a fall onto the support bar on her bicycle. You interview the woman alone and find out that her father has been sexually assaulting her. Which of the following statements best describes injuries related to sexual assault?

a. Most injuries are considered major and require surgical correction.
b. Most injuries require hospitalization.
c. More than 50% of victims will have an injury.
d. Most injuries occur after the assault has taken place.
e. Vaginal and vulvar lacerations are common in virginal victims.

Questions 467 to 472

467. You are evaluating a 19-year-old victim of sexual assault in the emergency department. As a physician, your legal requirement includes which of the following?

a. Identification of the attacker
b. Detailed notation of injuries
c. Delivery of evidence to a law enforcement facility
d. Treating patient even if she refuses
e. Writing the diagnosis of rape in the patient's chart

468. The patient is concerned that she may have been exposed to a sexually transmitted infection. Which of the following tests should be ordered?

a. HIV, HBsAg, Pap smear, RPR, and urine culture
b. HIV, HBsAg, Pap smear, RPR, and urine pregnancy test
c. Chlamydia and gonorrhea cultures, complete blood count, HIV, HBsAg, Pap smear, and RPR
d. Chlamydia and gonorrhea cultures, HIV, HBsAg, Pap smear, RPR, and urine pregnancy test
e. Chlamydia and gonorrhea cultures, DNA probe for trichomonas, HIV, HBsAg, and RPR

469. Which of the following antibiotic regimens do you recommend she take to prophylax against sexually transmitted infections?

a. Azithromycin 1 g orally plus ceftriaxone 250 mg IM plus metronidazole 2 g orally
b. Ceftriaxone 125 mg IM
c. Ciprofloxacin 500 mg PO twice daily x 7 days
d. Metronidazole 2 g orally in a single dose
e. No antibiotic prophylaxis is indicated

470. During your evaluation, the patient expresses fear of becoming pregnant due to the assault. Which of the following is the best method to recommend for emergency contraception?

a. None, because it will cause an abortion and is morally wrong.
b. None, because it will be ineffective if taken more than 12 hours after coitus.
c. An intrauterine device, because it is 99% effective.
d. Combination of estrogen and progestin contraceptive pills.
e. Plan B, a progestin only contraception.

471. After your evaluation and treatment has been completed, you discharge the patient to home. When is the best time to schedule a follow-up appointment?

a. 24 to 48 hours.
b. 1 week.
c. 6 weeks.
d. 12 weeks.
e. There is no need for the patient to have any additional follow-up as long as she feels well.

472. The patient returns to your office 2 months after the assault for a follow-up visit. She informs you that her sleep has improved and she can now be by herself without feeling anxious or panicked. She has also developed new friendships through her church. She tells you that she is changing jobs and moving to a new town. She feels that with this change she will be in control of her life. The best recommendation you can make for the recovery of this patient is which of the following?

a. Continue counseling.
b. Face her attacker to bring closure to this event.
c. Get her to accept responsibility for the attack.
d. Stop counseling since her recovery is now complete.
e. Take anxiolytic medication.

473. A family medicine physician refers a 19-year-old woman to you for abnormal findings during her well-woman examination. She emigrated to the United States with her family 6 years ago from West Africa. She is not sexually active at this time, but has had one partner 2 years ago. She has no history of sexually transmitted infections. She takes nitrofurantoin for recurrent urinary tract infections, but is otherwise healthy. She says she has not had any surgeries, but she remembers undergoing a special ceremony as young child in Africa. Lung, cardiac, breast, and abdominal examinations are within normal limits. On pelvic examination you note extensive scarring on the vulva, and the labia minora have been removed. The prepuce of the clitoris is missing and the clitoris is scarred over. Which of the following is most likely a result of the procedure the patient had in Africa?

a. Amenorrhea
b. Decreased vaginal infections
c. Easier vaginal deliveries
d. Enhanced sexual function
e. Psychosomatic symptoms

474. A 5-year-old girl is brought in to the emergency department by her mother. The mother is concerned that her daughter may have been sexually molested. She reports that her daughter has been complaining of abdominal pain, and has been particularly clingy. This morning, she noted some bloody discharge on her daughter's underwear. The child lives at home with her mother, 1-year-old brother, maternal aunt, and 18-year-old cousin. The child's father is dead, and her mother is not seeing anyone currently. Which of the following is the most likely abuser?

a. Male stranger
b. Female stranger
c. Male relative
d. Female relative
e. Mother

475. A mother brings in her 16-year-old daughter for an evaluation of chronic abdominal pain. You have seen the girl many times before for various vague complaints over the past year. She has regular cycles that last 4 days with medium to light flow. She reports no dysmenorrhea, gastrointestinal symptoms, or depression. She says she is not sexually active. The mother states that lately she has been doing poorly in school. She denies drug or alcohol use. Her mother thinks it may be related to recent changes at home since the mother's boyfriend moved in. Your examination and laboratory tests are normal.

A previous workup by a gastroenterologist was also negative. Which of the following is the best next step in the management of this patient's symptoms?

a. Initiate biofeedback therapy for chronic pain.
b. Order immediate psychiatric evaluation.
c. Prescribe antibiotics for chronic gastroenteritis.
d. Prescribe an antidepressant.
e. Question the patient about possible sexual abuse.

476. You are called to the pediatric emergency department to evaluate a 7-year-old girl for sexual assault. As a health care provider taking care of this girl, which of the following are you required to do?

a. Administer antibiotics only if testing for infection is positive.
b. Demand that the child be placed in foster care pending further investigation.
c. Hospitalize the child until the offender has been apprehended.
d. Inform the parents that they must notify the police.
e. Notify child welfare authorities.

Questions 477 and 478

477. A 25-year-old G1P0 presents to your office for a routine return OB visit at 30 weeks. When you listen to the fetal heart tones, you notice that the patient has a number of bruises on her abdomen. You ask her what happened, and she tells you the bruises resulted from a fall she suffered several days earlier, when she slipped on the stairs. The patient returns to your office 3 weeks later for another routine visit, and you note that she has a broken arm in a cast. She says that she fell again. You question her about physical abuse, and the patient begins crying, and reveals a long-standing history of abuse by her husband. Which of the following is the most likely reason for upper extremity injury in this patient?

a. Injury from being restrained
b. Defensive injury
c. Fall from being pushed
d. Injury related to striking back at her husband
e. Self-inflicted wounds

478. Which of the following is the normal course of an abusive relationship during pregnancy?

a. Abuse is uncommon during pregnancy.
b. An increase in abuse occurs in about 20% of relationships.
c. Abuse is usually directed away from the breast and abdomen.
d. Pregnant women who are abused usually have fewer complaints.
e. Abused women usually receive adequate prenatal care.

479. A 73-year-old woman is brought to your clinic for a gynecological examination by a neighbor for vaginal bleeding. She appears unkempt and frail. Her friend is concerned about abuse by the patient's family. You interview and examine the patient and make the appropriate referrals for social services. What is the common type of abuse of the elderly?

a. Emotional
b. Financial
c. Neglect
d. Physical
e. Sexual

Questions 480 and 482

480. You are evaluating a 36-year-old woman in the emergency department for a broken arm. She states that she slipped in the tub. This is the third time you have seen her for a trauma-related injury in the past 6 months. You suspect domestic violence. After treating her broken arm and evaluating her emotional status, which of the following is the next appropriate step in the management of this patient?

a. Confront the patient's partner.
b. Discharge her to home.
c. Offer counseling and resources.
d. Order her to leave her partner.
e. Provide an antidepressant.

481. Which of the following is a common characteristic of intimate partner violence (IPV)?

a. Victims repeatedly visit clinics and emergency departments for different complaints.
b. Victims are reluctant to reveal abuse when their physicians ask them about it.
c. The events are isolated and not associated with other abuses.
d. The head and neck are rare areas of injury.
e. Signs and symptoms are usually evident, and the correct diagnosis is made most of the time.

482. You are seeing a 37-year-old woman in your office for follow-up of an injury related to domestic violence. She states that her husband is over with his abusive behavior and is treating her like royalty. He has bought her a new necklace to show how sorry he is about the incident. She has changed her plans to seek counseling and to move out. Which of the following is the most likely outcome in this situation?

a. Abuser accepts responsibility for his behavior.
b. Cessation of all abuse.
c. Decreased episodes of violence.
d. Increasing severity of battering.
e. Role reversal with victim taking control of relationship.

Sexual Abuse and Intimate Domestic Violence

Answers

463. The answer is d. The physician's responsibility in the care of a rape victim includes medical, medical-legal, and emotional support. The physician's medical responsibilities include treatment of injuries, testing, and prevention and treatment of both infections and pregnancy. This patient has a normal examination, and a CT is not indicated. She should be tested for sexually transmitted infections and given prophylactic antibiotics to treat such diseases. A pregnancy test should be performed, and if negative, she should be offered emergency contraception. Since emergency contraception should be given within 72 hours of the event, this patient is not a candidate for emergency contraception. Even though there can be long-standing psychological consequences of rape, antidepressants are not indicated at this time for this patient.

464 and 465. The answers are 464-d, 465-d. Rape trauma syndrome is the medical term that refers to the response that survivors have to rape. It is considered to be the natural response of a psychologically well person to the traumatic event. As part of the rape trauma syndrome, victims of sexual assault may appear calm, tearful, or agitated, or they may demonstrate a combination of these emotions. In addition, victims of sexual assault may suffer an involuntary loss of cognition where they cannot think clearly or remember things. The immediate or acute phase of the rape trauma syndrome can last for hours to days. It is associated with a paralysis of the victim's usual coping mechanisms. The victim's response may be complete emotional breakdown or well-controlled behavior. The actual reaction of the victims will depend on many factors, including use of force, length of attack or how long they were held against their will, and their relationship to the attacker (stranger versus someone close to them). The victim is usually disorganized immediately after the assault and has both physical and emotional complaints.

466. The answer is e. Injuries occur in 12% to 40% of sexual assault victims. Most occur when the victim is restrained or physically coerced into the sexual act. Most are minor and require simple repair; only 1% require major surgical repair and hospitalization. The physician should evaluate for injuries such as abrasions, bruises, scratches, and lacerations on the neck, abdomen, back, buttocks, and extremities, as well as the genital area. Lacerations of the vagina and vulva are common in children, virginal victims, and postmenopausal women.

467 to 472. The answers are 467-b, 468-e, 469-a, 470-e, 471-a, 472-a. When possible, the acute evaluation of sexual assault victims should be undertaken by someone with specific training to care for victims of sexual assault. Complete evaluations are time intensive and require several hours. Your legal requirement as a physician evaluating a sexual assault victim includes documentation of history, examination and notation of injuries, and collection of clothing and vaginal, rectal, oropharynx, pubic hair samples, and fingernail scrapings, as appropriate, for testing. The history should focus on precise details of the sexual assault, and should be obtained in a sensitive and supportive environment. The examination should describe emotional state, and should document any evidence of trauma. The forensic evaluation requires informed consent. Forensic specimens must be submitted to the proper authorities in a timely manner. You must submit any specimens to forensic authorities and receive a receipt for the patient's chart. Since *rape* and *assault* are legally defined terms, they should not be stated as a diagnosis. The CDC recommends that the following laboratory tests be considered to evaluation for sexually transmitted infections in victims of sexual assault. These are as follows: gonorrhea and chlamydia nucleic acid amplification tests from the vagina, anus, and throat; DNA probe for trichomonas vaginalis; and serum testing for hepatitis B, syphilis, and HIV. Whether or not to test for these infections should be individualized. The CDC also recommends antibiotic prophylaxis, since many assault victims will not return for follow up. Prophylaxis should be directed at treating the most common infections, including gonorrhea, chlamydia, and trichomonas. The recommended treatment is ceftriaxone 250 mg intramuscularly in a single dose plus azithromycin 1 g orally in a single dose, plus metronidazole 2 g orally in a single dose. Post-exposure hepatitis B vaccination and HIV prophylaxis are also recommended. "Emergency contraception" (medication prophylaxis) to prevent pregnancy should be offered to women following sexual assault. A pregnancy test should be performed to exclude pregnancy.

Nausea is a very common side effect with combination estrogen/progestin pills used for emergency contraception. Plan B, a progestin-only form of emergency contraception, has a much lower rate of nausea and is better tolerated, making it the preferred choice. Prophylaxis can be given up to 72 hours after the assault, but has been shown to be effective up to 5 days after the rape. Emergency contraception has efficacy rates of 74% to 89%. Patients should be informed that their next menses may be delayed and counseled to get a pregnancy test if it is delayed more than 2 weeks. A copper IUD can be inserted for emergency contraception but should be avoided until active infection can be ruled out. Following the assault, the patient should receive follow-up counseling within 24 to 48 hours, and subsequent follow-up appointments can be arranged at 1 and 4 weeks. The patient should not leave without plans for follow-up. Psychosocial support is an important part of recovery for assault survivors. The reorganization phase of the rape trauma syndrome involves long-term adjustments and may last for months to years. Flashbacks and nightmares may continue and phobias may develop. Victims may also make many new lifestyle changes (eg, moving, making new friends, getting a new job). This is an attempt by victims to regain control over their lives. Medical and counseling care should remain nonjudgmental, sensitive, and attuned to the patient's overall well-being. It is important for the patient to continue counseling during this time for full recovery to be achieved.

473. The answer is e. Female genital mutilation, also known as female circumcision or female genital cutting, is a genital alteration performed on girls and young women for nontherapeutic reasons. It is primarily practiced in Africa, but variations are also found in the Middle East and Southeast Asia. Reasons given by families who perform female genital mutilation include psychosexual reasons (ie, attenuation of sexual desire in women to ensure chastity and virginity before marriage), cultural reasons (ie, initiation of girls into womanhood), myths about enhanced fertility or promotion of child survival, and religious reasons. It is often performed by untrained practitioners in unsterile conditions with crude instruments and without anesthesia. It is performed predominantly on girls in early childhood through 14 years of age. The most common type of female genital mutilation involves the removal of the clitoris and partial or total excision of the labia minora. Many complications can occur, such as infection, tetanus, shock, hemorrhage, and death. Long-term complications include chronic infection, scar and abscess formation, sterility, obstetrical complications, and incontinence.

Psychological problems related to sexual abuse may also be evident, such as anxiety, depression, and sexual dysfunction.

474. The answer is c. Perpetrators of sexual abuse in children are usually male, and are often trusted adults or family members. Approximately 40% of cases of sexual abuse of a child involve a family member; approximately half of these cases are attributed to the father, and about 5% to the mother. Perpetrators often gain access to children through caretaking.

475. The answer is e. Children who have been abused may exhibit a variety of behaviors, including guilt, anger, behavioral problems, unexplained physical symptoms, poor school performance, and sleep disturbances. Physicians who evaluate patients with vague chronic pain syndromes that show no evidence of physical etiology should investigate sexual abuse as a possible contributor. Counseling should be offered as part of the treatment if abuse is encountered.

476. The answer is e. Whenever possible, this evaluation should be undertaken by a member of an experienced child abuse team in a nonemergent setting, such as a child advocacy center. In evaluating a child of suspected sexual assault, you should carefully obtain a history and allow the child to say what happened. A careful history, physical examination, and forensic evidence collection should be taken. Techniques of examining a rape victim should be employed (collection of cultures, clothing, hair samples, etc.). The police and child protective services should be notified. Any injuries should be treated, and the child should be hospitalized only if needed based on injuries. Appropriate antibiotic prophylaxis should be given and counseling should be scheduled. The child should be returned to the home only if it is deemed safe.

477 and 478. The answers are 477-b and 478-b. IPV affects millions of women, regardless of age, ethnicity, economic status, religion, or sexual orientation. More than one in three women in the United States have experienced rape, physical violence, or stalking in their lifetime. There are 4.8 million incidents reported annually in the United States, but the true incidence is unknown, because victims are afraid to disclose their personal experience of violence. Physical abuse is common in pregnancy, occurring in up to 10% of pregnancies. In women who have been previously abused, about 20% will experience an increase in abuse during pregnancy. Abused women sometimes receive inadequate prenatal care and have more somatic complaints than those who have not been abused. Screening for IPV should be a core part of women's health visits. It should be done at the first prenatal visit, once per trimester, and at the postpartum visit. Battering is frequently directed toward the breasts and abdomen. Other common sites of injury are the head, neck, chest, and upper extremities. An upper extremity may be fractured as the woman attempts to defend herself.

479. The answer is c. As many as 1 in 10 older adults have been victims of elder abuse, and more than 65% of these are women. The U.S. Census data shows significant growth in the population of people older than 65 years, and as the population ages, the incidence of elder abuse is expected to increase. It is estimated that for every case of elder abuse that is reported, 23 cases go undetected. Elder abuse is defined as: "a single or repeated act, or lack of appropriate actions, which causes harm, risk of harm, or distress to a person age 60 or older, and occurs: (1) where there is a relationship with the expectation of trust, or (2) when the act is targeted toward an older person by virtue of age or disability." Elder abuse may be physical, emotional, sexual, financial exploitation, neglect, self-neglect, and miscellaneous. By far, neglect is the most common form of abuse. It most often occurs at the hands of family members and in the home of the elder. Risk factors include caregiver stress, cognitive impairment of the patient, need for assistance with activities of daily living, conflicts within the family, and poor social support.

480 and 481. The answers are 480-c and 481-a. Approximately 25% of women treated for injuries in emergency departments are victims of IPV. Victims of IPV sometimes make repeated visits to clinics and emergency rooms with a variety of somatic complaints. Physicians treating these patients correctly make the diagnosis in only 3% of the cases. Most women report that they would be willing to divulge their domestic abuse to a physician if the physician were to ask. Partner abuse may be seen in conjunction with other forms of abuse such as elder abuse and child abuse. Physical injury in cases of IPV usually involves the head and neck, trunk, skin, and extremities. As a physician, you should treat the injuries and assess the emotional needs of the patient from a psychiatric standpoint, such as possible depression or anxiety. If such a condition exists, you should refer the patient to a mental health worker. You should investigate the patient's own awareness of her situation and her willingness to take appropriate action. The physician's job is to recognize IPV, and to ensure counseling for the patient so that she understands her rights and options and can protect herself and her children. A victim of abuse may not leave her situation for economic reasons or fear of retribution.

482. The answer is d. IPV attacks often run in cycles of three phases. The first phase consists of a buildup of tension with an escalation of friction between family members. It includes name-calling, intimidation, and mild physical abuse. The second phase is the acute battering, which is an uncontrolled discharge of built-up tension. Verbal or physical abuse may occur. Alcohol is involved in two-thirds of cases. The third phase occurs after the abuse has taken place. At this time the batterer apologizes, begs forgiveness, and shows remorse. Abusers will offer gifts and make promises to the victim. They are often very charming in this phase. The cycles repeat themselves, with the first phase becoming longer and increasing in intensity; the battering is usually more severe, and the third phase usually decreases in both length and intensity.

Suggested Readings

American College of Obstetricians and Gynecologists. *Elder Abuse and Women's Health.* Committee Opinion Number 568, July 2013.

American College of Obstetricians and Gynecologists. *Emergency Contraception.* Practice Bulletin Number 112, May 2010.

American College of Obstetricians and Gynecologists. Female genital cutting. *Guidelines for Women's Health Care: A Resource Manual.* 4th ed. p. 510.

American College of Obstetricians and Gynecologists. *Intimate Partner Violence.* Committee Opinion Number 518, February 2012.

American College of Obstetricians and Gynecologists. *Sexual Assault.* Committee Opinion Number 592, April 2014.

Centers for Disease Control and Prevention. 2010 Sexually Transmitted Diseases Treatment Guidelines. www.cdc.gov.

Ethical and Legal Issues in Obstetrics and Gynecology

Questions

483. Which of the following is not a requirement for hospitals according to the Federal Patient Self-Determination Act?

a. To provide all adults with information about their right to accept or refuse treatment in the event of life-threatening conditions
b. To state the institution's policy on advanced directives
c. To prohibit discrimination in care provided to a patient on the basis of the patient's advanced directive
d. To require donation of organs after death
e. To allow patients to decide who has the right to make decisions for them

484. A 31-year-old G3P3 Jehovah's Witness begins to bleed heavily 2 days after a cesarean delivery. She refuses blood transfusion, and says that she would rather die than receive any blood or blood products. You personally feel that you cannot do anything and watch her die. Appropriate actions that you can take under these circumstances include which of the following?

a. Tell the patient to find another physician who will care for her
b. Transfuse her forcibly
c. Only provide supportive care
d. Obtain a court order for a blood transfusion
e. Have the patient's husband sign a release to forcibly transfuse her

485. A physician is being sued for malpractice by the parents of a baby born with cerebral palsy. Which of the following is not a prerequisite for finding the physician guilty of malpractice?

a. A doctor-patient relationship was established.
b. The physician owed a duty to the patient.
c. The physician breached a duty to the patient.
d. The breach of duty caused damage to the plaintiff.
e. The physician failed to give expert care to the patient.

486. A 27-year-old woman who has previously received no prenatal care presents at term. On ultrasound, she is shown to have a placenta previa, but refuses to have a cesarean delivery under any circumstances. Important points to consider in her management include which of the following?

a. The obstetrician's obligation to the supposedly normal fetus supersedes the obligation to the healthy mother.
b. The inclusion of several people in this complex situation raises the legal risk to the physician.
c. Child abuse statutes require the physician to get a court order to force a cesarean delivery.
d. Court-ordered cesarean deliveries have almost always been determined to achieve the best management.
e. A hospital ethics committee should be convened to evaluate the situation.

487. Your 36-year-old patient is admitted to the hospital for induction of labor at 42 weeks' gestation. She provides the hospital with her living will at the time of her admission. She signed the will 5 years ago, but she says to her nurse that she still wants to abide by the will. She has also signed an organ donor card allowing the harvesting of her organs in the event of her death. Why is her living will not valid for this hospitalization?

a. In the event that she becomes delirious during labor, she will be unable to change her mind.
b. She is pregnant.
c. It has been too many years since the signing of the will.
d. Signing an organ donor card automatically invalidates a living will.
e. Her husband may decide later on that he disagrees with her living will.

Questions 488 to 492

488. Your patient is a 44-year-old G4P4 with symptomatic uterine fibroids that have been unresponsive to medical therapy. The patient has severe menorrhagia to the point that when she menstruates, she cannot leave the house. Since she has failed medical management, you recommend a hysterectomy. You counsel her that she may need a blood transfusion if she has significant blood loss during the surgical procedure. Her current hematocrit is 25.0%. The patient is a Jehovah's Witness who adamantly refuses to have a blood transfusion, even if it results in her death. Which of the following is not an ethical concern that needs to be considered when working through this case?

a. Legal issues
b. Patient preferences
c. Quality-of-life issues
d. Medical indications
e. Comorbid conditions

489. The patient's insurance company refuses to pay for the surgical procedure. Which of the following ethical areas is involved?

a. Autonomy
b. Justice
c. Contextual issue
d. Patient preference
e. Quality of life

490. Respect for the patient's autonomy requires that which of the following be assessed?

a. The needs of society
b. The duty not to inflict harm
c. The impact that the treatment will have on the patient's quality of life
d. Consideration of what is the best treatment
e. The patient's personal values

491. Prior to performing the hysterectomy, you must obtain the patient's informed consent. Which of the following is not a key element of informed consent?

a. The patient must have the ability to comprehend medical information.
b. Alternatives to the procedure must be presented.
c. If the patient is incapable of providing consent, the procedure cannot be performed.
d. The risks of the procedure must be presented.
e. The benefits of the procedure must be presented.

492. The patient requests that you do not talk at all to her husband about her medical care. This request falls under which of the following ethical concepts?

a. Informed consent
b. Confidentiality
c. Nonmaleficence
d. Advanced directive

Questions 493 to 502

Match the ethical concern or principle with the appropriate definition. Each lettered option may be used once, more than once, or not at all.

a. Patient preferences
b. Beneficence
c. Quality of life
d. Nonmaleficence
e. Autonomy
f. Medical indication
g. Contextual issues
h. Justice

493. The duty not to inflict harm or injury

494. The duty to promote the good of the patient

495. Giving the patient his or her due

496. Respect of the patient's right to self-determination

497. What does the patient want?

498. What is the best treatment?

499. What impact will the proposed treatment have on the patient's life?

500. What are the needs of society?

501. What are the treatment alternatives?

502. What impact will lack of the proposed treatment have on the patient's life?

503. Ms Jones is a 28-year-old woman who has agreed to be a gestational surrogate for a couple who cannot bear children. She presents to your office for prenatal care. Which of the following is your responsibility as an obstetrician caring for a gestational surrogate?

a. Consult with intended parents regarding all clinical interventions and management of the pregnancy.
b. Discuss the health of the surrogate and progress of the pregnancy with the intended parents without consent of the surrogate mother.
c. Make recommendations for prenatal care in accordance with the agreement between the gestational surrogate and the intended parents.
d. Only provide prenatal care to her, if the adoptive mother is also your patient.
e. Provide appropriate care regardless of the patient's plans to keep or relinquish the future child.

504. A 24-year-old patient who you have been seeing for routine gynecological care reports that she is considering becoming a surrogate mother for a couple she knows at work. As her physician, what is your responsibility to her in preparing her to become a surrogate?

a. Contact the intended parents so that you can provide care for them also.
b. Explain to her that you will require an additional fee to care for her pregnancy since she will be a surrogate.
c. Recommend that she utilize the same legal counsel as the intended parents.
d. Refer her to mental health counseling.
e. Review the surrogate contract to ensure that she is being fully compensated.

Ethical and Legal Issues in Obstetrics and Gynecology

Answers

483. The answer is d. The Patient Self-Determination Act (PSDA) took effect in 1991, and is intended to promote awareness and discussion to prepare for medical decisions at the end of life. It requires hospitals to inform patients upon admission of state laws concerning self-determination. Hospitals must inform patients about their rights to accept or refuse terminal care, and this information has to be documented in the patient's chart. The patient has the option to make a clear assignment of who can make medical decisions if the patient is unable. Patients are not required to allow organ donation.

484. The answer is c. Determination of ethical conduct in doctor-patient relationships can sometimes be very difficult for the physician who is confronted with a patient's autonomy in making a decision that the physician finds incomprehensible. However, the autonomy of the patient who is oriented and alert must be respected even if it means that the patient is refusing potentially lifesaving therapy. Attempting to obtain a court order to transfuse an adult against his or her will is almost never an acceptable option, and leads to a tremendously slippery slope of the doctor's control of the patient's behavior. A patient's spouse also does not have legal authority to make decisions for the patient if the patient is competent, awake, and alert. The situation is different when a child is involved, in which case societal interests can occasionally override parental autonomy. It would be inappropriate for a physician to abandon a patient without obtaining suitable coverage from another qualified physician. Transfusing forcibly is assault and battery; thus, in this case, the physician must adhere to the patient's wishes and, if need be, let her die.

485. The answer is e. Negligence law governs conduct and embraces acts of both commission and omission (ie, what a person did or failed to do). In general, the law expects all persons to conduct themselves in a fashion that does not expose others to an unreasonable risk of harm. In a fiduciary relationship such as the physician-patient relationship, the physician is held to a higher standard of behavior because of the imbalance of knowledge. In general, the real gist of negligence is not carelessness or ineptitude, but rather, how unreasonable was the risk of harm to the patient caused by the physician's action? Thus physicians are held accountable to a standard of care that asks the question, "What would the reasonable physician do under this specific set of circumstances?" The physician is not held accountable to the level of the leading experts in any given field, but rather to the prevailing standards among average practitioners. When a doctor-patient relationship is established, the defendant (doctor) owes a duty to the patient. If the defendant breaches that duty—that is, acts in a way that is inconsistent with the standard of care and that can be shown to have caused damage directly to the patient (*proximate damage*)—then the physician may be held liable for compensation.

486. The answer is e. When confronted by a complex situation in which there are conflicting values and rights, getting the most qualified people involved is the best approach to reduce risk and to come up with the best, most defensible answer under the current circumstances. The obstetrician should employ whatever departmental or hospital resources are available. A standing ethics committee or an ad hoc committee to deal with such complex situations is often available, and will minimize the ultimate medicolegal problems that can ensue when bad outcomes seem likely. The obstetrician must further recognize that he or she has two patients, but that it is not clear, nor is it legislated, whose interests take priority. However, general ethical opinion is that the mother usually should come first. Most court-ordered cesarean deliveries have been performed on patients who were estranged from the medical system, and this sets a very bad precedent for further state intervention in doctor-patient relationships and maternal rights. Child abuse statutes do not, at this point, require a court order to force a cesarean delivery, even for a healthy fetus.

487. The answer is b. Living wills present the opportunity for patients to declare their wishes in advance of situations in which they become no longer competent to do so. They are revocable by the patient at any time, and are automatically invalid if the patient is pregnant, as another being is involved. Living wills can be set aside if a long period has elapsed since their drafting and the wishes are not known to be current. Also, there is the potential for conflict if the patient has signed a donor card and prolongation of life would be needed to carry out those wishes. Generally, such action would not be honored unless relatively expeditious arrangements were possible.

488 to 492. The answers are 488-a, 489-b, 490-e, 491-c, 492-b. Patient preferences, quality-of-life issues, and medical indications are all examples of ethical concerns that must be taken into account when working through ethical dilemmas. Consideration of legal issues is not a factor in ethical decision-making. If the patient's insurance company refuses to pay for the indicated procedure (in this case, hysterectomy), the ethical principle of justice (the patient should be given her due) is being challenged. Autonomy is the ethical principle whereby the patient has the right to self-determination. Therefore, the needs of society (a contextual issue) are not considered as a factor of autonomy. Informed consent requires that the patient be able to understand the risks, benefits, indications, and alternatives of a particular medical procedure. If the patient is unable to understand the medical information, a legal guardian can be assigned to make those decisions for him or her. A patient's desire not to have his or her medical history discussed with anyone else involves the ethical concept of confidentiality.

493 to 502. The answers are 493-d, 494-b, 495-h, 496-e, 497-a, 498-f, 499-c, 500-g, 501-f, 502-c.

503. The answer is e. When a pregnant surrogate seeks medical care for an established pregnancy, the obstetrician should explore with the surrogate her understanding of her legal agreement with the intended parents. She should be cared for as any other obstetrical patient. The obstetrician's professional obligation is to support the well-being of the pregnant woman and her fetus, and to provide appropriate care regardless of her plans to keep or give up the baby. The pregnant surrogate should be the one to give consent regarding treatment of the pregnancy in the clinic or on labor and delivery. The obstetrician should make treatment decisions that are in the best interest of the surrogate and her fetus, regardless of the agreement between her and the intended parents. Patient confidentiality should be maintained. The patient's medical information should only be given to the intended parents with the surrogate's explicit consent. The obstetrician should avoid conflicts of interest and should not facilitate a woman's becoming a gestational surrogate for a couple for whom the physician is treating.

504. The answer is d. When approached by a patient considering becoming a surrogate mother, the physician should address medical risks and benefits, along with ethical and legal concerns. Recommendations for independent legal counsel and explicit written preconditions and contingency agreements should be made. The physician should not treat the couple for whom the patient will become a surrogate. Referral for mental health counseling should be provided prior to initiation of pregnancy to explore potential psychological risks and effects on the surrogate mother. Compensation to the surrogate should not be determined by the physician or be contingent on the successful delivery of a healthy infant. The physician should receive only usual fees for medical services; other payments for financial gain are inappropriate.

Suggested Readings

American College of Obstetricians and Gynecologists. *Guidelines for Women's Health Care: A Resource Manual.* 4th ed, 2014.

American College of Obstetricians and Gynecologists. *Maternal Decision Making, Ethics, and the Law.* Committee Opinion Number 321, November 2005.

American College of Obstetricians and Gynecologists. *Surrogate Motherhood.* Committee Opinion Number 397, February 2008.

American College of Obstetricians and Gynecologists. *The Limits of Conscientious Refusal in Reproductive Medicine.* Committee Opinion Number 385, November 2007, reaffirmed 2013.

Koch KA. Patient self determination act. *J Fla Med Assoc.* Apr 1992; 79(4):240-243.

Index